Molecular Pathology Library

Series editor

Philip T. Cagle, MD

More information about this series at http://www.springer.com/series/7723

Michael T. Deavers · Donna M. Coffey
Editors

Precision Molecular Pathology of Uterine Cancer

Springer

Editors
Michael T. Deavers
Department of Pathology and Genomic Medicine
Houston Methodist Hospital
Houston, TX
USA

Donna M. Coffey
Department of Pathology and Genomic Medicine
Houston Methodist Hospital
Houston, TX
USA

ISSN 1935-987X ISSN 1935-9888 (electronic)
Molecular Pathology Library
ISBN 978-3-319-57983-2 ISBN 978-3-319-57985-6 (eBook)
DOI 10.1007/978-3-319-57985-6

Library of Congress Control Number: 2017943170

Printed on acid-free paper

This Springer imprint is published by Springer Nature
The registered company is Springer International Publishing AG
The registered company address is: Gewerbestrasse 11, 6330 Cham, Switzerland

Contents

Part I Introduction

1 **Endometrial Carcinoma: Precursor Lesions and Molecular Profiles** 3
Sudeshna Bandyopadhyay and Rouba Ali-Fehmi

Part II Endometrial Carcinoma

2 **Classification of Endometrial Carcinoma** 21
Sigurd F. Lax

3 **Immunohistochemical Markers in Endometrial Carcinoma** 43
Bojana Djordjevic and Russell R. Broaddus

4 **Molecular Pathology of Endometrioid Adenocarcinoma** 65
Katherine C. Kurnit, Bojana Djordjevic and Russell R. Broaddus

5 **The Molecular Pathology of Serous Endometrial Cancer** 87
Mary Ellen Urick, Meghan L. Rudd and Daphne W. Bell

6 **Uterine Clear Cell Carcinoma** 123
Melissa K. McConechy, Cheng-Han Lee and Blaise A. Clarke

7 **Mucinous Adenocarcinoma of the Endometrium** 143
Kyu-Rae Kim and Stanley J. Robboy

8 **Molecular Pathology of Uterine Carcinosarcoma** 155
Susanna Leskelä, Belen Pérez-Mies, Juan Manuel Rosa-Rosa, Eva Cristóbal, Michele Biscuola and José Palacios

9 **Hereditary Endometrial Carcinoma** 169
Anne M. Mills and Teri A. Longacre

10 **Targeted Therapy and Prevention of Endometrial Cancer** 187
Takaya Shiozaki and Shannon N. Westin

Part III Uterine Mesenchymal Tumors

11 Molecular Pathology of Uterine Mesenchymal Tumors 227
Brooke E. Howitt and Marisa R. Nucci

Part IV Cervical Carcinomas

12 Molecular Pathology of Cervical Dysplasia and Carcinoma 253
Yimin Ge and Ming Guo

Index 279

Contributors

Rouba Ali-Fehmi, MD Department of Pathology, Wayne State University School of Medicine, Harper University Hospital, Detroit, MI, USA

Sudeshna Bandyopadhyay, MD Department of Pathology, Harper University Hospital, Wayne State University School of Medicine, Detroit, MI, USA

Daphne W. Bell, MD Cancer Genetics and Comparative Genomics Branch, National Human Genome Research Institute, National Institutes of Health, Bethesda, MD, USA

Michele Biscuola, PhD Department of Pathology, Instituto de Biomedicina de Sevilla (IBiS), Hospital Universitario Virgen del Rocío/CSIC/Universidad de Sevilla, Seville, Spain

Russell R. Broaddus, MD, PhD Department of Pathology, University of Texas MD Anderson Cancer Center, Houston, TX, USA; Unit 85, Department of Pathology, University of Texas MD Anderson Cancer Center, Houston, TX, USA

Blaise A. Clarke, FRCPC, MSc Department of Laboratory Medicine and Pathobiology, University of Toronto, University Health Network, Toronto, ON, Canada

Eva Cristóbal, PhD Servicio de Anatomía Patológica, Hospital Universitario Ramón y Cajal (IRYCIS), Departamento de Medicina y Especialidades Médicas, Universidad de Alcalá, Madrid, Spain; Red Temática de Investigación Cooperativa en Cáncer (RTICC), CIBERONC, Madrid, Spain

Bojana Djordjevic, MD Department of Anatomic Pathology, Department of Laboratory Medicine and Pathobiology, Sunnybrook Health Sciences Centre, University of Toronto, Toronto, ON, Canada

Yimin Ge, MD Department of Pathology and Genomic Medicine, Houston Methodist Hospital, Houston, TX, USA

Ming Guo, MD Department of Pathology, University of Texas MD Anderson Cancer Center, Houston, TX, USA

Brooke E. Howitt, MD Department of Pathology, Harvard Medical School, Brigham and Women's Hospital, Boston, MA, USA

Kyu-Rae Kim, MD, PhD Department of Pathology, Asan Medical Center, Songpa-gu, Seoul, Republic of Korea

Katherine C. Kurnit, MD Unit 1362, Department of Gynecologic Oncology and Reproductive Medicine, University of Texas MD Anderson Cancer Center, Houston, TX, USA

Sigurd F. Lax, MD, PhD Department of Pathology, Hospital Graz Sued-West, Academic Teaching Hospital of the Medical University, Graz, Austria

Cheng-Han Lee Department of Laboratory Medicine and Pathology, University of Alberta, Edmonton, AB, Canada

Susanna Leskelä, PhD Servicio de Anatomía Patológica, Hospital Universitario Ramón y Cajal (IRYCIS), Departamento de Medicina y Especialidades Médicas, Universidad de Alcalá, Madrid, Spain; Red Temática de Investigación Cooperativa en Cáncer (RTICC), CIBERONC, Madrid, Spain

Teri A. Longacre, MD Department of Pathology, Stanford Medicine, Stanford, CA, USA

Melissa K. McConechy Department of Human Genetics, Research Institute of the McGill University Health Centre, McGill University, Montreal, QC, Canada

Anne M. Mills, MD Department of Pathology, University of Virginia, Charlottesville, VA, USA

Marisa R. Nucci, MD Department of Pathology, Harvard Medical School, Brigham and Women's Hospital, Boston, MA, USA

José Palacios, MD, PhD Servicio de Anatomía Patológica, Hospital Universitario Ramón y Cajal (IRYCIS), Departamento de Medicina y Especialidades Médicas, Universidad de Alcalá, Madrid, Spain; Red Temática de Investigación Cooperativa en Cáncer (RTICC), CIBERONC, Madrid, Spain

Belen Pérez-Mies, MD. PhD Servicio de Anatomía Patológica, Hospital Universitario Ramón y Cajal (IRYCIS), Departamento de Medicina y Especialidades Médicas, Universidad de Alcalá, Madrid, Spain; Red Temática de Investigación Cooperativa en Cáncer (RTICC), CIBERONC, Madrid, Spain

Stanley J. Robboy, MD Department of Pathology, Duke University Medical Center, Durham, NC, USA

Juan Manuel Rosa-Rosa, PhD Servicio de Anatomía Patológica, Hospital Universitario Ramón y Cajal (IRYCIS), Departamento de Medicina y

Especialidades Médicas, Universidad de Alcalá, Madrid, Spain; Red Temática de Investigación Cooperativa en Cáncer (RTICC), CIBERONC, Madrid, Spain

Meghan L. Rudd, MS Cancer Genetics and Comparative Genomics Branch, National Human Genome Research Institute, National Institutes of Health, Bethesda, MD, USA

Takaya Shiozaki, MD, PhD Department of Obstetrics and Gynecology, Kinan Hospital, Minamimurogun, Mie, Japan

Mary Ellen Urick, PhD Cancer Genetics and Comparative Genomics Branch, National Human Genome Research Institute, National Institutes of Health, Bethesda, MD, USA

Shannon N. Westin, MD, MPH Department of Gynecologic Oncology and Reproductive Medicine, University of Texas MD Anderson Cancer Center, Houston, TX, USA

Part I
Introduction

Chapter 1
Endometrial Carcinoma: Precursor Lesions and Molecular Profiles

Sudeshna Bandyopadhyay and Rouba Ali-Fehmi

Introduction

Endometrial carcinoma is the most common gynecological malignancy. Approximately 54,870 endometrial carcinomas were diagnosed in 2015 with 10,170 deaths [1]. It has been categorized into 2 groups based on histopathology, clinical findings, and outcome and molecular findings. The biology of these tumors is underpinned by genetic and molecular features. This dichotomy in clinical, pathological, and molecular features validates a dualistic classification of endometrial carcinoma, which includes Type I and Type II cancers. Type I lesions include endometrioid carcinoma and its subtypes, while serous carcinoma is a prototype of Type II. These differences have also been identified at the precursor level, whereas uterine serous carcinomas (USCs) comprise less than 10% of all endometrial carcinomas, but paradoxically cause a high proportion of relapses and endometrial cancer-related deaths.

Endometrioid Carcinoma (Type 1)

Endometrioid carcinoma is the prototype of Type I endometrial cancer. These tumors have been linked to increased and prolonged estrogenic stimulation, occur in pre- and perimenopausal women, and occur in a background of hyperplasia [2]. Typically, they are diagnosed at a lower stage and have a good prognosis.

S. Bandyopadhyay · R. Ali-Fehmi (✉)
Department of Pathology, Wayne State University School of Medicine,
Harper University Hospital, 4160 John R, Detroit, MI 48201 USA
e-mail: rali@med.wayne.edu

S. Bandyopadhyay
e-mail: sbandyop@med.wayne.edu

M.T. Deavers and D.M. Coffey (eds.), *Precision Molecular Pathology of Uterine Cancer*, Molecular Pathology Library,
DOI 10.1007/978-3-319-57985-6_1

Precursor Lesions

Endometrioid adenocarcinoma occurs in a background of endometrial hyperplasia which is characterized morphologically by architectural complexity, cytological atypia, or both. The architectural patterns include cystic dilatation of the endometrial glands and a spectrum of more complex changes including glandular out pouching with back-to-back glandular proliferation, papillary infolding into the gland lumen with budding, villoglandular patterns, and cribriform architecture. An increase in the gland to stromal ratio of approximately 3:1 is also noted in hyperplasia [3]. Simple hyperplasia indicates an increased gland to stroma ratio, while complex hyperplasia denotes back-to-back glands with a more complex architecture. Based on the degree of architectural atypia (simple versus complex) and superimposed cytological atypia characterized by nuclear rounding and pleomorphism, vesicular chromatin with prominent nucleoli, increased N:C ratio, and loss of polarity, these lesions are classified as follows:

1. Simple hyperplasia without atypia;
2. Simple hyperplasia with atypia;
3. Complex hyperplasia without atypia;
4. Complex hyperplasia with atypia [4].

These morphological variations each have been assigned a different attributable risk of progression to carcinoma. The maximum risk of progression to endometrial carcinoma is associated with complex atypical hyperplasia, estimated to be 29%, while complex hyperplasia without atypia has an estimated risk of about 3% [5]. In another study, it was shown that the risk of progression to carcinoma in women with non-atypical endometrial hyperplasia was <5%, while almost 30% of women with atypical endometrial hyperplasia were diagnosed with endometrial carcinoma [6].

Up to 50% of women with atypical hyperplasia on the endometrial biopsy have endometrial carcinoma in the resection specimen [7–9].

The progression of hyperplasia to adenocarcinoma has common underlying molecular abnormalities detected in both these lesions. These have been described in a later section.

Uterine Serous Carcinoma (Type 2)

USC comprises less than 10% of all endometrial carcinomas, but paradoxically cause a high proportion of relapses and endometrial cancer-related deaths, which is a testimony to its biologically aggressive nature [10, 11]. Advanced stage disease (Stage III and IV) has a dismal prognosis with a 3-year survival of about 56% [12]. USC was first recognized by Lauchlan [13] and then described by Hendrickson as an endometrial carcinoma with histology similar to ovarian serous carcinoma [10]. Its defining histological features and distinctive behavior have been validated in subsequent studies [14–16].

USC usually occurs in postmenopausal women, in the milieu of an atrophic endometrium [17]. Although it was traditionally considered to be estrogen independent (as opposed to the endometrioid type), it has become increasingly evident that estrogen production continues after menopause from extra-ovarian sources, and therefore, it is fair to say that USC is more likely estrogen deficient than estrogen independent (reviewed in [18]). High-grade histological features characterize USC. These tumors exhibit severe nuclear pleomorphism, hyperchromasia, prominent nucleoli, increased mitotic activity, and single cell apoptosis, akin to ovarian serous carcinoma (Figs. 1.1 and 1.2). Additionally, the cells are dyshesive and lack cell polarity. Contrary to the high-grade cytology, these tumors tend to form glands (lined by these highly atypical cells). In addition, areas of papillary and solid architecture are also seen. Also seen are characteristic slit-like spaces and budding/micropapillae. These tumors, diagnosed later in life, often arise in a background of atrophic endometrium [10, 16, 19]. Clinically, the aggressive biology of USC has been well established, and this underlies the interest that has been generated in this disease. These tumors are biologically distinct with a poorer

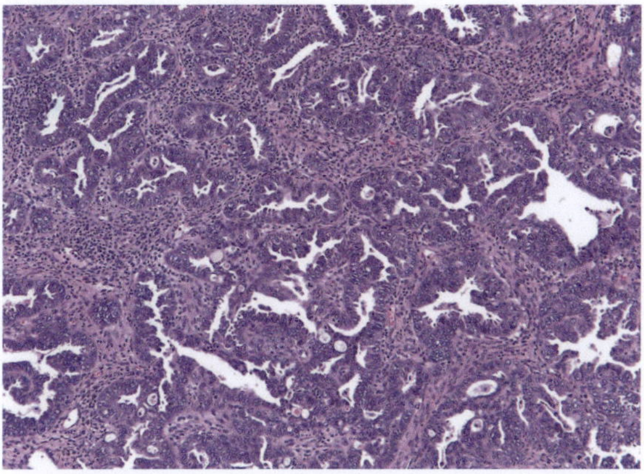

Fig. 1.1 Low power section from endometrial serous carcinoma glandular pattern

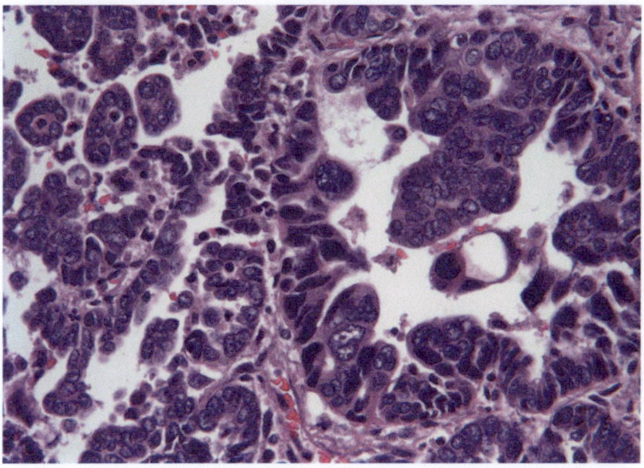

Fig. 1.2 High power illustration of endometrial serous carcinoma presenting the significant cytologic atypia and the floating papillae

prognosis compared to stage-matched endometrioid carcinomas [11, 20, 21]. Sherman et al. had argued that a diagnosis of serous carcinoma is used when at least 25% of the tumor is serous in nature [16]; however, other investigators have reported that any serous component in mixed tumors will confer a worse prognosis compared to endometrioid carcinomas [22, 23]. Also, it has been determined that the usual risk factors to predict recurrence in endometrioid carcinomas may not be useful to assess the risk of recurrence in USC [23]. At clinical presentation, these tumors are more commonly diagnosed at a high stage with evidence of extrauterine spread [24, 25]. Slomovitz and colleagues have reported a significant frequency of extrauterine disease (37%) and a poor prognosis [26] in patients with small endometrial lesions that do not invade the myometrium. Wheeler et al. [27] looked at a subset of "minimal USC" which included a cohort of EIC and superficial serous carcinoma, characterized as USC without myometrial or lymphovascular invasion. In their experience, 25% of the EIC cases and 26% of the superficial serous carcinoma cases had extrauterine disease. In another series of patients diagnosed with "minimal USC," Hui et al. [28] found extrauterine disease in 45% of the patients. In a more recent study which included a cohort of USC without myometrial invasion, Semaan et al. [29] reported that 1.8% of the cases had Stage II disease, 1.8% had Stage IIIA, and 16.4% of the cases had stage IVB disease.

The association of serous carcinoma with endometrial polyps was first described by Silva and Jenkins [30]. In their study, they described 16 patients with USC involving a polyp with minimal or no myometrial invasion. Six of these 16 (37.5%) patients also had extrauterine disease. Involvement of an endometrial polyp was also found in 30.9% of cases in series of USC limited to the endometrium, reported by Semaan et al. [29], and of these, 29.4% had stage IVB disease. Numerous studies have also identified a high risk of lymph node metastasis (ranging from 13 to 36%) in patients with uterine serous carcinoma without myometrial invasion [20, 26, 31]. These findings underline the fact that the traditional risk factors associated with endometrial carcinomas may not be applicable in USC.

Precursor Lesions

Serous endometrial intraepithelial carcinoma (EIC) also known as "endometrial carcinoma in situ," "surface serous carcinoma," and "minimal USC" is considered to be the precursor to USC, first recognized as intraepithelial carcinoma present adjacent to serous carcinoma [14, 16, 32]. This lesion is described as composed of cytologically malignant cells, similar to those seen in USC, lining the surface of the endometrium or endometrial glands without invasion of endometrial stroma, myometrium, or lymphovascular spaces [33]. It is often seen in conjunction with USC, which raises the possibility that this might be a precursor lesion. Pure EIC is a rare disease. Although technically noninvasive in appearance, these tumors have been associated with extrauterine disease, reflecting their aggressive biology [25–27, 31]. Identical p53 mutations in EIC and the pelvic serous component have been described by various studies [34, 35]. One of the mechanisms of spread that have been postulated is that there is dissemination of dyshesive neoplastic cells shed from the surface of the endometrium and glands through the fallopian tubes into the peritoneal cavity [36, 37]. Another possibility is development of multifocal disease, as synchronous primaries involving various foci in the Mullerian epithelium [38].

Molecular Signature

The concept of a dualistic model of carcinogenesis for endometrial carcinomas was first introduced by Jan Bokhman in 1982 [39] based on the widely varied clinical presentation and behavior of various types of endometrial carcinoma. This hypothesis has subsequently been validated by various studies, which have identified varying molecular aspects underlying the morphological and clinical differences between Type I and Type II carcinomas. Type I endometrial carcinomas comprise close to 80% of all endometrial cancers and are related to unopposed estrogen stimulation. Common molecular alterations seen in those tumors are PTEN mutations, microsatellite instability, K-ras, and β-catenin mutations [40–45]. Type II tumors include serous and clear cell carcinomas. Chromosomal instability, characterized as extensive genetic alterations which include loss or gain of chromosome arms and/or whole chromosomes [46], is frequently seen in serous carcinoma [47], while microsatellite instability is reportedly uncommon [19]. The most frequently detected genetic alterations are p53 mutations, Her-2/neu amplification, negative or reduced E-cadherin expression, and inactivation of p16. Below is a review of these common genetic alterations encountered in endometrial carcinoma.

Molecular Alterations in Endometrioid Carcinoma

A. PTEN:

This is a tumor suppressor gene that is present on the long arm of chromosome 10 at locus 10q23. This codes a phosphatase, which works on both protein and lipid substrates. An important substrate is phosphatidyl inositol [3–5] phosphate (PIP3). Increased PIP3 results in the activation of protein kinase Akt, which mediates cell survival and proliferation. PTEN gene product is a phosphatase and limits the amount of PIP3 available, thereby putting a check on cell proliferation. PTEN mutation or deletion does not appear to increase cell proliferation and rather results in anti-apoptosis [48, 49].

Differences in PTEN expression have been illustrated in normal cycling endometrium, being highest in the proliferative phase where a significant regulatory need is anticipated [50]. PTEN null endometrial glands have been detected in morphologically normal appearing endometrial glands with intact estrogen and progesterone receptors [51]. This suggests that these PTEN null glands may be perpetuated and are the starting point for neoplastic transformation. Only a small subset of these glands do eventually progress to carcinoma which implies that while the loss of PTEN function may be an early step in transformation, it is by no means the determining step for carcinogenesis. PTEN mutations have been detected in up to 55% of endometrial hyperplasia and endometrioid carcinoma [43, 52, 53]. Also, increased detection of PTEN mutation was seen in cases of atypical hyperplasia versus endometrial hyperplasia without atypia. This indicates that PTEN mutation is most likely an early event in endometrial carcinogenesis. Although some studies have ascribed a better prognosis to endometrial carcinoma with PTEN mutations, this most likely is a reflection of its association with Type 1 tumors.

B. K-ras:

K-ras gene belongs to the ras family of oncogenes, involved in encoding proteins which act as signal transducers. The gene product is a membrane-based signal transducer which acts upon adenylate cyclase and modulates the cell cycle. Mutations in codons 12, 13, and 61 are required for activation and results in loss of its GTPase activity, stimulating neoplastic transformation.

K-ras gene activation has been reported in 38% of endometrioid carcinomas. The majority of the mutations have been identified in codon 12 of the K-ras gene. Another study by Caduff et al. [40] identified the K-ras codon 12 mutation is a smaller proportion of cases (12%) of endometrioid carcinomas while it was not present in any serous/clear cell carcinomas included in the study (0/17).

In contrast to similar frequencies of K-ras mutations in colonic adenomas and carcinomas, these mutations were discovered at a much lower frequency in endometrial hyperplasia. Enomoto et al. [54] reported K-ras mutations in 12.5% of atypical hyperplasia (in contrast to 34% of endometrioid carcinoma). No mutations were identified in non-atypical hyperplasia. In contrast, Sasaki et al. [55] reported the presence of such mutations in non-atypical hyperplasia. No significant correlations with grade, stage, or clinical outcomes have been reported.

C. Microsatellite instability:

Aberrations in mismatch repair genes (hMLH1, hMSH2, hMSH6, and hPMS) have been reported in 15–20% of sporadic endometrioid carcinomas [56, 57]. Such aberrations result in size variations in the nucleotide repeat sequences which arise as defects during the cell cycle. In non-inherited sporadic endometrioid carcinoma, these aberrations predominantly arise secondary to hypermethylation of the hMSH1 promoter gene [58]. These changes have been identified in histologically normal appearing non-neoplastic endometrial glands in patients who subsequently developed endometrial carcinoma [59]. In contrast, these changes are rare or undetectable in random benign endometrial samples. Microsatellite instability has also been reported in complex atypical hyperplasia, suggesting that these changes occur early in the process of carcinogenesis [60].

Molecular Alterations in Serous Carcinoma

A. TP53:

The most common mutations seen in uterine serous carcinoma are those involving the p53 gene and include missense mutation followed by insertion mutation. The majority of the mutations in the p53 gene occur in exons 5–8 [61]. These mutations lead to an accumulation of abnormal intranuclear protein, which is more stable than the normal protein and therefore easily identified by immunohistochemistry. Rarely, a nonsense mutation may result in a truncated protein, which is not compatible with immunohistochemistry and therefore results in negative staining pattern [62, 63]. Loss of the normal protein prevents apoptosis and promotes tumor progression [64]. Mutations in the p53 gene have been reported in up to 90% of serous carcinomas [63]. Additionally, these mutations have also been documented in EIC adjacent to uterine serous carcinoma and EIC without associated USC, implying that these mutations occur early in the pathogenesis. The similarity in mutations between EIC and coexistent USC supports the hypothesis that EIC is linked to the development of USC. It has been postulated that the p53 mutation occurs early in one gene resulting in EIC; this is then followed by loss of heterozygosity affecting the remaining wild-type gene and resulting in progression to USC [63]. There exists a strong correlation between strong p53 protein expression (strong immunohistochemistry) and p53 missense mutations. Rarely insertion mutations may result in a more unstable protein, which may not be stained by immunohistochemistry. Identical mutations have also been reported in USC and extrauterine serous carcinoma, supporting a monoclonal origin for these tumors [34, 35].

There are reports in the literature, which have attempted to establish "preprecursors" of USC. Zheng et al. [65] have reported an entity, "endometrial glandular dysplasia" (EmGD), composed of single or a group of atypical appearing glands or surface epithelium, with enlarged, hyperchromatic nuclei and rare mitoses. The nuclear atypia described is less than that seen in EIC. These glands have an "intermediate" level of p53 and Ki-67 expression. In subsequent molecular studies [66], approximately a third of the foci of EmGD identified showed LOH at TP53 in a pattern concordant with the coexistent EIC and USC. Concordant p53 mutations have also been reported in EmGD and coexisting EIC and USC lesions [67].

The identification of the "p53 signature" in the fallopian tube in association with in situ carcinoma [68] has generated a search for a similar lesion in the endometrium. Jarboe et al. reported the increased expression of p53 in cytologically benign appearing glands adjacent to EIC involving endometrial polyps and in benign endometrial polyps. The Ki-67 labeling index in these foci ranged from 0 to 20% (often <5%), akin to the p53 signature described in fallopian tubes. Concurrent mutation analysis of the p53 gene from both the "p53 signature" and the adjacent EIC showed similar mutations in a subset of cases, suggesting biological clonality [69]. Based on these findings, the authors suggest that there might exist a latent precursor of EIC in the endometrial lining, similar to the "p53 signature" lesions seen in the fallopian tube. Multiple such events with varying mutations might occur early on with only a subset progressing to malignancy [69].

It has been postulated that the hypoxic environment of atrophic endometrium promotes selection of cells able to overcome apoptosis, thereby selecting for cells with p53 mutations.

B. Her-2/neu:

Her-2 receptor is a membrane-bound protein encoded by the Her-2/neu gene, located on chromosome 17p. It belongs to the Her family of tyrosine kinase receptors which include Her-1, Her-3, and Her-4. It is a tyrosine kinase receptor with an extracellular ligand-binding domain, a trans-membrane component, and an intracellular component related to tyrosine kinase enzyme [70, 71]. There is no known ligand for the Her-2 receptor; activation occurs by homodimerization or heterodimerization with other Her family receptors with Her-2/Her-3 heterodimer forming the most potent combination for mitogenesis [72]. Her-2 receptors are normally present on the cell membrane of non-neoplastic epithelial cells, but not in enough numbers to result in dimerization and activation of the tyrosine kinase enzyme. Her-2/neu gene amplification results in overexpression of the receptors with homo- and heterodimerization and ultimately in activation of the tyrosine kinase enzyme and related pathways resulting ultimately in increased cell proliferation, survival, and migration [73].

Variable levels of Her-2/neu protein expression have been reported in USC [74–77], and the concordance level with Her-2/neu gene amplification by Fluorescent In Situ Hybridization (FISH) assay has also been variable. While Santin et al. [74] found a high level of concordance between protein expression and gene amplification, Mentrikoski and colleagues reported concordance between protein expression and gene expression in about 1/3rd of the cases. This is far short of the concordance level of >95%, that is, mandated in breast carcinoma for this marker to be clinically relevant. The heterogeneity of Her-2/neu protein expression reported in the above studies might be attributed to small sample size, lack of standardized Her-2/neu scoring system, different histological subtypes of cancer included, and variation in the antibodies used.

Overexpression of Her-2 protein has been associated with poor prognosis and shorter overall survival [75, 78, 79]. Santin and colleagues [80] have also reported a significantly shorter survival in patients with Her-2/neu gene amplification, compared to those without. However, other studies have failed to show such correlation [81]. One of the explanations for this could be that the cases included in this study were already high stage or recurrent.

Interest in the role of Her-2/neu gene in endometrial carcinoma increased after the discovery of successful targeted therapy in patients with Her-2/neu-positive breast carcinoma. The same efficacy has not been established in endometrial carcinoma yet. The utility and therapeutic efficiency of Her-2/neu-targeted therapy in endometrial carcinoma may follow accurate and optimal patient selection.

C. EGFR:

Epidermal Growth Factor Receptor (EGFR/Her-1) is a trans-membrane tyrosine kinase receptor (belonging to the Her family receptors). It is composed of an extracellular ligand-binding domain, intracellular tyrosine kinase activity and a portion spanning the cell membrane. Ligands associated with EGFR are EGF and transforming growth factor α. Mutant variants of EGFR, while do not bind a ligand, have activated tyrosine kinase resulting in increased cell progression and inhibition of apoptosis. Although the studies are limited in the literature, EGFR overexpression has been reported in a significant subset of serous carcinomas; however, concomitant EGFR mutations in these cases were not documented [82, 83]. Downstream PIK3CA mutations were identified in a small proportion of these cases [83].

D. E-cadherin:

This is a cell adhesion molecule, which is present on the cell membrane and is calcium-dependent. This molecule maintains the cell-to-cell adhesion by interacting with the actin cytoskeleton of the cell and β-catenin. Reduced or negative expression of E-cadherin has been attributed to loss of heterozygosity of the CDH1 tumor suppressor gene in serous carcinomas [84]. Decreased or aberrant E-cadherin function has been implicated in the epithelial to myoepithelial transformation pathway [85], which results in dyshesion of the affected neoplastic cells, increased invasive and metastatic potential with tumor dedifferentiation. Decreased E-cadherin expression has been associated with higher grade endometrial carcinoma, increasing depth of invasion and increased lymph node metastasis [86]. Aberrant E-cadherin protein also results in cytosolic accumulation of β-catenin with subsequent translocation to the nucleus. β-catenin is a key player in the Wnt signaling pathway. By immunohistochemistry, E-cadherin and β-catenin expressions are membranous, in non-neoplastic epithelium. Defective expression of the E-cadherin protein results in aberrant staining pattern described as reduced and patchy or negative, while β-catenin is seen to be cytosolic or nuclear. In uterine serous carcinoma, authors have shown decreased E-cadherin expression in at least a proportion of serous carcinoma [44, 84, 87, 88], suggesting that dysfunction of this molecule may at least in part contribute to the aggressive behavior of these tumors. Increased expression of E-cadherin in Stage I–III endometrial carcinomas has been associated with a better prognosis [84]. A concurrent nuclear localization of β-catenin is not observed in serous carcinomas, suggesting that the abnormalities of this molecule are more relevant in the Type I carcinogenesis.

E. P16 (INK4a):

This is a tumor suppressor gene present on the 9p21 gene locus. It controls the G1-S transition of the cell cycle via the pRB pathway. Any damage to p16 by mutation or hypermethylation will result in defective tumor suppressor function of the pRB gene, and this may result in overexpression of p16 protein, presumable due to an aberrant negative feedback mechanism. Loss of p16 function in various neoplasms

Table 1.1 Differential involvement of genes in endometrioid and serous carcinoma of the endometrium

Genes	Function	Endometrioid cancer (%)	Serous cancer
PTEN	Tumor suppressor gene	37–61	10%
K-ras	Signal transducer	10–30	Almost absent
MSI	Mismatch repair gene	17–30	Rare
TP53	Tumor suppressor gene	10–20	90%
Her2/neu	Tyrosine kinase receptor	1–47	14–80%
E-Cad	Calcium-dependent cell adhesion molecule	20	62–90%
P16	Tumor suppressor gene		45% inactivation

Reviewed in [91–94]

has been well documented including head and neck squamous cell carcinoma, pulmonary neuroendocrine carcinomas and pulmonary squamous, and adenocarcinomas. High expression of p16 is also seen in cervical adenocarcinoma and adenocarcinoma in situ, in these cases being used as a marker for high-risk HPV infection. Although limited, studies have shown that a significantly higher proportion of USCs are diffusely positive for p16 by immunohistochemistry when compared to non-serous USC [89, 90]. These studies also demonstrated a lack of high-risk HPV DNA in these cases of USC, suggesting alternate molecular mechanisms might be involved in carcinogenesis. Table 1.1 summarizes the differential involvement of various genes in Type I and Type II endometrial cancers.

Genomic Characterization of USC

Most recently, The Cancer Genome Atlas Research Network published its findings from the genomic characterization of 373 endometrial carcinomas, which included 66 cases of USC. By unsupervised hierarchical clustering, they found that endometrial carcinomas could be grouped into 4 distinct clusters. USC (along with a subset of the FIGO 3 endometrioid carcinomas) formed a separate cluster which was characterized by a high frequency of TP53 mutations (90%), fewer PTEN mutations (11%), and MSI (6%). This cluster also included other gene amplifications, which included ERRB2, MYC, CCNE1, FGFR3, and SOX17. Tumors in this "serous-like" cluster had a worse prognosis compared to the "endometrioid-like" tumors [95].

Conclusion

USC is an aggressive variant of endometrial carcinoma with poor prognosis in even seemingly limited or early-stage disease. This highlights the need to understand the pathogenesis of this disease and identify novel therapeutic treatments. Continued appraisal of its molecular alterations may help identify precursor lesions that may be easier to cure. Furthermore, such understanding will identify specific changes that can be targeted with novel approaches and drugs.

References

1. Society AC. Cancer facts and figures. Am Cancer Soc. 2015;p. 1–70.
2. Al Kushi A, Lim P, Aquino-Parsons C, Gilks CB. Markers of proliferative activity are predictors of patient outcome for low-grade endometrioid adenocarcinoma but not papillary serous carcinoma of endometrium. Mod Pathol Off J U S Can Acad Pathol Inc. 2002;15 (4):365–71.
3. Longacre TA, Atkins KA, Kempson RL, et al. The Uterine Corpus. In: Mills S, editor. Sternberg's Diagnostic Surgical Pathology, vol. 2. 5th ed. New York, NY: Lippincott Williams & Wilkins; 2009. p. 2184–277.
4. Scully RE, Bonfiglio TA, Kurman RJ, Silverberg SG, Wilkinson EJ. Histological typing of female genital tract tumours. New York: Springer; 2012.
5. Kurman RJ, Kaminski PF, Norris HJ. The behavior of endometrial hyperplasia. A long-term study of "untreated" hyperplasia in 170 patients. Cancer. 1985;56(2):403–12.
6. Lacey JV Jr, Ioffe OB, Ronnett BM, Rush BB, Richesson DA, Chatterjee N, et al. Endometrial carcinoma risk among women diagnosed with endometrial hyperplasia: the 34-year experience in a large health plan. Br J Cancer. 2008;98(1):45–53.
7. Silverberg SG. Problems in the differential diagnosis of endometrial hyperplasia and carcinoma. Mod Pathol off J U S Can Acad Pathol Inc. 2000;13(3):309–27.
8. Pennant S, Manek S, Kehoe S. Endometrial atypical hyperplasia and subsequent diagnosis of endometrial cancer: a retrospective audit and literature review. J Obstet Gynaecol J Inst Obstet Gynaecol. 2008;28(6):632–3.
9. Trimble CL, Kauderer J, Zaino R, Silverberg S, Lim PC, Burke JJ 2nd, et al. Concurrent endometrial carcinoma in women with a biopsy diagnosis of atypical endometrial hyperplasia: a Gynecologic Oncology Group Study. Cancer. 2006;106(4):812–9.
10. Hendrickson M, Ross J, Eifel P, Martinez A, Kempson R. Uterine papillary serous carcinoma: a highly malignant form of endometrial adenocarcinoma. Am J Surg Pathol. 1982;6(2):93–108.
11. Slomovitz BM, Caputo TA, Gretz HF 3rd, Economos K, Tortoriello DV, Schlosshauer PW, et al. A comparative analysis of 57 serous borderline tumors with and without a noninvasive micropapillary component. Am J Surg Pathol. 2002;26(5):592–600.
12. Sovak MA, Hensley ML, Dupont J, Ishill N, Alektiar KM, Abu-Rustum N, et al. Paclitaxel and carboplatin in the adjuvant treatment of patients with high-risk stage III and IV endometrial cancer: a retrospective study. Gynecol Oncol. 2006;103(2):451–7.
13. Lauchlan SC. Tubal (serous) carcinoma of the endometrium. Acrch Pathol Lab Med. 1981;105:615–8.
14. Ambros RA, Sherman ME, Zahn CM, Bitterman P, Kurman RJ. Endometrial intraepithelial carcinoma: a distinctive lesion specifically associated with tumors displaying serous differentiation. Hum Pathol. 1995;26(11):1260–7.

15. Lachance JA, Everett EN, Greer B, Mandel L, Swisher E, Tamimi H, et al. The effect of age on clinical/pathologic features, surgical morbidity, and outcome in patients with endometrial cancer. Gynecol Oncol. 2006;101(3):470–5.
16. Sherman ME, Bitterman P, Rosenshein NB, Delgado G, Kurman RJ. Uterine serous carcinoma. A morphologically diverse neoplasm with unifying clinicopathologic features. Am J Surg Pathol. 1992;16(6):600–10.
17. Kurman RJ, Ellenson LH, Ronnett BM, editors. Blaustein's pathology of the female genital tract. 6th ed. 2011. p. 393–452.
18. Sivridis E, Giatromanolaki A. The pathogenesis of endometrial carcinomas at menopause: facts and figures. J Clin Pathol. 2011;64(7):553–60.
19. Tashiro H, Lax SF, Gaudin PB, Isacson C, Cho KR, Hedrick L. Microsatellite instability is uncommon in uterine serous carcinoma. Am J Pathol. 1997;150(1):75–9.
20. Cirisano FD Jr, Robboy SJ, Dodge RK, Bentley RC, Krigman HR, Synan IS, et al. The outcome of stage I–II clinically and surgically staged papillary serous and clear cell endometrial cancers when compared with endometrioid carcinoma. Gynecol Oncol. 2000; 77(1):55–65.
21. Hamilton CA, Cheung MK, Osann K, Balzer B, Berman ML, Husain A, et al. The effect of adjuvant chemotherapy versus whole abdominopelvic radiation on the survival of patients with advanced stage uterine papillary serous carcinoma. Gynecol Oncol. 2006;103(2):679–83.
22. Boruta DM 2nd, Gehrig PA, Groben PA, Bae-Jump V, Boggess JF, Fowler WC Jr, et al. Uterine serous and grade 3 endometrioid carcinomas: is there a survival difference? Cancer. 2004;101(10):2214–21.
23. Fader AN, Starks D, Gehrig PA, Secord AA, Frasure HE, O'Malley DM, et al. An updated clinicopathologic study of early-stage uterine papillary serous carcinoma (UPSC). Gynecol Oncol. 2009;115(2):244–8.
24. Trope C, Kristensen GB, Abeler VM. Clear-cell and papillary serous cancer: treatment options. Best Pract Res Clin obstet Gynaecol. 2001;15(3):433–46.
25. Soslow RA, Pirog E, Isacson C. Endometrial intraepithelial carcinoma with associated peritoneal carcinomatosis. Am J Surg Pathol. 2000;24(5):726–32.
26. Slomovitz BM, Burke TW, Eifel PJ, Ramondetta LM, Silva EG, Jhingran A, et al. Uterine papillary serous carcinoma (UPSC): a single institution review of 129 cases. Gynecol Oncol. 2003;91(3):463–9.
27. Wheeler DT, Bell KA, Kurman RJ, Sherman ME. Minimal uterine serous carcinoma: diagnosis and clinicopathologic correlation. Am J Surg Pathol. 2000;24(6):797–806.
28. Hui P, Kelly M, O'Malley DM, Tavassoli F, Schwartz PE. Minimal uterine serous carcinoma: a clinicopathological study of 40 cases. Mod Pathol Off J U S Can Acad Pathol Inc. 2005; 18(1):75–82.
29. Semaan A, Mert I, Munkarah AR, Bandyopadhyay S, Mahdi HS, Winer IS, et al. Clinical and pathologic characteristics of serous carcinoma confined to the endometrium: a multi-institutional study. Int J Gynecol Pathol Off J Int Soc Gynecol Pathol. 2013; 32(2):181–7.
30. Silva EG, Jenkins R. Serous carcinoma in endometrial polyps. Mod Pathol Off J U S Can Acad Pathol Inc. 1990;3(2):120–8.
31. Goff BA, Kato D, Schmidt RA, Ek M, Ferry JA, Muntz HG, et al. Uterine papillary serous carcinoma: patterns of metastatic spread. Gynecol Oncol. 1994;54(3):264–8.
32. Spiegel GW. Endometrial carcinoma in situ in postmenopausal women. Am J Surg Pathol. 1995;19(4):417–32.
33. Sherman ME, Bur ME, Kurman RJ. p53 in endometrial cancer and its putative precursors: evidence for diverse pathways of tumorigenesis. Hum Pathol. 1995;26(11):1268–74.
34. Baergen RN, Warren CD, Isacson C, Ellenson LH. Early uterine serous carcinoma: clonal origin of extrauterine disease. Int J Gynecol Pathol Off J Int Soc Gynecol Pathol. 2001; 20(3):214–9.

35. Kupryjanczyk J, Thor AD, Beauchamp R, Poremba C, Scully RE, Yandell DW. Ovarian, peritoneal, and endometrial serous carcinoma: clonal origin of multifocal disease. Mod Pathol Off J U S Can Acad Pathol Inc. 1996;9(3):166–73.
36. Snyder MJ, Bentley R, Robboy SJ. Transtubal spread of serous adenocarcinoma of the endometrium: an underrecognized mechanism of metastasis. Int J Gynecol Pathol Off J Int Soc Gynecol Pathol. 2006;25(2):155–60.
37. Stewart CJ, Doherty DA, Havlat M, Koay MH, Leung YC, Naran A, et al. Transtubal spread of endometrial carcinoma: correlation of intra-luminal tumour cells with tumour grade, peritoneal fluid cytology, and extra-uterine metastasis. Pathology. 2013;45(4):382–7.
38. Muto MG, Welch WR, Mok SC, Bandera CA, Fishbaugh PM, Tsao SW, et al. Evidence for a multifocal origin of papillary serous carcinoma of the peritoneum. Can Res. 1995;55(3): 490–2.
39. Bokhman JV. Two pathogenetic types of endometrial carcinoma. Gynecol Oncol. 1983; 15(1):10–7.
40. Caduff RF, Johnston CM, Frank TS. Mutations of the Ki-ras oncogene in carcinoma of the endometrium. Am J Pathol. 1995;146(1):182–8.
41. Caduff RF, Johnston CM, Svoboda-Newman SM, Poy EL, Merajver SD, Frank TS. Clinical and pathological significance of microsatellite instability in sporadic endometrial carcinoma. Am J Pathol. 1996;148(5):1671–8.
42. Enomoto T, Inoue M, Perantoni AO, Terakawa N, Tanizawa O, Rice JM. K-ras activation in neoplasms of the human female reproductive tract. Can Res. 1990;50(19):6139–45.
43. Mutter GL, Lin MC, Fitzgerald JT, Kum JB, Baak JP, Lees JA, et al. Altered PTEN expression as a diagnostic marker for the earliest endometrial precancers. J Natl Cancer Inst. 2000;92(11):924–30.
44. Schlosshauer PW, Ellenson LH, Soslow RA. Beta-catenin and E-cadherin expression patterns in high-grade endometrial carcinoma are associated with histological subtype. Mod Pathol Off J U S Can Acad Pathol Inc. 2002;15(10):1032–7.
45. Palacios J, Catasus L, Moreno-Bueno G, Matias-Guiu X, Prat J, Gamallo C. Beta- and gamma-catenin expression in endometrial carcinoma. Relationship with clinicopathological features and microsatellite instability. Virchows Arch Int J Pathol. 2001;438(5):464–9.
46. Lengauer C, Kinzler KW, Vogelstein B. Genetic instability in colorectal cancers. Nature. 1997;386(6625):623–7.
47. Nordstrom B, Strang P, Lindgren A, Bergstrom R, Tribukait B. Endometrial carcinoma: the prognostic impact of papillary serous carcinoma (UPSC) in relation to nuclear grade, DNA ploidy and p53 expression. Anticancer Res. 1996;16(2):899–904.
48. Cantley LC, Neel BG. New insights into tumor suppression: PTEN suppresses tumor formation by restraining the phosphoinositide 3-kinase/AKT pathway. Proc Natl Acad Sci U S A. 1999;96(8):4240–5.
49. Besson A, Robbins SM, Yong VW. PTEN/MMAC1/TEP1 in signal transduction and tumorigenesis. Eur J Biochem FEBS. 1999;263(3):605–11.
50. Mutter GL, Lin MC, Fitzgerald JT, Kum JB, Eng C. Changes in endometrial PTEN expression throughout the human menstrual cycle. J Clin Endocrinol Metab. 2000; 85(6):2334–8.
51. Mutter GL, Ince TA, Baak JP, Kust GA, Zhou XP, Eng C. Molecular identification of latent precancers in histologically normal endometrium. Can Res. 2001;61(11):4311–4.
52. Levine RL, Cargile CB, Blazes MS, van Rees B, Kurman RJ, Ellenson LH. PTEN mutations and microsatellite instability in complex atypical hyperplasia, a precursor lesion to uterine endometrioid carcinoma. Can Res. 1998;58(15):3254–8.
53. Maxwell GL, Risinger JI, Gumbs C, Shaw H, Bentley RC, Barrett JC, et al. Mutation of the PTEN tumor suppressor gene in endometrial hyperplasias. Can Res. 1998;58(12):2500–3.
54. Enomoto T, Inoue M, Perantoni AO, Buzard GS, Miki H, Tanizawa O, et al. K-ras activation in premalignant and malignant epithelial lesions of the human uterus. Can Res. 1991; 51(19):5308–14.

55. Sasaki H, Nishii H, Takahashi H, Tada A, Furusato M, Terashima Y, et al. Mutation of the Ki-ras protooncogene in human endometrial hyperplasia and carcinoma. Can Res. 1993; 53(8):1906–10.
56. O'Hara AJ, Bell DW. The genomics and genetics of endometrial cancer. Adv Genomics Genet. 2012;2012(2):33–47.
57. Samarnthai N, Hall K, Yeh IT. Molecular profiling of endometrial malignancies. Obstet Gynecol Int. 2010;2010:162363.
58. Esteller M, Levine R, Baylin SB, Ellenson LH, Herman JG. MLH1 promoter hypermethylation is associated with the microsatellite instability phenotype in sporadic endometrial carcinomas. Oncogene. 1998;17(18):2413–7.
59. Faquin WC, Fitzgerald JT, Lin MC, Boynton KA, Muto MG, Mutter GL. Sporadic microsatellite instability is specific to neoplastic and preneoplastic endometrial tissues. Am J Clin Pathol. 2000;113(4):576–82.
60. Mutter GL, Boynton KA, Faquin WC, Ruiz RE, Jovanovic AS. Allelotype mapping of unstable microsatellites establishes direct lineage continuity between endometrial precancers and cancer. Can Res. 1996;56(19):4483–6.
61. Harris CC. 1995 Deichmann Lecture—p53 tumor suppressor gene: at the crossroads of molecular carcinogenesis, molecular epidemiology and cancer risk assessment. Toxicol Lett. 1995;82–83:1–7.
62. Lax SF, Kendall B, Tashiro H, Slebos RJ, Hedrick L. The frequency of p53, K-ras mutations, and microsatellite instability differs in uterine endometrioid and serous carcinoma: evidence of distinct molecular genetic pathways. Cancer. 2000;88(4):814–24.
63. Tashiro H, Isacson C, Levine R, Kurman RJ, Cho KR, Hedrick L. p53 gene mutations are common in uterine serous carcinoma and occur early in their pathogenesis. Am J Pathol. 1997;150(1):177–85.
64. Kuerbitz SJ, Plunkett BS, Walsh WV, Kastan MB. Wild-type p53 is a cell cycle checkpoint determinant following irradiation. Proc Natl Acad Sci USA. 1992;89(16):7491–5.
65. Zheng W, Liang SX, Yu H, Rutherford T, Chambers SK, Schwartz PE. Endometrial glandular dysplasia: a newly defined precursor lesion of uterine papillary serous carcinoma. Part I: morphologic features. Int J Surg Pathol. 2004;12(3):207–23.
66. Liang SX, Chambers SK, Cheng L, Zhang S, Zhou Y, Zheng W. Endometrial glandular dysplasia: a putative precursor lesion of uterine papillary serous carcinoma. Part II: molecular features. Int J Surg Pathol. 2004;12(4):319–31.
67. Jia L, Liu Y, Yi X, Miron A, Crum CP, Kong B, et al. Endometrial glandular dysplasia with frequent p53 gene mutation: a genetic evidence supporting its precancer nature for endometrial serous carcinoma. Clin Cancer Res Off J Am Assoc Cancer Res. 2008; 14(8):2263–9.
68. Crum CP, Drapkin R, Miron A, Ince TA, Muto M, Kindelberger DW, et al. The distal fallopian tube: a new model for pelvic serous carcinogenesis. Curr Opin Obstet Gynecol. 2007;19(1):3–9.
69. Jarboe EA, Pizer ES, Miron A, Monte N, Mutter GL, Crum CP. Evidence for a latent precursor (p53 signature) that may precede serous endometrial intraepithelial carcinoma. Mod Pathol Off J U S Can Acad Pathol Inc. 2009;22(3):345–50.
70. Hung MC, Lau YK. Basic science of HER-2/neu: a review. Semin Oncol. 1999;26(4 Suppl 12):51–9.
71. Busse D, Doughty RS, Arteaga CL. HER-2/neu (erbB-2) and the cell cycle. Semin oncol. 2000;27(6 Suppl 11):3–8; discussion 92–100.
72. Graus-Porta D, Beerli RR, Daly JM, Hynes NE. ErbB-2, the preferred heterodimerization partner of all ErbB receptors, is a mediator of lateral signaling. EMBO J. 1997;16(7): 1647–55.
73. Reese DM, Slamon DJ. HER-2/neu signal transduction in human breast and ovarian cancer. Stem Cells. 1997;15(1):1–8.
74. Santin AD, Bellone S, Van Stedum S, Bushen W, De Las Casas LE, Korourian S, et al. Determination of HER2/neu status in uterine serous papillary carcinoma: comparative

analysis of immunohistochemistry and fluorescence in situ hybridization. Gynecol Oncol. 2005;98(1):24–30.
75. Slomovitz BM, Broaddus RR, Burke TW, Sneige N, Soliman PT, Wu W, et al. Her-2/neu overexpression and amplification in uterine papillary serous carcinoma. J Clin Oncol Off J Am Soc Clin Oncol. 2004;22(15):3126–32.
76. Halperin R, Zehavi S, Habler L, Hadas E, Bukovsky I, Schneider D. Comparative immunohistochemical study of endometrioid and serous papillary carcinoma of endometrium. Eur J Gynaecol Oncol. 2001;22(2):122–6.
77. Mentrikoski MJ, Stoler MH. HER2 immunohistochemistry significantly overestimates HER2 amplification in uterine papillary serous carcinomas. Am J Surg Pathol. 2014;38(6):844–51.
78. Diaz-Montes TP, Ji H, Smith Sehdev AE, Zahurak ML, Kurman RJ, Armstrong DK, et al. Clinical significance of Her-2/neu overexpression in uterine serous carcinoma. Gynecol Oncol. 2006;100(1):139–44.
79. Togami S, Sasajima Y, Oi T, Ishikawa M, Onda T, Ikeda S, et al. Clinicopathological and prognostic impact of human epidermal growth factor receptor type 2 (HER2) and hormone receptor expression in uterine papillary serous carcinoma. Cancer Sci. 2012;103(5):926–32.
80. Santin AD, Bellone S, Van Stedum S, Bushen W, Palmieri M, Siegel ER, et al. Amplification of c-erbB2 oncogene: a major prognostic indicator in uterine serous papillary carcinoma. Cancer. 2005;104(7):1391–7.
81. Fleming GF, Sill MW, Darcy KM, McMeekin DS, Thigpen JT, Adler LM, et al. Phase II trial of trastuzumab in women with advanced or recurrent, HER2-positive endometrial carcinoma: a gynecologic oncology group study. Gynecol Oncol. 2010;116(1):15–20.
82. Konecny GE, Santos L, Winterhoff B, Hatmal M, Keeney GL, Mariani A, et al. HER2 gene amplification and EGFR expression in a large cohort of surgically staged patients with nonendometrioid (type II) endometrial cancer. Br J Cancer. 2009;100(1):89–95.
83. Hayes MP, Douglas W, Ellenson LH. Molecular alterations of EGFR and PIK3CA in uterine serous carcinoma. Gynecol Oncol. 2009;113(3):370–3.
84. Moreno-Bueno G, Hardisson D, Sarrio D, Sanchez C, Cassia R, Prat J, et al. Abnormalities of E- and P-cadherin and catenin (beta-, gamma-catenin, and p120ctn) expression in endometrial cancer and endometrial atypical hyperplasia. J Pathol. 2003;199(4):471–8.
85. Kang Y, Massague J. Epithelial-mesenchymal transitions: twist in development and metastasis. Cell. 2004;118(3):277–9.
86. Sakuragi N, Nishiya M, Ikeda K, Ohkouch T, Furth EE, Hareyama H, et al. Decreased E-cadherin expression in endometrial carcinoma is associated with tumor dedifferentiation and deep myometrial invasion. Gynecol Oncol. 1994;53(2):183–9.
87. Yalta T, Atay L, Atalay F, Caydere M, Gonultas M, Ustun H. E-cadherin expression in endometrial malignancies: comparison between endometrioid and non-endometrioid carcinomas. J Int Med Res. 2009;37(1):163–8.
88. Holcomb K, Delatorre R, Pedemonte B, McLeod C, Anderson L, Chambers J. E-cadherin expression in endometrioid, papillary serous, and clear cell carcinoma of the endometrium. Obstet Gynecol. 2002;100(6):1290–5.
89. Yemelyanova A, Ji H, Shih Ie M, Wang TL, Wu LS, Ronnett BM. Utility of p16 expression for distinction of uterine serous carcinomas from endometrial endometrioid and endocervical adenocarcinomas: immunohistochemical analysis of 201 cases. Am J Surg Pathol. 2009; 33(10):1504–14.
90. Chiesa-Vottero AG, Malpica A, Deavers MT, Broaddus R, Nuovo GJ, Silva EG. Immunohistochemical overexpression of p16 and p53 in uterine serous carcinoma and ovarian high-grade serous carcinoma. Int J Gynecol Pathol Off J Int Soc Gynecol Pathol. 2007;26(3):328–33.
91. Matias-Guiu X, Prat J. Molecular pathology of endometrial carcinoma. Histopathology. 2013;62(1):111–23.
92. Buza N, Roque DM, Santin AD. HER2/neu in endometrial cancer: a promising therapeutic target with diagnostic challenges. Arch Pathol Lab Med. 2014;138(3):343–50.

93. Doll A, Abal M, Rigau M, Monge M, Gonzalez M, Demajo S, et al. Novel molecular profiles of endometrial cancer-new light through old windows. J Steroid Biochem Mol Biol. 2008; 108(3–5):221–9.
94. Silva JL, Paulino E, Dias MF, Melo AC. Endometrial cancer: redefining the molecular-targeted approach. Cancer Chemother Pharmacol. 2015;76(1):1–11.
95. Cancer Genome Atlas Research N, Kandoth C, Schultz N, Cherniack AD, Akbani R, Liu Y, et al. Integrated genomic characterization of endometrial carcinoma. Nature. 2013; 497(7447):67–73.

Part II
Endometrial Carcinoma

Chapter 2
Classification of Endometrial Carcinoma

Sigurd F. Lax

A Putative Pathogenetic Model for Endometrial Carcinoma

A simplified model has been developed based on clinicopathologic and molecular parameters in order to better understand endometrial tumorigenesis. According to this model, (Table 2.1) there are two types of endometrial carcinoma that are characterized by distinct features and that develop along different pathways (Table 2.2). Type I carcinomas, which account for the great majority of endometrial carcinomas (approximately 80–90%), are characterized by low stage at diagnosis and a favorable clinical course. They typically develop in a normal-sized or a myohyperplastic uterus and are associated with disordered proliferative or hyperplastic endometrium. The latter reflects unopposed estrogenic stimulation, which may be caused by persistent follicles due to anovulatory cycles, an estrogen producing tumor such as adult granulosa cell tumor, endogenous estrogen production by the aromatase of adipose tissue in the setting of high body mass index, or hormone replacement therapy by pure estrogens. Thus, the typical age of a patient with type I carcinoma is in the peri- and postmenopausal period. The patients also have elevated levels of free estrogen in the serum [5]. Histologically, type I carcinomas are endometrioid adenocarcinoma, including its variants and mucinous carcinoma, and are mostly low histological grade (good or moderate histopathologic differentiation). Atypical endometrial hyperplasia/endometrioid intraepithelial neoplasia (EIN) is considered the precursor lesion. The fact that these carcinomas usually highly express estrogen (ER) and progesterone receptors (PR) further underlines their relationship to an estrogenic pathway.

S.F. Lax (✉)
Department of Pathology, Hospital Graz Sued-West,
Academic Teaching Hospital of the Medical University,
LKH Graz Süd-West, Standort West,
Göstingerstrasse 22, 8020 Graz, Austria
e-mail: sigurd.lax@kages.at

M.T. Deavers and D.M. Coffey (eds.), *Precision Molecular Pathology of Uterine Cancer*, Molecular Pathology Library,
DOI 10.1007/978-3-319-57985-6_2

Table 2.1 Histopathologic classification of endometrial carcinoma (WHO 2014) [1]

Histological type	ICD-O
Endometrioid adenocarcinoma	8380/3
Endometrioid adenocarcinoma-variants	
With squamous differentiation	
Secretory variant	8570/3
Villoglandular variant	8263/3
Ciliated cell variant	8382/3
Mucinous adenocarcinoma	8480/3
Serous endometrial intraepithelial carcinoma (SEIC)	8441/2
Serous adenocarcinoma	8441/3
Clear cell adenocarcinoma	8310/3
Mixed cell adenocarcinoma	8323/3
Undifferentiated carcinoma	8020/3
Monomorphic type Dedifferentiated type (dedifferentiated carcinoma)	
Neuroendocrine tumors	
Well differentiated neuroendocrine tumor (carcinoid tumor)	8240/3
Poorly differentiated small cell neuroendocrine carcinoma	80412/3
Poorly differentiated large cell neuroendocrine carcinoma	8013/3

Table 2.2 An expanded dualistic model for endometrial carcinoma

Features	Type I carcinoma	Type II carcinoma
Estrogen-related	Yes	No
Endometrial histology	Usually hyperplastic or disordered proliferative	Usually atrophic
Estrogen- and progesterone receptors	Usually positive	Usually negative or weakly positive
Age (median)	55–65 years	65–75 years
Stage	Mostly stage I	Mostly stages II–IV
Prognosis	Favorable	Unfavorable
Histological type	Endometrioid + variants; Mucinous	Serous, clear cell
Molecular alterations	PTEN inactivation Microsatellite instability ß-catenin mutations K-ras mutations	P53 mutations E-cadherin inactivation
Molecular type according to TCGA	Hypermutated, copy number low (endometrioid-like)	Copy number high (serous like)

In contrast, type II carcinomas are diagnosed at high stage and are aggressive tumors with a poor outcome. The histologic prototype is serous carcinoma, but clear cell and undifferentiated carcinomas are also considered type II carcinomas. These tumors are usually not related to estrogenic stimulation, as reflected by the following features: they usually occur in an atrophic uterus and are associated with atrophic or inactive endometrium; they may occur in atrophic polyps; serum estrogen is low in these patients; in addition, ER and PR immunoreactivity is weak or negative. Serous endometrial intraepithelial carcinoma (SEIC) had been considered the precursor of serous carcinoma. Recently, our concept of SEIC has transitioned to a non-invasive carcinoma, since it is frequently associated with extensive extrauterine disease. In this setting, SEIC may be part of pelvic serous carcinoma without a clear site of origin. For other type II carcinomas putative precursors are unknown, although EIC has been found in a subset of clear cell carcinomas. In addition to SEIC, a less atypical lesion has been characterized and described as dysplasia [6–9].

Type I and type II carcinomas are also distinct on the molecular level [3]. Most type I carcinomas are characterized by minor changes in the genome as evidenced by a low number of somatic copy number alterations, whereas most type II carcinomas are characterized by major changes in the genome, such as a high number of somatic copy number alterations and aneuploidy. Frequent mutations of *PTEN* (>50%), *K-RAS* (20–30%), *ARID1A* (40% of low grade endometrioid carcinomas), *CTNNB1* (ß-catenin) (30%) and *PIK3R1* (20–45%) are typical for type I carcinomas, whereas mutations of *TP53* (80–90%), *FBXW7* (20–30%) and *PPP2R1A* (20–30%) are more frequently found in type II carcinomas [10–16]. In addition, a mutator phenotype leading to microsatellite instability (MSI) is found in 25–40% of type I carcinomas, but is very rare in type II carcinomas (<5%). Microsatellite instability leads to frameshift mutations in repetitive sequences, which may be located in crucial genes such as Bax, an apoptosis related gene [17]. On the other hand, mutations of PIK3CA are almost equally found in type I and type II carcinomas [18–20], and TP53 mutations can found in a subset of type I carcinomas, grade 3 endometrioid adenocarcinoma (30%) [13].

The studies of The Cancer Genome Atlas (TCGA) project revealed four prognostic groups of endometrial carcinoma, of which tumors with "serous-like" genomic changes, particularly high copy number changes, had the worst prognosis. Tumors with mutations in the polymerase E gene (*POLE*) had an excellent prognosis; the prognosis of tumors with low copy number changes and of hypermutated tumors was in between [21]. Recent studies reported *POLE* mutations in endometrial carcinomas with serous and high grade endometrioid phenotypes that had an excellent prognosis [22]. Subsequently, a novel molecular based classification system for endometrial carcinoma has been proposed, including immunohistochemistry for p53 and mismatch repair proteins, as well as mutational analysis for *POLE* [23].

Although clear cell carcinoma is considered biologically and clinically a type II carcinoma, it shares some molecular alterations with type I carcinoma, in particular *PTEN* mutations (30–40%) and loss of *ARID1A* expression, but without mutations

(25%) [24, 25]. A recent study found a serous-like mutation profile of clear cell carcinoma with concurrent mutations in *TP53* and *PPP2R1A*, but wild type *ARID1A*, *PTEN*, *CTNNB1* and *POLE* [26].

In summary, type I carcinoma seems to follow an adenoma-carcinoma sequence, developing from atypical hyperplasia/EIN and progressing from low grade to high grade carcinoma. Some of the molecular changes, such as mutations in PTEN, K-RAS and ARID1A, seem to occur early, particularly in atypical hyperplasia and grade 1 endometrioid adenocarcinoma; others, such as TP53 mutations, seem to represent late events since they occur in high grade endometrioid adenocarcinoma [13, 14, 27]. In contrast, serous carcinoma seems to develop de novo from atrophic endometrium through SEIC [28]. Mutations of *TP53, PIK3CA*, *FBXW7* and *PPP2R1A* as well as overexpression of *cyclin E1* are considered early events in the development of serous carcinoma since they are present in SEIC [16, 29, 30]. Some of these genetic alterations seem to be strong drivers of tumorigenesis. In particular, mutated *TP53* seems to be a strong driver for growth in serous carcinoma that leads to a strong selective advantage. The diffuse strong or flat negative immunoreactivity, briefly called "all or null pattern", is characteristic for *TP53* mutations and seems to reflect an early clonal expansion that involves the whole tumor.

Histopathologic Classification

Endometrioid Adenocarcinoma

Endometrioid adenocarcinoma is by the far most frequent histologic type of endometrial carcinoma [1, 31, 32]. It typically displays glandular, papillary or solid patterns (Fig. 2.1). The glandular structures are typically well formed and show regular luminal borders resembling the glands of non-neoplastic endometrium. The nuclei are elongated and pseudostratified or round. Villous and papillary structures are commonly found and need to be distinguished from the papillae of serous carcinoma.

Endometrioid adenocarcinoma may be associated with various types of cellular differentiation that do not have clinical significance. Nevertheless, it is important to be aware of these histologic features, and they should be included in the pathology report since they may help in recognition of a local recurrence or metastasis. **Squamous differentiation** occurs in about 10–25% of endometrioid adenocarcinomas and may present as focal morular structures within glandular lumens (Figs. 2.1 and 2.2) or as confluent sheets [33]. Squamous differentiation may be characterized by polygonal or spindle cells resembling squamous differentiation in the uterine cervix. Other characteristics include intercellular bridges and the formation of squamous pearls. The squamous areas often have bland or slightly polymorphic nuclei, but the degree of atypia usually concurs with the histopathologic grade of the tumor [34]. Extensive immature squamous differentiation may

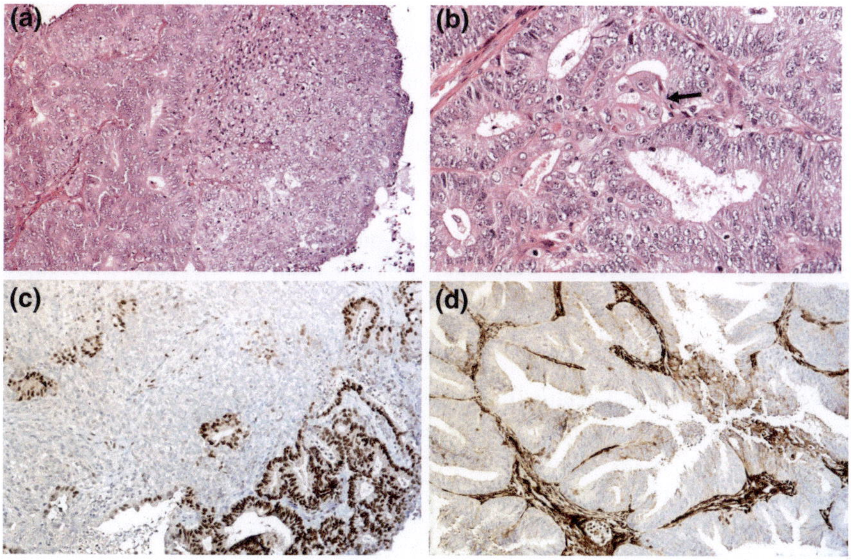

Fig. 2.1 FIGO grade 2 endometrioid adenocarcinoma with glandular and solid patterns (**a**). The glands are well formed and have regular luminal borders (**b**). A small focus of squamous differentiation is present (*arrow*). Estrogen receptor immunoreactivity is strong in the glandular area and weak in the solid area (**c**), PTEN immunoreactivity is lost in the tumor, but present in the stromal cells (**d**)

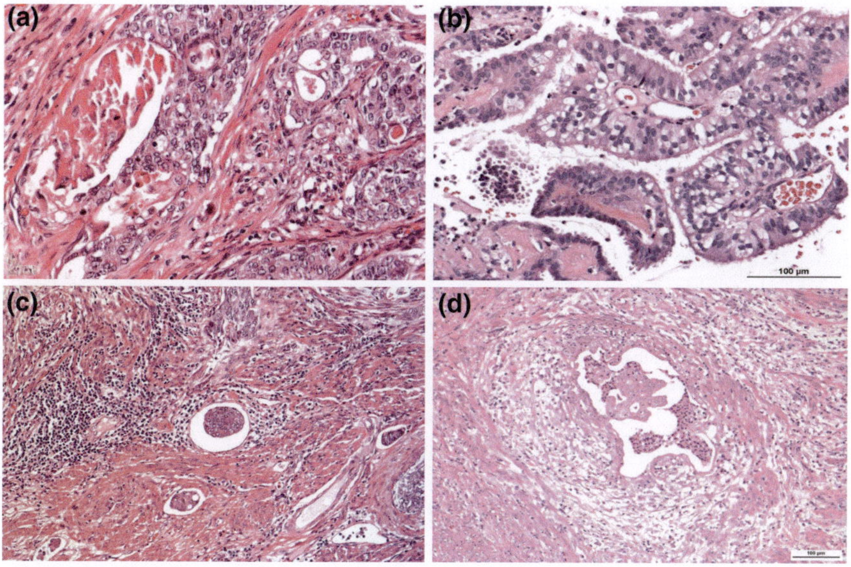

Fig. 2.2 Endometrioid adenocarcinoma with squamous differentiation (**a**). Secretory variant of endometrioid adenocarcinoma with cytoplasmic vacuoles resembling early secretory phase (**b**). Lymphvascular space involvement (*LVSI*) (**c**) and a microcystic elongated and fragmented glandular pattern (**d**) as poor prognostic factors in histologically low grade endometrioid adenocarcinomas

significantly influence the histopathologic grade of a carcinoma if it is not recognized and is misinterpreted as solid non-squamous growth [35]. For the differentiation of these two, it is helpful to take into account the nuclear atypia of the solid area. Ki-67 can be used as an adjunct since its labeling index is low in low grade "metaplastic" squamous areas, but high in solid non-squamous structures. Poorly differentiated endometrioid adenocarcinoma with squamous differentiation (the former "adenosquamous carcinoma") may infiltrate as small nests of atypical squamous cells or grow in sheets of atypical spindle cells resembling a sarcomatoid carcinoma [33]. Extensive keratinization is rare, but can be associated with keratin granulomas at various sites outside the uterus [36]. Mucinous differentiation associated with squamous differentiation in endometrioid adenocarcinoma is not unusual.

The **villoglandular variant** is usually low grade and composed of glands and delicate papillae, covered by columnar epithelium with mild to moderate nuclear atypia [37]. It often presents with low stage and superficial myometrial invasion. The prognosis of the villoglandular variant with myoinvasion is controversial and has been under debate [37, 38]. Differentiating it from serous carcinoma is crucial and may be challenging in some cases; criteria are detailed in the serous carcinoma section.

The **secretory variant** or **variant with secretory differentiation** resembles early secretory phase endometrium with glands containing sub- and/or supranuclear vacuoles (Fig. 2.2). The secretory changes may be focal or diffuse, and they may be associated with the secretory phase or with exogenous progestins, and thus represent a transient change. If the changes occur in premenopausal women, the adjacent endometrium may show similar changes. The secretory variant is usually low grade and predominantly glandular, but if it contains solid areas it must not be misinterpreted as clear cell carcinoma. In contrast to clear cell carcinoma, the secretory variant of endometrioid adenocarcinoma lacks significant nuclear atypia and other characteristic features of clear cell carcinoma [39, 40].

The **ciliated variant** is rare, although cells with apical cilia are not unusual in typical endometrioid adenocarcinoma. These are usually low grade and low stage tumors, and there is some evidence of association with estrogens [41].

Endometrioid adenocarcinoma may also have variant growth patterns. An unusual pattern of invasion contains microcystic, elongated and fragmented glands (MELF) (Fig. 2.2) and seems to be frequently associated with LVSI [42]. Extensive lymph vascular space involvement (LVSI) is a prognostic factor for increased risk of recurrence (Fig. 2.2). Myometrial invasion may be clearly recognizable, particularly when it contains haphazardly distributed glands or diffusely arranged cords and clusters of cells or individual cells. The infiltrated myometrium frequently has a desmoplastic reaction, or less often an inflammatory response. In other cases of endometrial carcinoma, myometrial invasion may have a smooth, pushing border and lack desmoplasia, akin to adenoma malignum of the cervix [43]. A similar pattern can be found when endometrial carcinoma extends into adenomyosis. The distinction from true myometrial invasion is important, since prognosis is not adversely influenced by involvement of adenomyosis. The presence of clearly recognizable adenomyosis on H&E sections is required for the diagnosis of carcinoma involving adenomyosis. This may be difficult, particularly when the glands in adenomyosis are sparse and the stroma is atrophic or fibrotic. Similarly, the diagnosis of superficial myometrial invasion can be problematic because of irregularity of the endomyometrial junction [44]. For the diagnosis of myometrial invasion, clear evidence of irregularly distributed tumor nests within the myometrium, without proximity to residual non-neoplastic glands or endometrial stroma, is needed.

The proportion of the solid, non-squamous component of the tumor determines the FIGO histologic grade of endometrioid adenocarcinoma (Table 2.3) (Fig. 2.1). In FIGO grade 1 carcinomas, solid areas account for less than 5%, in FIGO grade 2 carcinomas 6–50% and FIGO grade 3 carcinomas have more than 50% of non-squamous solid areas. Solid areas of squamous differentiation are not considered for grading purposes. There are several problems with FIGO grading, such as the recognition of small areas with solid growth, the distinction between solid squamous and non-squamous areas and the interobserver reproducibility of bizarre nuclear atypia. Finally, the reproducibility of a three-tier system may have its weaknesses. Alternative grading systems using only two tiers and considering patterns of growth have been proposed and subsequently validated, but have not been generally accepted [45–48].

The differential diagnosis of endometrioid adenocarcinoma includes atypical hyperplasia and atypical polypoid adenomyoma (APAM). Distinction from atypical hyperplasia may be particularly difficult in biopsies and curettage specimens. The best proof of carcinoma is evidence of invasion into adjacent stroma or myometrium. A confluent glandular or cribriform pattern resulting in a complex labyrinth- or maze-like appearance is considered invasive as it reflects loss of stroma [49]. Other criteria for invasion are a desmoplastic stromal response, and extensive papillary architecture [50]. APAM consists of crowded glands, often with squamous morules, surrounded by spindle cell stroma [51]. If the arrangement of the glands is complex, the differential diagnosis may be difficult, particularly since the stromal cells are of myofibroblastic origin and may suggest a desmoplastic reaction. Immunohistochemistry may not helpful for the differential diagnosis between APAM and myoinvasive endometrioid adenocarcinoma [52]. In contrast to endometrioid adenocarcinoma, APAM has an organoid pattern with a mixture of the glandular and mesenchymal components, and a lobulated appearance of the glandular component. Rarely, endometrioid adenocarcinoma may arise in APAM and is characterized by a confluent glandular growth pattern.

Table 2.3 FIGO grading of endometrioid carcinoma of the endometrium

FIGO grade	Amount of solid non-squamous, non-morular growth (%)
FIGO grade 1[a]	≤ 5
FIGO grade 2[a]	6–50
FIGO grade 3	>50

[a]The presence of bizarre nuclear atypia raises the grade by 1

Serous and clear cell carcinoma are by definition high grade (grade 3) and not further graded. According to UICC carcinosarcoma (MMMT) is also by definition grade 3

Table 2.4 Immunohistochemical typing of endometrial carcinoma

Histologic type	Typical immunohistochemical findings
Endometrioid G1/2 incl. variants	ER++/+++, PR++/+++, p53 wild type[a], Ki67+/++, PTEN−/+, p16 heterogeneous
Endometrioid G3 incl. variants	ER++/+, PR+/++, p53 heterogeneous, Ki67++/+++, PTEN−/+
Mucinous	ER++/+++, PR++/+++, p53 wild type, Ki67+/++, PTEN−/+, p16 + ++(diffuse)
Serous	ER+, PR+, p53 mutant[a], Ki67+++, PTEN++, p16+++
Clear cell	ER−/+, PR−/+, p53 heterogeneous, PTEN+/−, p16+/−, HNF1ß ++, Napsin A++, Rcemase++, ARID1A−/+

[a]P53 immunoreactivity: A diffuse positive or flat negative (all or null) pattern is associated with p53 mutation and therefore considered mutant. A heterogeneous pattern with at least a third strong positive nuclei is also associated with p53 mutations. A weak to moderate staining pattern is considered "wild type" [13]

Immunohistochemical staining for ER and PR is usually intense in low grade endometrioid adenocarcinoma, but may be absent in areas of squamous differentiation (Table 2.4). ß-catenin often shows aberrant (nuclear) staining, and PTEN and PAX-2 staining is reduced or lost (Fig. 2.1) [53, 54]. Ki-67 staining is variable. p53 immunoreactivity shows heterogenous, mostly weak to moderate nuclear staining with interspersed intense or negative nuclei, which is considered a "wild type pattern" [13]. P16 immunoreactivity is negative or patchy with focal staining [55]. High-grade endometrioid adenocarcinomas may partially show intense nuclear immunoreactivity for p53, suggestive of mutated TP53 [13]. ER and PR immunoreactivity is weak to moderate, or may be negative; the Ki-67 labeling index is usually 30–50% [56, 57].

Mucinous Carcinoma

Pure mucinous carcinoma of the endometrium is rare. By definition, more than 50% of cells contain PAS positive diastase resistant intracytoplasmic mucin [1]. More commonly, focal mucinous differentiation is found in endometrioid adenocarcinoma, often in combination with squamous differentiation. Cribriform or microglandular areas may resemble microglandular hyperplasia of the uterine endocervix, which should be considered in the differential diagnosis in biopsy specimens. The histological grade (assessed according to FIGO) and stage are usually low. Its association with exogenous estrogen has been reported [58]. Immunohistochemical staining shows diffuse positivity for ER and PR, and positivity for vimentin, which can be helpful in its differentiation from endocervical adenocarcinoma [59]. The Ki-67 labeling index is low (Table 2.4). An potential pitfall to note is the frequently high and diffuse immunoreactivity for p16, which is unrelated to HPV [60].

Serous Carcinoma

Serous carcinoma is considered a distinctive tumor, both histologically and at the molecular level [28, 61]. The diagnostic hallmark of serous carcinoma is the combination of low grade, often papillary architecture, and high nuclear grade [1]. However, the histologic pattern may vary by containing both short thick, and thin elongated papillae, but also glandular and solid structures (Fig. 2.3). Therefore, the term serous "papillary" carcinoma is misleading and should be avoided. Serous carcinomas are by definition high grade (grade 3). The tumor cells are usually polygonal and characterized by highly atypical nuclei, often with prominent nucleoli and frequent mitoses. Furthermore, the tumor cells are irregularly arranged and form buds and tufts, and are detached in small groups. The luminal borders of the glands and the surface of the papillae are scalloped. Serous carcinoma often occurs in a small uterus with atrophic endometrium and may be found within endometrial polyps. It may be associated with extensive LVSI.

The typical patient's median age is around 65–70 years. About one half of the patients are diagnosed at an advanced stage (stage >I). Serous carcinoma requires full surgical staging, since stage I uterine serous carcinoma can be associated with an excellent outcome [62, 63].

The differential diagnosis of serous carcinoma includes the papillary variant of endometrioid adenocarcinoma and clear cell carcinoma (detailed in Table 2.5). The

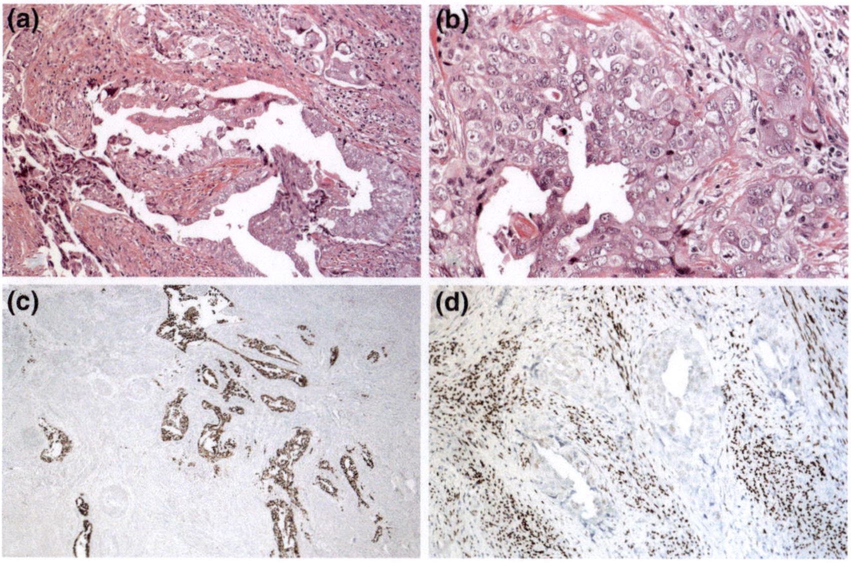

Fig. 2.3 Serous carcinoma with papillary, glandular, and solid growth patterns (**a**, **b**). Diffuse and strong p53 immunoreactivity (**c**) and weak ER immunoreactivity (**d**) are typical

Table 2.5 Differential diagnosis between serous, clear cell and endometrioid adenocarcinoma (papillary variant)

	Serous carcinoma	Papillary variant	Clear cell carcinoma
Papillae	Variable: short, thick, densely fibrotic or thin	Uniform, thin and delicate or broad	Short, thick with hyaline bodies
Cells	Columnar/polygonal; proliferation with tufting and budding; detached cell clusters	Columnar, pseudostratified; cohesive	Polygonal or hobnail shaped; slightly detached
Luminal borders	Scalloped	Regular, smooth ("straight")	Irregular
Nuclear features	Marked pleomorphism, frequent mitoses	Mild pleomorphism, infrequent mitoses	At least focal marked pleomorphism, frequent mitoses
Immuno-histochemistry	P53 diffusely positive or flat negative ER and PR negative/focal positive Ki-67 high	P53 negative/focally positive ER diffusely or heterogenously positive Ki-67 low/moderate	P53 focally positive ER and PR negative or mildly positive Ki-67 moderate to high

papillary variant of endometrioid adenocarcinoma usually has thin papillae and lacks marked nuclear atypia. Clear cell carcinoma usually contains at least focally cells with clear cytoplasm, hyalinized bodies, and eosinophilic globules.

Serous endometrial intraepithelial carcinoma (SEIC) consists of highly atypical cells replacing the endometrial surface and glands that do not invade the myometrium. SEIC has been considered an immediate precursor of serous carcinoma [64]. Biologically, SEIC is now considered a non-myoinvasive carcinoma since it may be associated with extensive extrauterine disease involving the peritoneum (e.g. omentum), the ovaries, and the fallopian tube [65]. (Endometrial glandular dysplasia was not adopted by the recent WHO classification.) In the setting of extensive pelvic serous carcinoma, it may be difficult to determine a site of origin. WT-1 immunohistochemistry may be helpful in the distinction between uterine and extra-uterine origin, since it is negative in about 90% of uterine serous carcinomas and positive in 70–100% of serous carcinomas originating from the ovary, fallopian tube, and peritoneum [66–68].

Immunohistochemistry shows a typical "all or null" or "mutant" immunoreactive pattern for p53 that correlates well with TP53 mutations (Table 2.4) (Fig. 2.3). Flat negative immunostaining is associated with frameshift mutations or a stop codon leading to a truncated protein that is not detectable with the usual p53 antibodies

[29]. ER immunoreactivity is usually weak or negative, and PR is often negative [56]. In cases with extensive extrauterine disease and a putative ovarian/tubal origin, ER and PR immunoreactivity may be moderate to strong.

Clear Cell Carcinoma

Clear cell carcinoma is composed of polygonal or hob-nail shaped cells with clear or eosinophilic cytoplasm and high grade nuclear features [69]. The architectural pattern may be tubulo-cystic, papillary, or solid (Fig. 2.4). The papillae are short and branching with hyalinized stroma. Other typical features are densely eosinophilic extracellular globules and hyaline bodies. Like serous carcinoma, clear cell carcinoma can occur in atrophic endometrium, within endometrial polyps, and is by definition high grade (grade 3) [1].

Immunohistochemical staining (Table 2.4) shows negativity or mild positivity for ER and PR, a Ki-67 proliferation index of at least 25–30%, and frequent positivity for HNF-1ß, Napsin A and racemase (AMACR) [57, 70–72]. Focal strong positivity for p53 is found in about one third of the cases and correlates with TP53 mutations on the genomic level (Fig. 2.4) [25]. About 30% of the cases show loss of PTEN [25]. Approximately 50% of the patients are diagnosed at stages II–IV and have a poor outcome, with a 5-year survival rate of less than 50% [69, 73, 74]. In contrast, an excellent prognosis is reported for stage I, particularly IA tumors [75].

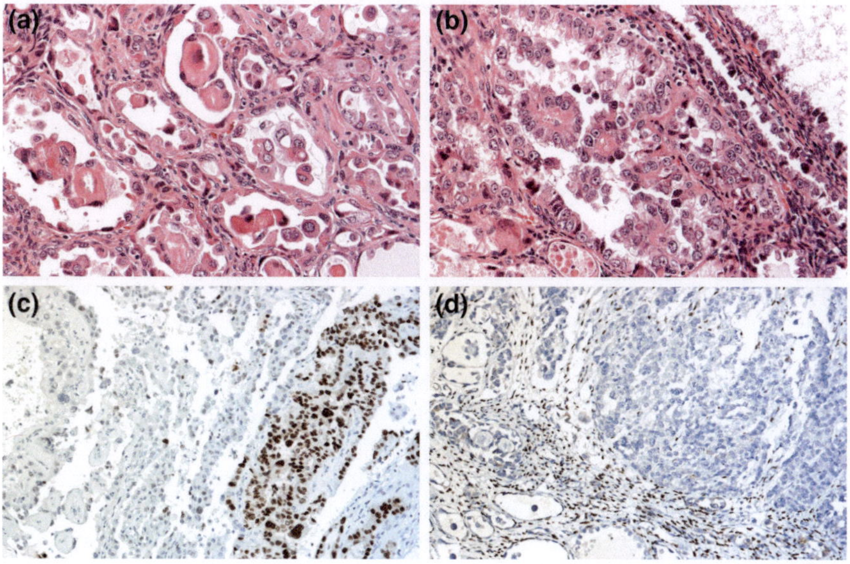

Fig. 2.4 Clear cell carcinoma with glandular (**a**) and papillary architecture (**b**). The cells are hob-nail shaped and the glands contain eosinophilic material. The typical immunoprofile is heterogeneous for p53 (**c**) and negative for ER (**d**)

Mixed Carcinoma

The recent WHO consensus defined mixed carcinoma as a composition of two or more different histologic types of endometrial carcinoma, of which at least one is of the type II category, particularly serous and clear cell carcinoma [1]. These different tumor types should be clearly visible on H&E stained sections and the minimum percentage of the minor component has been arbitrarily set at 5%. The most frequent combinations are endometrioid and serous carcinoma, and endometrioid and clear cell carcinoma. Immunohistochemistry can help support the diagnosis [76]. The high grade carcinoma determines the prognosis, even if it is present as a minor component (i.e. 5%) [77]. It was suggested that progression from endometrioid to serous carcinoma could lead to a mixed serous and endometrioid carcinoma [11, 78].

Undifferentiated Carcinoma

Undifferentiated carcinoma is a rare tumor that is defined by its lack of specific differentiation. The recent WHO classification distinguishes between monomorphic and dedifferentiated undifferentiated carcinoma [1]. The **monomorphic type** is composed of small to intermediate sized, relatively uniform cells usually arranged in sheets. The nuclei are hyperchromatic with frequent mitoses and may exhibit focal pleomorphism. The stroma may contain myxoid matrix resembling a carcinosarcoma, but in contrast to the latter a biphasic histological pattern is absent. The differential diagnosis includes other high grade neoplasms, such as high grade sarcomas, lymphoma and neuroendocrine carcinoma [79].

The **dedifferentiated type** is characterized by a sharply demarcated second component that consists of a low grade (FIGO grade 1 or 2) endometrioid adenocarcinoma [80]. Typically, the undifferentiated component infiltrates the myometrium, whereas the low grade component lines the endometrial cavity (Fig. 2.5). The undifferentiated component may have a sarcomatous appearance and lack immunoreactivity or have focal staining for cytokeratin and EMA, whereas vimentin is usually diffusely positive (Fig. 2.5). ER and PR are negative. Focal positivity for synaptophysin and chromogranin may be found and should not by itself lead to a diagnosis of neuroendocrine carcinoma [81]. The median patient age is about 55 years, which may reflect the fact that a subset of undifferentiated carcinomas occurs in patients with Lynch syndrome. The prognosis is poor with more than 50% of cases having a fatal outcome.

The differential diagnosis includes any high grade neoplasm of the endometrium, including carcinosarcoma (mixed malignant Mullerian tumor/MMMT). Carcinosarcoma has been considered an epithelial neoplasm with a special kind of epithelial-mesenchymal transition during its pathogenesis [82]. The pattern of metastatic spread resembles that seen in carcinoma, and the metastases of carcinosarcoma often contain predominantly or purely the carcinomatous component

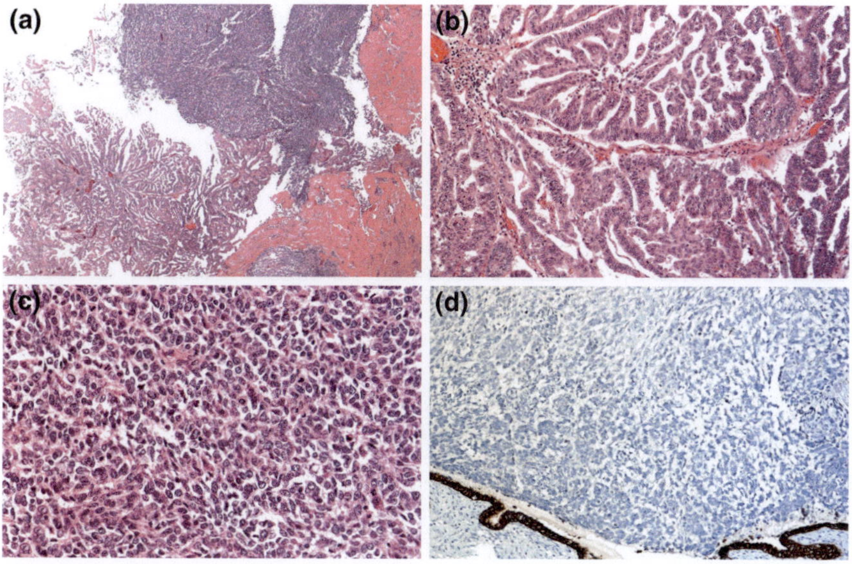

Fig. 2.5 Dedifferentiated type of undifferentiated carcinoma containing well differentiated endometrioid (**a**, **b**) and undifferentiated components (**a**, **c**). The latter consists of small, loosely cohesive cells (**c**) that are not immunoreactive with antibodies against cytokeratins (AE1/AE3) (**d**). The undifferentiated component was strongly immunoreactive for vimentin (not shown)

[83]. Carcinosarcoma is by definition a grade 3 tumor and is treated as an endometrial carcinoma for FIGO staging. However, in the WHO classification carcinosarcoma is categorized among the mixed tumors [1]. Histologically, carcinosarcoma is characterized by a biphasic pattern containing a variety of homologous or heterologous malignant mesenchymal tissues that are mixed with the malignant epithelial component [84]. The tumor components are often, but not necessarily, high grade [85]. The outcome is poor, comparable to high grade endometrioid adenocarcinoma, and seems to be influenced by the presence of heterologous elements. This biphasic intermixed histologic pattern differs from that seen in dedifferentiated carcinoma, which resembles collision tumors with large areas of demarcation between the two components. In addition, the components of dedifferentiated carcinoma are less heterogeneous as compared to those in carcinosarcoma.

Neuroendocrine Tumors

Neuroendocrine tumors were newly defined in the recent WHO classification (Table 2.1) [81]. They are very rare and occur at a median age of between 60 and 65 years. So far, only a few cases of low grade neuroendocrine tumor (carcinoid tumor) have been reported [86–88]. **Small cell neuroendocrine carcinoma (SCNEC)** resembles its counterparts at other sites (e.g. lung, gastrointestinal tract) [89, 90], grows diffusely or in nests, and may have trabecular and rosette-like structures. **Large cell neuroendocrine carcinoma (LCNEC)** consists of highly atypical cells with frequent mitoses that grow in well-demarcated nests, trabeculae and cords with palisading at the periphery. Extensive tumor cell necrosis is typical. A neuroendocrine growth pattern is generally present in at least a part of the tumor [91]. Immunohistochemistry with positivity for at least synaptophysin or chromogranin A is necessary to confirm the diagnosis of low grade neuroendocrine tumors. In poorly differentiated neuroendocrine carcinomas, chromogranin A is usually negative; CD56 (NCAM) may be positive, but is considered less specific. SCNEC shows a dot-like staining pattern for cytokeratins. The differential diagnosis includes other high grade neoplasms, in particular undifferentiated carcinoma. The prognosis for SCNEC and LCNEC is poor.

Staging of Endometrial Carcinoma

Endometrial carcinoma is surgically staged and, therefore, final staging is arrived at postoperatively. The current staging system as proposed by both FIGO and UICC in 2009 is detailed in Table 2.6. Several changes were made from the prior system, particularly for stages I and II. Stage IA now includes both carcinomas without invasion and those with invasion of the inner half of the myometrium, which helps in cases with difficult assessment of myometrial invasion. Stage II is now confined to tumors with invasion of cervical stroma; tumors that involve endocervical glands only are now grouped under stage I. This revised staging system provides a simplified approach, but has been challenged [92–97].

Prognostic Factors

The strongest prognostic factor for endometrial carcinoma is stage. Carcinomas that are confined to the uterine corpus (stage I) generally have a favorable prognosis [98]. Histologic type and grade, depth of myometrial invasion, and the presence of (lymph) vascular invasion stratify this group for prognosis [99, 100]. Although peritoneal cytology has been excluded from staging, positivity for tumor cells has been demonstrated as an adverse prognostic factor in multivariate analysis [101]. Three different risk groups for recurrence and distant metastases of endometrial carcinomas confined to the uterus have been developed by radiation oncologists [99, 102, 103]. The TCGA project resulted in a molecular based stratification with three major prognostic groups, of which the serous-like had the worst prognosis [21].

Table 2.6 2009 FIGO/UICC staging of endometrial carcinoma (including carcinosarcoma/MMMT)

Stage	pTNM	Definition
I		Tumor confined to the uterine corpus
IA	pT1a	No or less than one half myometrial invasion
IB	pT1b	Invasion equal to or more than one half of the myometrium
II	pT2	Tumor invades cervical stroma but does not extend beyond uterus
III		Local and/or regional spread of the tumor
IIIA	pT3a	Tumor invades the serosa of the uterus and/or adnexa
IIIB	pT3b	Vaginal and/or parametrial involvement
IIIC		Metastases to pelvic and/or para-aortic lymph nodes
IIIC1	pN1	Positive pelvic nodes
IIIC2	pN2	Positive para-aortic nodes with or without positive pelvic nodes
IV		Tumor invades bladder and/or bowel mucosa; distant metastases
IVA	pT4	Tumor invasion bladder and/or bowel mucosa
IVB	pM1	Distant metastases including intra-abdominal metastases and/or inguinal nodes

Hereditary Endometrial Carcinoma

Hereditary non-polyposis colorectal cancer (HNPCC)/Lynch syndrome and Cowden syndrome are heritable syndromes associated with increased risk for endometrial carcinoma [104, 105]. Lynch syndrome is characterized by germline mutations in the mismatch repair proteins MLH1, MSH2, MSH6 or PMS2 and is associated with carcinomas of the colon and rectum, and the endometrium. Additionally, transitional cell carcinoma of the urogenital tract and ovarian carcinoma (particularly the clear cell type) may occur. Approximately 2% of all endometrial carcinomas are associated with Lynch syndrome, most of which are endometrioid histotype [106]. Recently, other histologic types have been described in patients with Lynch syndrome, particularly the dedifferentiated variant of undifferentiated carcinoma. There is evidence that a subset of these tumors arises from the lower uterine segment. In patients with Lynch syndrome there is a 20–60% lifetime risk of developing atypical hyperplasia and endometrial carcinoma [105, 106]. Endometrial carcinoma may be the sentinel event or follow colorectal carcinoma in these individuals. Late onset of either endometrial or colorectal carcinoma is not unusual for Lynch syndrome, since the median age for both cancers is slightly above 60 years. Secondary to the late onset of disease and recent smaller family sizes, the selection criteria for Lynch mutation carriers such as Amsterdam II and Bethesda II are considered increasingly less reliable. Therefore, screening of all newly detected endometrial carcinomas by immunohistochemistry has been proposed [107].

Cowden syndrome is much less frequent than Lynch syndrome. Patients with Cowden syndrome harbor germline mutations for PTEN and may be affected by carcinomas of various organs such as the uterus (endometrium), the thyroid, and the breast.

References

1. Kurman RJ, Carcangiu ML, Herrington S, Young RH (eds) (2014) Tumours of the female reproductive organs. WHO classification of tumours. IARC Press, Lyon.
2. Bokhman JV. Two pathogenetic types of endometrial carcinoma. Gynecol Oncol. 1983;15 (1):10–7.
3. Lax SF. Molecular genetic pathways in various types of endometrial carcinoma: from a phenotypical to a molecular-based classification. Virchows Arch. 2004;444(3):213–23.
4. Sherman ME. Theories of endometrial carcinogenesis: a multidisciplinary approach. Mod Pathol. 2000;13(3):295–308. doi:10.1038/modpathol.3880051.
5. Sherman ME, Sturgeon S, Brinton LA, Potischman N, Kurman RJ, Berman ML, Mortel R, Twiggs LB, Barrett RJ, Wilbanks GD. Risk factors and hormone levels in patients with serous and endometrioid uterine carcinomas. Mod Pathol. 1997;10(10):963–8.
6. Jia L, Liu Y, Yi X, Miron A, Crum CP, Kong B, Zheng W. Endometrial glandular dysplasia with frequent p53 gene mutation: a genetic evidence supporting its precancer nature for endometrial serous carcinoma. Clin Cancer Res. 2008;14(8):2263–9. doi:10.1158/1078-0432.CCR-07-4837.
7. Liang SX, Chambers SK, Cheng L, Zhang S, Zhou Y, Zheng W. Endometrial glandular dysplasia: a putative precursor lesion of uterine papillary serous carcinoma. Part II: molecular features. Int J Surg Pathol. 2004;12(4):319–31.
8. Zheng W, Liang SX, Yi X, Ulukus EC, Davis JR, Chambers SK. Occurrence of endometrial glandular dysplasia precedes uterine papillary serous carcinoma. Int J Gynecol Pathol. 2007;26(1):38–52. doi:10.1097/01.pgp.0000228138.56222.4e.
9. Zheng W, Liang SX, Yu H, Rutherford T, Chambers SK, Schwartz PE. Endometrial glandular dysplasia: a newly defined precursor lesion of uterine papillary serous carcinoma. Part I: morphologic features. Int J Surg Pathol. 2004;12(3):207–23.
10. Yeramian A, Moreno-Bueno G, Dolcet X, Catasus L, Abal M, Colas E, Reventos J, Palacios J, Prat J, Matias-Guiu X. Endometrial carcinoma: molecular alterations involved in tumor development and progression. Oncogene. 2013;32(4):403–13. doi:10.1038/onc.2012.76.
11. Matias-Guiu X, Prat J. Molecular pathology of endometrial carcinoma. Histopathology. 2013;62(1):111–23. doi:10.1111/his.12053.
12. Djordjevic B, Barkoh BA, Luthra R, Broaddus RR. Relationship between PTEN, DNA mismatch repair, and tumor histotype in endometrial carcinoma: retained positive expression of PTEN preferentially identifies sporadic non-endometrioid carcinomas. Mod Pathol. 2013;26(10):1401–12. doi:10.1038/modpathol.2013.67.
13. Lax SF, Kendall B, Tashiro H, Slebos RJ, Hedrick L. The frequency of p53, K-ras mutations, and microsatellite instability differs in uterine endometrioid and serous carcinoma: evidence of distinct molecular genetic pathways. Cancer. 2000;88(4):814–24.
14. Tashiro H, Blazes MS, Wu R, Cho KR, Bose S, Wang SI, Li J, Parsons R, Ellenson LH. Mutations in PTEN are frequent in endometrial carcinoma but rare in other common gynecological malignancies. Cancer Res. 1997;57(18):3935–40.
15. Guan B, Mao TL, Panuganti PK, Kuhn E, Kurman RJ, Maeda D, Chen E, Jeng YM, Wang TL, Shih Ie M. Mutation and loss of expression of ARID1A in uterine low-grade endometrioid carcinoma. Am J Surg Pathol. 2011;35(5):625–32. doi:10.1097/PAS.0b013e318212782a.

16. Kuhn E, Wu RC, Guan B, Wu G, Zhang J, Wang Y, Song L, Yuan X, Wei L, Roden RB, Kuo KT, Nakayama K, Clarke B, Shaw P, Olvera N, Kurman RJ, Levine DA, Wang TL, Shih Ie M. Identification of molecular pathway aberrations in uterine serous carcinoma by genome-wide analyses. J Natl Cancer Inst. 2012;104(19):1503–13. doi:10.1093/jnci/djs345.
17. Catasus L, Matias-Guiu X, Machin P, Munoz J, Prat J. BAX somatic frameshift mutations in endometrioid adenocarcinomas of the endometrium: evidence for a tumor progression role in endometrial carcinomas with microsatellite instability. Lab Invest. 1998;78(11):1439–44.
18. Oda K, Stokoe D, Taketani Y, McCormick F. High frequency of coexistent mutations of PIK3CA and PTEN genes in endometrial carcinoma. Cancer Res. 2005;65(23):10669–73. doi:10.1158/0008-5472.CAN-05-2620.
19. Bashir S, Jiang G, Joshi A, Miller C Jr, Matrai C, Yemelyanova A, Caputo TA, Holcomb KM, Ellenson LH, Gupta D. Molecular alterations of PIK3CA in uterine carcinosarcoma, clear cell, and serous tumors. Int J Gynecol Cancer. 2014;24(7):1262–7. doi:10.1097/IGC.0000000000000183.
20. Rudd ML, Price JC, Fogoros S, Godwin AK, Sgroi DC, Merino MJ, Bell DW. A unique spectrum of somatic PIK3CA (p110alpha) mutations within primary endometrial carcinomas. Clin Cancer Res. 2011;17(6):1331–40. doi:10.1158/1078-0432.CCR-10-0540.
21. Cancer Genome Atlas Research N, Kandoth C, Schultz N, Cherniack AD, Akbani R, Liu Y, Shen H, Robertson AG, Pashtan I, Shen R, Benz CC, Yau C, Laird PW, Ding L, Zhang W, Mills GB, Kucherlapati R, Mardis ER, Levine DA. Integrated genomic characterization of endometrial carcinoma. Nature. 2013;497(7447):67–73. doi:10.1038/nature12113.
22. Hussein YR, Weigelt B, Levine DA, Schoolmeester JK, Dao LN, Balzer BL, Liles G, Karlan B, Kobel M, Lee CH, Soslow RA. Clinicopathological analysis of endometrial carcinomas harboring somatic POLE exonuclease domain mutations. Mod Pathol. 2015;28(4):505–14. doi:10.1038/modpathol.2014.143.
23. Talhouk A, McConechy MK, Leung S, Li-Chang HH, Kwon JS, Melnyk N, Yang W, Senz J, Boyd N, Karnezis AN, Huntsman DG, Gilks CB, McAlpine JN. A clinically applicable molecular-based classification for endometrial cancers. Br J Cancer. 2015;113(2):299–310. doi:10.1038/bjc.2015.190.
24. Wiegand KC, Lee AF, Al-Agha OM, Chow C, Kalloger SE, Scott DW, Steidl C, Wiseman SM, Gascoyne RD, Gilks B, Huntsman DG. Loss of BAF250a (ARID1A) is frequent in high-grade endometrial carcinomas. J Pathol. 2011;224(3):328–33. doi:10.1002/path.2911.
25. An HJ, Logani S, Isacson C, Ellenson LH. Molecular characterization of uterine clear cell carcinoma. Mod Pathol. 2004;17(5):530–7. doi:10.1038/modpathol.3800057.
26. Hoang LN, McConechy MK, Meng B, McIntyre JB, Ewanowich C, Gilks CB, Huntsman DG, Kobel M, Lee CH. Targeted mutation analysis of endometrial clear cell carcinoma. Histopathology. 2015;66(5):664–74. doi:10.1111/his.12581.
27. Guan B, Wang TL, Shih le M. ARID1A, a factor that promotes formation of SWI/SNF-mediated chromatin remodeling, is a tumor suppressor in gynecologic cancers. Cancer Res. 2011;71(21):6718–27. doi:10.1158/0008-5472.CAN-11-1562.
28. Sherman ME, Bitterman P, Rosenshein NB, Delgado G, Kurman RJ. Uterine serous carcinoma. A morphologically diverse neoplasm with unifying clinicopathologic features. Am J Surg Pathol. 1992;16(6):600–10.
29. Tashiro H, Isacson C, Levine R, Kurman RJ, Cho KR, Hedrick L. p53 gene mutations are common in uterine serous carcinoma and occur early in their pathogenesis. Am J Pathol. 1997;150(1):177–85.
30. Kuhn E, Bahadirli-Talbott A, Shih Ie M. Frequent CCNE1 amplification in endometrial intraepithelial carcinoma and uterine serous carcinoma. Mod Pathol. 2014;27(7):1014–9. doi:10.1038/modpathol.2013.209.
31. Ferlay J, Shin HR, Bray F, Forman D, Mathers C, Parkin DM. Estimates of worldwide burden of cancer in 2008: GLOBOCAN 2008. Int J Cancer. 2010;127(12):2893–917. doi:10.1002/ijc.25516.

32. Abeler VM, Kjorstad KE. Endometrial adenocarcinoma in Norway. A study of a total population. Cancer. 1991;67(12):3093–103.
33. Zaino RJ, Kurman R, Herbold D, Gliedman J, Bundy BN, Voet R, Advani H. The significance of squamous differentiation in endometrial carcinoma. Data from a Gynecologic Oncology Group study. Cancer. 1991;68(10):2293–302.
34. Abeler VM, Kjorstad KE. Endometrial adenocarcinoma with squamous cell differentiation. Cancer. 1992;69(2):488–95.
35. Zaino RJ, Kurman RJ. Squamous differentiation in carcinoma of the endometrium: a critical appraisal of adenoacanthoma and adenosquamous carcinoma. Semin Diagn Pathol. 1988;5 (2):154–71.
36. Kim KR, Scully RE. Peritoneal keratin granulomas with carcinomas of endometrium and ovary and atypical polypoid adenomyoma of endometrium. A clinicopathological analysis of 22 cases. Am J Surg Pathol. 1990;14(10):925–32.
37. Zaino RJ, Kurman RJ, Brunetto VL, Morrow CP, Bentley RC, Cappellari JO, Bitterman P. Villoglandular adenocarcinoma of the endometrium: a clinicopathologic study of 61 cases: a gynecologic oncology group study. Am J Surg Pathol. 1998;22(11):1379–85.
38. Malpica A. How to approach the many faces of endometrioid carcinoma. Mod Pathol. 2016;29(Suppl 1):S29–44. doi:10.1038/modpathol.2015.142.
39. Christopherson WM, Alberhasky RC, Connelly PJ. Carcinoma of the endometrium: I. A clinicopathologic study of clear-cell carcinoma and secretory carcinoma. Cancer. 1982;49 (8):1511–23.
40. Tobon H, Watkins GJ. Secretory adenocarcinoma of the endometrium. Int J Gynecol Pathol. 1985;4(4):328–35.
41. Hendrickson MR, Kempson RL. Ciliated carcinoma—a variant of endometrial adenocarcinoma: a report of 10 cases. Int J Gynecol Pathol. 1983;2(1):1–12.
42. Han G, Lim D, Leitao MM Jr, Abu-Rustum NR, Soslow RA. Histological features associated with occult lymph node metastasis in FIGO clinical stage I, grade I endometrioid carcinoma. Histopathology. 2014;64(3):389–98. doi:10.1111/his.12254.
43. Mai KT, Perkins DG, Yazdi HM, Thomas J. Endometrioid carcinoma of the endometrium with an invasive component of minimal deviation carcinoma. Hum Pathol. 2002;33(8): 856–8.
44. Ali A, Black D, Soslow RA. Difficulties in assessing the depth of myometrial invasion in endometrial carcinoma. Int J Gynecol Pathol. 2007;26(2):115–23. doi:10.1097/01.pgp. 0000233165.56385.0b.
45. Sagae S, Saito T, Satoh M, Ikeda T, Kimura S, Mori M, Sato N, Kudo R. The reproducibility of a binary tumor grading system for uterine endometrial endometrioid carcinoma, compared with FIGO system and nuclear grading. Oncology. 2004;67(5–6):344–50. doi:10.1159/ 000082917.
46. Lax SF, Kurman RJ, Pizer ES, Wu L, Ronnett BM. A binary architectural grading system for uterine endometrial endometrioid carcinoma has superior reproducibility compared with FIGO grading and identifies subsets of advance-stage tumors with favorable and unfavorable prognosis. Am J Surg Pathol. 2000;24(9):1201–8.
47. Guan H, Semaan A, Bandyopadhyay S, Arabi H, Feng J, Fathallah L, Pansare V, Qazi A, Abdul-Karim F, Morris RT, Munkarah AR, Ali-Fehmi R. Prognosis and reproducibility of new and existing binary grading systems for endometrial carcinoma compared to FIGO grading in hysterectomy specimens. Int J Gynecol Cancer. 2011;21(4):654–60. doi:10.1097/ IGC.0b013e31821454f1.
48. Alkushi A, Abdul-Rahman ZH, Lim P, Schulzer M, Coldman A, Kalloger SE, Miller D, Gilks CB. Description of a novel system for grading of endometrial carcinoma and comparison with existing grading systems. Am J Surg Pathol. 2005;29(3):295–304.
49. Longacre TA, Chung MH, Jensen DN, Hendrickson MR. Proposed criteria for the diagnosis of well-differentiated endometrial carcinoma. A diagnostic test for myoinvasion. Am J Surg Pathol. 1995;19(4):371–406.

50. Kurman RJ, Norris HJ. Evaluation of criteria for distinguishing atypical endometrial hyperplasia from well-differentiated carcinoma. Cancer. 1982;49(12):2547–59.
51. Heatley MK. Atypical polypoid adenomyoma: a systematic review of the English literature. Histopathology. 2006;48(5):609–10. doi:10.1111/j.1365-2559.2005.02315.x.
52. Soslow RA, Chung MH, Rouse RV, Hendrickson MR, Longacre TA. Atypical polypoid adenomyofibroma (APA) versus well-differentiated endometrial carcinoma with prominent stromal matrix: an immunohistochemical study. Int J Gynecol Pathol. 1996;15(3):209–16.
53. Monte NM, Webster KA, Neuberg D, Dressler GR, Mutter GL. Joint loss of PAX2 and PTEN expression in endometrial precancers and cancer. Cancer Res. 2010;70(15):6225–32. doi:10.1158/0008-5472.CAN-10-0149.
54. Moreno-Bueno G, Hardisson D, Sarrio D, Sanchez C, Cassia R, Prat J, Herman JG, Esteller M, Matias-Guiu X, Palacios J. Abnormalities of E- and P-cadherin and catenin (beta-, gamma-catenin, and p120ctn) expression in endometrial cancer and endometrial atypical hyperplasia. J Pathol. 2003;199(4):471–8. doi:10.1002/path.1310.
55. Ansari-Lari MA, Staebler A, Zaino RJ, Shah KV, Ronnett BM. Distinction of endocervical and endometrial adenocarcinomas: immunohistochemical p16 expression correlated with human papillomavirus (HPV) DNA detection. Am J Surg Pathol. 2004;28(2):160–7.
56. Lax SF, Pizer ES, Ronnett BM, Kurman RJ. Clear cell carcinoma of the endometrium is characterized by a distinctive profile of p53, Ki-67, estrogen, and progesterone receptor expression. Hum Pathol. 1998;29(6):551–8.
57. Lax SF, Pizer ES, Ronnett BM, Kurman RJ. Comparison of estrogen and progesterone receptor, Ki-67, and p53 immunoreactivity in uterine endometrioid carcinoma and endometrioid carcinoma with squamous, mucinous, secretory, and ciliated cell differentiation. Hum Pathol. 1998;29(9):924–31.
58. Ross JC, Eifel PJ, Cox RS, Kempson RL, Hendrickson MR. Primary mucinous adenocarcinoma of the endometrium. A clinicopathologic and histochemical study. Am J Surg Pathol. 1983;7(8):715–29.
59. Staebler A, Sherman ME, Zaino RJ, Ronnett BM. Hormone receptor immunohistochemistry and human papillomavirus in situ hybridization are useful for distinguishing endocervical and endometrial adenocarcinomas. Am J Surg Pathol. 2002;26(8):998–1006.
60. Chekmareva M, Ellenson LH, Pirog EC. Immunohistochemical differences between mucinous and microglandular adenocarcinomas of the endometrium and benign endocervical epithelium. Int J Gynecol Pathol. 2008;27(4):547–54. doi:10.1097/PGP.0b013e318177eadc.
61. Hendrickson M, Ross J, Eifel P, Martinez A, Kempson R. Uterine papillary serous carcinoma: a highly malignant form of endometrial adenocarcinoma. Am J Surg Pathol. 1982;6(2):93–108.
62. Giuntoli RL 2nd, Gerardi MA, Yemelyanova AV, Ueda SM, Fleury AC, Diaz-Montes TP, Bristow RE. Stage I noninvasive and minimally invasive uterine serous carcinoma: comprehensive staging associated with improved survival. Int J Gynecol Cancer. 2012;22(2):273–9. doi:10.1097/IGC.0b013e318238df4d.
63. Seward S, Ali-Fehmi R, Munkarah AR, Semaan A, Al-Wahab ZR, Elshaikh MA, Cote ML, Morris RT, Bandyopadhyay S. Outcomes of patients with uterine serous carcinoma using the revised FIGO staging system. Int J Gynecol Cancer. 2012;22(3):452–6. doi:10.1097/IGC.0b013e31823de6dd.
64. Ambros RA, Sherman ME, Zahn CM, Bitterman P, Kurman RJ. Endometrial intraepithelial carcinoma: a distinctive lesion specifically associated with tumors displaying serous differentiation. Hum Pathol. 1995;26(11):1260–7.
65. Wheeler DT, Bell KA, Kurman RJ, Sherman ME. Minimal uterine serous carcinoma: diagnosis and clinicopathologic correlation. Am J Surg Pathol. 2000;24(6):797–806.
66. Al-Hussaini M, Stockman A, Foster H, McCluggage WG. WT-1 assists in distinguishing ovarian from uterine serous carcinoma and in distinguishing between serous and endometrioid ovarian carcinoma. Histopathology. 2004;44(2):109–15.

67. Goldstein NS, Uzieblo A. WT1 immunoreactivity in uterine papillary serous carcinomas is different from ovarian serous carcinomas. Am J Clin Pathol. 2002;117(4):541–5. doi:10.1309/K84K-005F-TCB8-FV4B.
68. Hirschowitz L, Ganesan R, McCluggage WG. WT1, p53 and hormone receptor expression in uterine serous carcinoma. Histopathology. 2009;55(4):478–82. doi:10.1111/j.1365-2559.2009.03390.x.
69. Kurman RJ, Scully RE. Clear cell carcinoma of the endometrium: an analysis of 21 cases. Cancer. 1976;37(2):872–82.
70. Fadare O, Desouki MM, Gwin K, Hanley KZ, Jarboe EA, Liang SX, Quick CM, Zheng W, Parkash V, Hecht JL. Frequent expression of napsin A in clear cell carcinoma of the endometrium: potential diagnostic utility. Am J Surg Pathol. 2014;38(2):189–96. doi:10.1097/PAS.0000000000000085.
71. Fadare O, Parkash V, Gwin K, Hanley KZ, Jarboe EA, Liang SX, Quick CM, Zheng W, Rawish KR, Hecht JL, Desouki MM. Utility of alpha-methylacyl-coenzyme-A racemase (p504s) immunohistochemistry in distinguishing endometrial clear cell carcinomas from serous and endometrioid carcinomas. Hum Pathol. 2013;44(12):2814–21. doi:10.1016/j.humpath.2013.07.033.
72. Hoang LN, Han G, McConechy M, Lau S, Chow C, Gilks CB, Huntsman DG, Kobel M, Lee CH. Immunohistochemical characterization of prototypical endometrial clear cell carcinoma–diagnostic utility of HNF-1beta and oestrogen receptor. Histopathology. 2014;64(4):585–96. doi:10.1111/his.12286.
73. Abeler VM, Kjorstad KE. Clear cell carcinoma of the endometrium: a histopathological and clinical study of 97 cases. Gynecol Oncol. 1991;40(3):207–17.
74. Webb GA, Lagios MD. Clear cell carcinoma of the endometrium. Am J Obstet Gynecol. 1987;156(6):1486–91.
75. Carcangiu ML, Chambers JT. Early pathologic stage clear cell carcinoma and uterine papillary serous carcinoma of the endometrium: comparison of clinicopathologic features and survival. Int J Gynecol Pathol. 1995;14(1):30–8.
76. Alkushi A, Kobel M, Kalloger SE, Gilks CB. High-grade endometrial carcinoma: serous and grade 3 endometrioid carcinomas have different immunophenotypes and outcomes. Int J Gynecol Pathol. 2010;29(4):343–50. doi:10.1097/PGP.0b013e3181cd6552.
77. Quddus MR, Sung CJ, Zhang C, Lawrence WD. Minor serous and clear cell components adversely affect prognosis in "mixed-type" endometrial carcinomas: a clinicopathologic study of 36 stage-I cases. Reprod Sci. 2010;17(7):673–8. doi:10.1177/1933719110368433.
78. McConechy MK, Ding J, Cheang MC, Wiegand KC, Senz J, Tone AA, Yang W, Prentice LM, Tse K, Zeng T, McDonald H, Schmidt AP, Mutch DG, McAlpine JN, Hirst M, Shah SP, Lee CH, Goodfellow PJ, Gilks CB, Huntsman DG. Use of mutation profiles to refine the classification of endometrial carcinomas. J Pathol. 2012;228(1):20–30. doi:10.1002/path.4056.
79. Tafe LJ, Garg K, Chew I, Tornos C, Soslow RA. Endometrial and ovarian carcinomas with undifferentiated components: clinically aggressive and frequently underrecognized neoplasms. Mod Pathol. 2010;23(6):781–9. doi:10.1038/modpathol.2010.41.
80. Silva EG, Deavers MT, Bodurka DC, Malpica A. Association of low-grade endometrioid carcinoma of the uterus and ovary with undifferentiated carcinoma: a new type of dedifferentiated carcinoma? Int J Gynecol Pathol. 2006;25(1):52–8.
81. Altrabulsi B, Malpica A, Deavers MT, Bodurka DC, Broaddus R, Silva EG. Undifferentiated carcinoma of the endometrium. Am J Surg Pathol. 2005;29(10):1316–21.
82. Seidman JD, Chauhan S. Evaluation of the relationship between adenosarcoma and carcinosarcoma and a hypothesis of the histogenesis of uterine sarcomas. Int J Gynecol Pathol. 2003;22(1):75–82.
83. Nordal RR, Kristensen GB, Stenwig AE, Nesland JM, Pettersen EO, Trope CG. An evaluation of prognostic factors in uterine carcinosarcoma. Gynecol Oncol. 1997;67(3):316–21. doi:10.1006/gyno.1997.4875.

84. de Brito PA, Silverberg SG, Orenstein JM. Carcinosarcoma (malignant mixed mullerian (mesodermal) tumor) of the female genital tract: immunohistochemical and ultrastructural analysis of 28 cases. Hum Pathol. 1993;24(2):132–42.
85. Silverberg SG, Major FJ, Blessing JA, Fetter B, Askin FB, Liao SY, Miller A. Carcinosarcoma (malignant mixed mesodermal tumor) of the uterus. A Gynecologic Oncology Group pathologic study of 203 cases. Int J Gynecol Pathol. 1990;9(1):1–19.
86. Gonzalez-Bosquet E, Gonzalez-Bosquet J, Garcia Jimenez A, Gil A, Xercavins J. Carcinoid tumor of the uterine corpus. A case report. J Reprod Med. 1998;43(9):844–6.
87. Chetty R, Clark SP, Bhathal PS. Carcinoid tumour of the uterine corpus. Virchows Arch A Pathol Anat Histopathol. 1993;422(1):93–5.
88. Starzynski S, Kubicka-Pertkiewicz M. Carcinoid of the uterine corpus. Patol Pol. 1978;29 (2):237–40.
89. Huntsman DG, Clement PB, Gilks CB, Scully RE. Small-cell carcinoma of the endometrium. A clinicopathological study of sixteen cases. Am J Surg Pathol. 1994;18 (4):364–75.
90. van Hoeven KH, Hudock JA, Woodruff JM, Suhrland MJ. Small cell neuroendocrine carcinoma of the endometrium. Int J Gynecol Pathol. 1995;14(1):21–9.
91. Deodhar KK, Kerkar RA, Suryawanshi P, Menon H, Menon S. Large cell neuroendocrine carcinoma of the endometrium: an extremely uncommon diagnosis, but worth the efforts. J Cancer Res Ther. 2011;7(2):211–3. doi:10.4103/0973-1482.82942.
92. Zaino RJ. FIGO staging of endometrial adenocarcinoma: a critical review and proposal. Int J Gynecol Pathol. 2009;28(1):1–9. doi:10.1097/PGP.0b013e3181846c6d.
93. Abu-Rustum NR, Zhou Q, Iasonos A, Alektiar KM, Leitao MM Jr, Chi DS, Sonoda Y, Soslow R, Hensley M, Barakat RR. The revised 2009 FIGO staging system for endometrial cancer: should the 1988 FIGO stages IA and IB be altered? Int J Gynecol Cancer. 2011;21 (3):511–6. doi:10.1097/IGC.0b013e31820cc305.
94. Haltia UM, Butzow R, Leminen A, Loukovaara M. FIGO 1988 versus 2009 staging for endometrial carcinoma: a comparative study on prediction of survival and stage distribution according to histologic subtype. J Gynecol Oncol. 2014;25(1):30–5. doi:10.3802/jgo.2014. 25.1.30.
95. Kim HS, Kim HY, Park CY, Lee JM, Lee JK, Cho CH, Kim SM, Kim JW. Lymphadenectomy increases the prognostic value of the revised 2009 FIGO staging system for endometrial cancer: a multi-center study. Eur J Surg Oncol. 2012;38(3):230–7. doi:10. 1016/j.ejso.2011.12.023.
96. Werner HM, Trovik J, Marcickiewicz J, Tingulstad S, Staff AC, Amant F, Salvesen HB, MoMa TECsg. Revision of FIGO surgical staging in 2009 for endometrial cancer validates to improve risk stratification. Gynecol Oncol. 2012;125(1):103–8. doi:10.1016/j.ygyno. 2011.11.008.
97. Korczynski J, Jesionek-Kupnicka D, Gottwald L, Piekarski J. Comparison of FIGO 1989 and 2009 recommendations on staging of endometrial carcinoma: pathologic analysis and cervical status in 123 consecutive cases. Int J Gynecol Pathol. 2011;30(4):328–34. doi:10. 1097/PGP.0b013e3182069c30.
98. Morrow CP, Bundy BN, Kurman RJ, Creasman WT, Heller P, Homesley HD, Graham JE. Relationship between surgical-pathological risk factors and outcome in clinical stage I and II carcinoma of the endometrium: a Gynecologic Oncology Group study. Gynecol Oncol. 1991;40(1):55–65.
99. Bosse T, Peters EE, Creutzberg CL, Jurgenliemk-Schulz IM, Jobsen JJ, Mens JW, Lutgens LC, van der Steen-Banasik EM, Smit VT, Nout RA. Substantial lymph-vascular space invasion (LVSI) is a significant risk factor for recurrence in endometrial cancer—a pooled analysis of PORTEC 1 and 2 trials. Eur J Cancer. 2015;51(13):1742–50. doi:10. 1016/j.ejca.2015.05.015.
100. Hachisuga T, Kaku T, Fukuda K, Eguchi F, Emoto M, Kamura T, Iwasaka T, Kawarabayashi T, Sugimori H, Mori M. The grading of lymphovascular space invasion in endometrial carcinoma. Cancer. 1999;86(10):2090–7.

101. Han KH, Park NH, Kim HS, Chung HH, Kim JW, Song YS. Peritoneal cytology: a risk factor of recurrence for non-endometrioid endometrial cancer. Gynecol Oncol. 2014;134 (2):293–6. doi:10.1016/j.ygyno.2014.05.010.
102. Group AES, Blake P, Swart AM, Orton J, Kitchener H, Whelan T, Lukka H, Eisenhauer E, Bacon M, Tu D, Parmar MK, Amos C, Murray C, Qian W. Adjuvant external beam radiotherapy in the treatment of endometrial cancer (MRC ASTEC and NCIC CTG EN.5 randomised trials): pooled trial results, systematic review, and meta-analysis. Lancet. 2009;373(9658):137–46. doi:10.1016/S0140-6736(08)61767-5.
103. Creutzberg CL, van Putten WL, Warlam-Rodenhuis CC, van den Bergh AC, de Winter KA, Koper PC, Lybeert ML, Slot A, Lutgens LC, Stenfert Kroese MC, Beerman H, van Lent M. Outcome of high-risk stage IC, grade 3, compared with stage I endometrial carcinoma patients: the postoperative radiation therapy in endometrial carcinoma trial. J Clin Oncol. 2004;22(7):1234–41. doi:10.1200/JCO.2004.08.159.
104. Tan MH, Mester JL, Ngeow J, Rybicki LA, Orloff MS, Eng C. Lifetime cancer risks in individuals with germline PTEN mutations. Clin Cancer Res. 2012;18(2):400–7. doi:10.1158/1078-0432.CCR-11-2283.
105. Bonadona V, Bonaiti B, Olschwang S, Grandjouan S, Huiart L, Longy M, Guimbaud R, Buecher B, Bignon YJ, Caron O, Colas C, Nogues C, Lejeune-Dumoulin S, Olivier-Faivre L, Polycarpe-Osaer F, Nguyen TD, Desseigne F, Saurin JC, Berthet P, Leroux D, Duffour J, Manouvrier S, Frebourg T, Sobol H, Lasset C, Bonaiti-Pellie C, French Cancer Genetics N. Cancer risks associated with germline mutations in MLH1, MSH2, and MSH6 genes in Lynch syndrome. JAMA. 2011;305(22):2304–10. doi:10.1001/jama.2011.743.
106. Hampel H, Frankel W, Panescu J, Lockman J, Sotamaa K, Fix D, Comeras I, La Jeunesse J, Nakagawa H, Westman JA, Prior TW, Clendenning M, Penzone P, Lombardi J, Dunn P, Cohn DE, Copeland L, Eaton L, Fowler J, Lewandowski G, Vaccarello L, Bell J, Reid G, de la Chapelle A. Screening for Lynch syndrome (hereditary nonpolyposis colorectal cancer) among endometrial cancer patients. Cancer Res. 2006;66(15):7810–7. doi:10.1158/0008-5472.CAN-06-1114.
107. Mills AM, Liou S, Ford JM, Berek JS, Pai RK, Longacre TA. Lynch syndrome screening should be considered for all patients with newly diagnosed endometrial cancer. Am J Surg Pathol. 2014;38(11):1501–9. doi:10.1097/PAS.0000000000000321.

Chapter 3
Immunohistochemical Markers in Endometrial Carcinoma

Bojana Djordjevic and Russell R. Broaddus

Endometrial Carcinoma Versus Extramüllerian Primaries

Endometrial involvement by extragenital metastatic tumors is relatively infrequent. Most commonly, these are carcinomas [1, 2]. Morphologic clues that suggest the presence of a metastasis in the endometrium include an absence of a mass-forming tumor and an absence of pre-neoplastic endometrial lesions. Metastatic tumors tend to infiltrate endometrial stroma in the form of islands, small cell clusters or single malignant cells. Endometrial glands are typically not involved [3–5]. Breast carcinoma is the most common extragenital metastasis to the endometrium, followed by colon and gastric carcinoma [1, 2]. Rare cases of lung [6, 7], renal [8], and pancreatobiliary [9, 10] metastases have also been reported.

While expression rates vary depending upon tumor histotype, a large proportion of breast and endometrial neoplasms are estrogen receptor (ER) positive [11, 12]. Similarly, most breast and endometrial carcinomas express cytokeratin 7 (CK 7) and are negative for cytokeratin 20 (CK20). In endometrial tumors with mismatch repair deficiency, a lower percentage of cells express CK 7, which may cause diagnostic confusion [13]. The most useful panel for distinguishing breast from endometrial carcinoma consists of gross cystic disease fluid protein-15 (GCDFP-15), GATA binding protein 3 (GATA 3) and Pax 8. While GCDFP-15, expressed in the cytoplasm, is specific for breast, it has poor sensitivity, identifying

B. Djordjevic (✉)
Department of Anatomic Pathology, Sunnybrook Health Sciences Centre, University of Toronto, 2075 Bayview Ave, room E4-27b, Toronto, ON M4N 3M5, Canada
e-mail: bojanadjordjevicmd@gmail.com

R.R. Broaddus
Department of Pathology, University of Texas M.D. Anderson Cancer Center, 1515 Holcombe Blvd., Box 85, Houston, TX 77030, USA
e-mail: rbroaddus@mdanderson.org

M.T. Deavers and D.M. Coffey (eds.), *Precision Molecular Pathology of Uterine Cancer*, Molecular Pathology Library,
DOI 10.1007/978-3-319-57985-6_3

no more than 55% of breast tumors [14–16]. Mammaglobin is a more sensitive breast marker, expressed in up to 71% of breast tumors [15], but it lacks specificity with respect to endometrial carcinomas as up to 40% can be mammaglobin positive [17]. GATA 3, a nuclear marker that is also expressed in urothelium [18], stains over 90% of ductal and lobular breast neoplasms [19], but only 7% of endometrial cancers [20]. Pax 8, a nuclear marker, stains over 90% of endometrial endometrioid, serous and clear cell histotypes, and about 40% of mucinous endometrial carcinomas [21, 22]. Pax 8 is not expressed in breast carcinoma [22] (Fig. 3.1).

It may be challenging on occasion to distinguish a colorectal metastasis from an endometrial endometrioid primary, as both endometrial endometrioid tumors and colorectal adenocarcinomas of the usual type can have glands with pseudostratified columnar cells and areas of mucinous differentiation. This problem may occur not only in biopsy specimens, but also in some resection specimens, particularly when the tumor transmurally involves the uterus, producing a fistula between the uterine and the colonic lumens. While endometrial carcinomas are typically CK7 positive and CK20 negative, and colorectal carcinomas are typically CK7 negative and CK20 positive, it is important to note that a subset of colorectal tumors, particularly those that are microsatellite instability high, may express CK7, which can lead to diagnostic confusion [23]. Similarly, while CDX2 staining is typically ascribed to colorectal primaries, CDX2 may be expressed in endometrial tumors, particularly in areas of mucinous metaplasia or squamous morule formation [24, 25]. Additional markers helpful for this differential diagnosis are Pax 8 and ER, both of which stain endometrial endometrioid adenocarcinomas but not colorectal adenocarcinomas [12, 22, 26].

As gastric adenocarcinomas may assume any variation of the CK7/CK20 immunoprofile, those markers are not particularly useful when a gastric metastasis is considered. Again, Pax 8 and ER may be most helpful. In pancreatic carcinomas, loss of DPC4 and expression of insulin-like growth factor II mRNA binding protein 3 (IMP 3) in 44% [27] and 97% [28] pancreatic carcinomas may be of use.

When a lung or thyroid metastasis to the endometrium is suspected, the CK7/CK20 panel is not helpful. Caution is also needed with TTF-1, as up to 19% of endometrial carcinomas may have at least focal expression of TTF-1 [29]. Similarly, thyroid carcinomas and renal tumors are generally Pax 8 positive [22]. Therefore, ER may be the most useful marker for endometrial tumors in this setting, while Napsin A identifies 80% of lung adenocarcinomas [30] and thyroglobulin may be used to identify thyroid primaries.

In the rare instances when a urothelial carcinoma metastasis to the endometrium needs to be excluded, GATA 3 and CK20 (expressed in urothelial carcinoma), and ER, Pax 8, and CK7 (expressed in endometrial carcinoma) may be helpful.

Consideration of endometrial versus extramüllerian primaries is also relevant in the differential diagnosis of an unknown primary, especially when the first diagnosis of malignancy is made in a biopsy of an involved lymph node (Fig. 3.2). In this context, it is particularly important to consider the endometrial tumor histotype

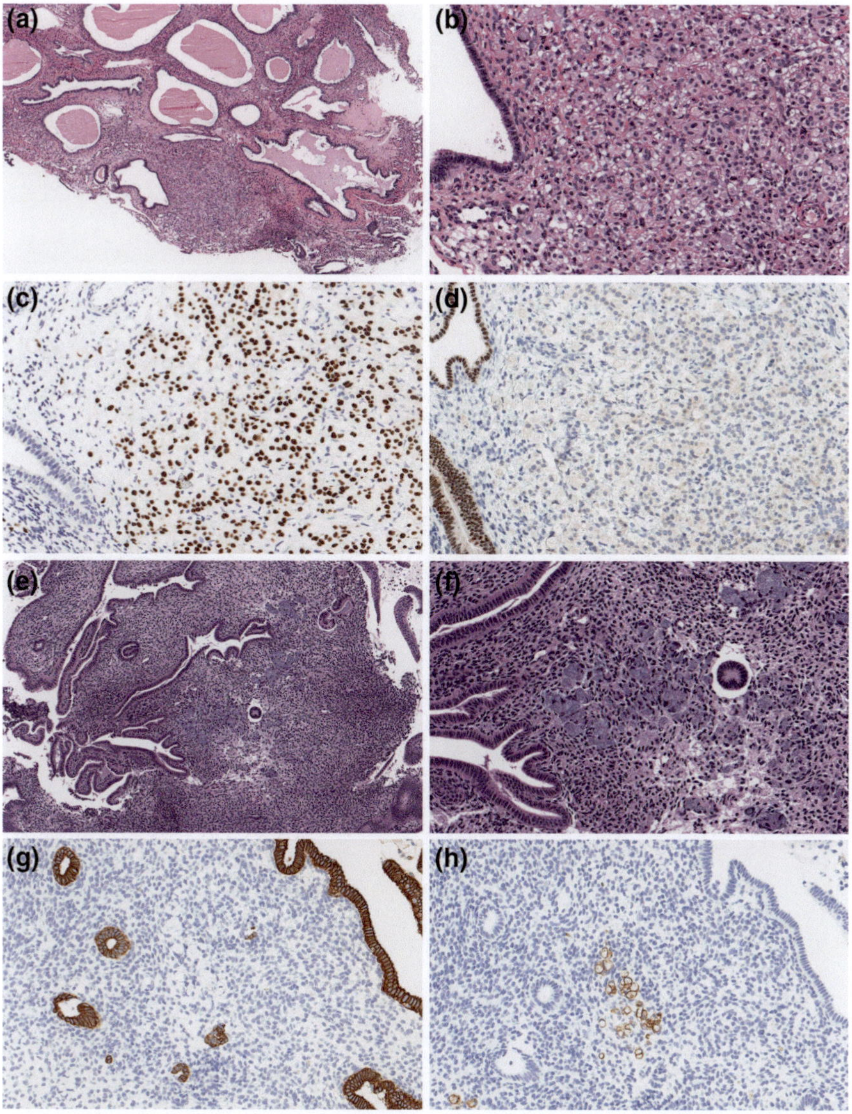

Fig. 3.1 a–d Breast carcinoma with metastasis to the endometrium. Tumor cells appear as islands and clusters of epithelial cells in the endometrial stroma, while the endometrial glands are uninvolved (**a** and **b**, H&E, low and high power). Tumor cells are highlighted by GATA 3 immunohistochemistry (**c**). Pax 8 is negative (**d**). **e–h** Colonic signet ring cell carcinoma with metastasis to the endometrium. **e** and **f** Tumor cells infiltrate endometrial stroma as cell clusters and single cells. Again, endometrial glandular architecture is undisturbed. The tumor cells are negative for CK7 (**g**), but do stain for CK20 (**h**)

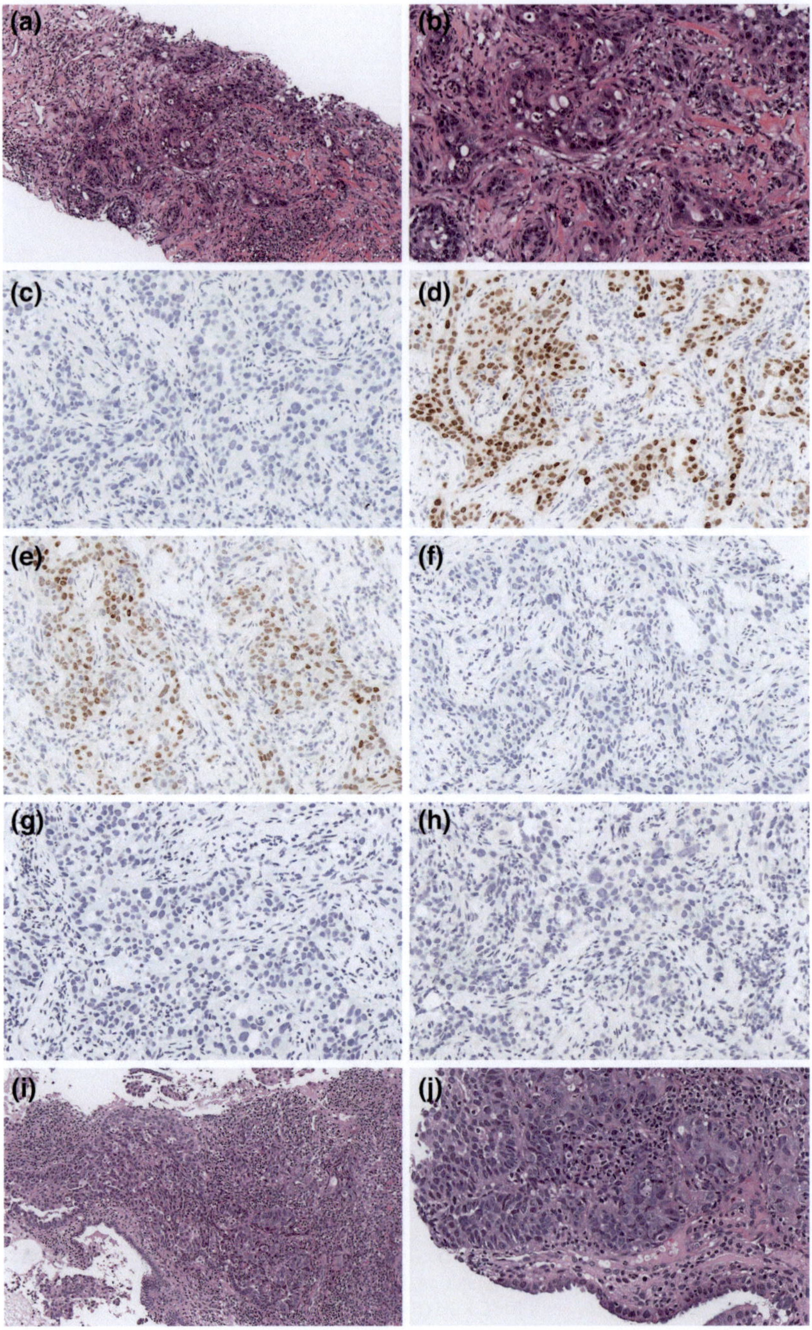
(a)
(b)
(c)
(d)
(e)
(f)
(g)
(h)
(i)
(j)

◀**Fig. 3.2 a–h** Work up of endometrial carcinoma as an unknown primary. Patient presented with axillary lymphadenopathy without any history of malignancy. **a** and **b** H&E sections (low and high power) show infiltrating glands and cords of carcinoma with high-grade nuclei in desmoplastic stroma. No lymphoid tissue is evident. By immunohistochemistry, the tumor cells are negative for ER (**c**), but do stain for Pax 8 (**d**) and GATA 3 (**e**). WT-1 (**f**), GCDFP-15 (**g**), and mammaglobin (**h**) are negative. Other stains (not shown) included a positive CK7 and negative CK20 and TTF-1. Diagnosis of high-grade carcinoma, favor Müllerian origin, was rendered on the basis of positive Pax 8 and negative GCDFP-15 and mammaglobin. **i** and **j** The patient was subsequently found to have an endometrial mass by imaging. Biopsy showed serous carcinoma with an immunohistochemical profile similar to the tumor in the axillary lymph node. Note that serous carcinomas of the endometrium are often negative (or weakly and focally positive) for ER and negative for WT-1. In this regard, they differ from ovarian, fallopian tube and peritoneal serous carcinomas that are typically positive for these markers. Note also that a small percentage of endometrial carcinomas may stain for GATA 3

in the interpretation of immunohistochemical results in order to avoid diagnostic confusion. For instance, in the majority of clear cell carcinomas and many serous carcinomas of the endometrium, ER expression may be reduced or absent [12, 31, 32]. In addition, histotype-specific endometrial tumor markers may be a useful adjunct under particular circumstances. These markers are discussed in detail in Sect. 3.

Endometrial Carcinoma Versus Other Müllerian Primaries

Differentiation of endometrial and endocervical primaries on biopsy is a common problem in routine gynecologic pathology practice and requires the use of immunohistochemistry. This distinction is clinically relevant, as it determines the type of subsequent treatment. Endometrial hyperplasia and/or squamous morules, particularly in a post menopausal patient, favor endometrial origin, while premenopausal age and presence of concurrent cervical squamous dysplasia or adenocarcinoma in situ favor endocervical origin.

The most helpful immunohistochemical panel in this differential diagnosis includes ER, vimentin, monoclonal carcinoembryonic antigen (mCEA), and p16. Diffuse staining for p16 (cytoplasmic and nuclear) and diffuse membranous staining for mCEA favor endocervical origin, while ER and vimentin staining favor an endometrioid endometrial primary [33–36] (Fig. 3.3). Squamous morules in endometrial carcinoma usually stain for mCEA and should not be included in the interpretation. Similarly, the majority of endometrial tumors have patchy staining for p16. Endocervical adenocarcinoma and adenocarcinoma in situ, however, have diffuse, strong p16 expression (a surrogate marker of HPV infection at this site) [37, 38]. HPV in situ hybridization (ISH) is another test that can be used in conjunction with the four marker immunohistochemical panel. It should be noted, however, that false negative HPV ISH results may arise due to DNA degradation. ProExC is another marker that has been shown to perform comparatively to p16 [39].

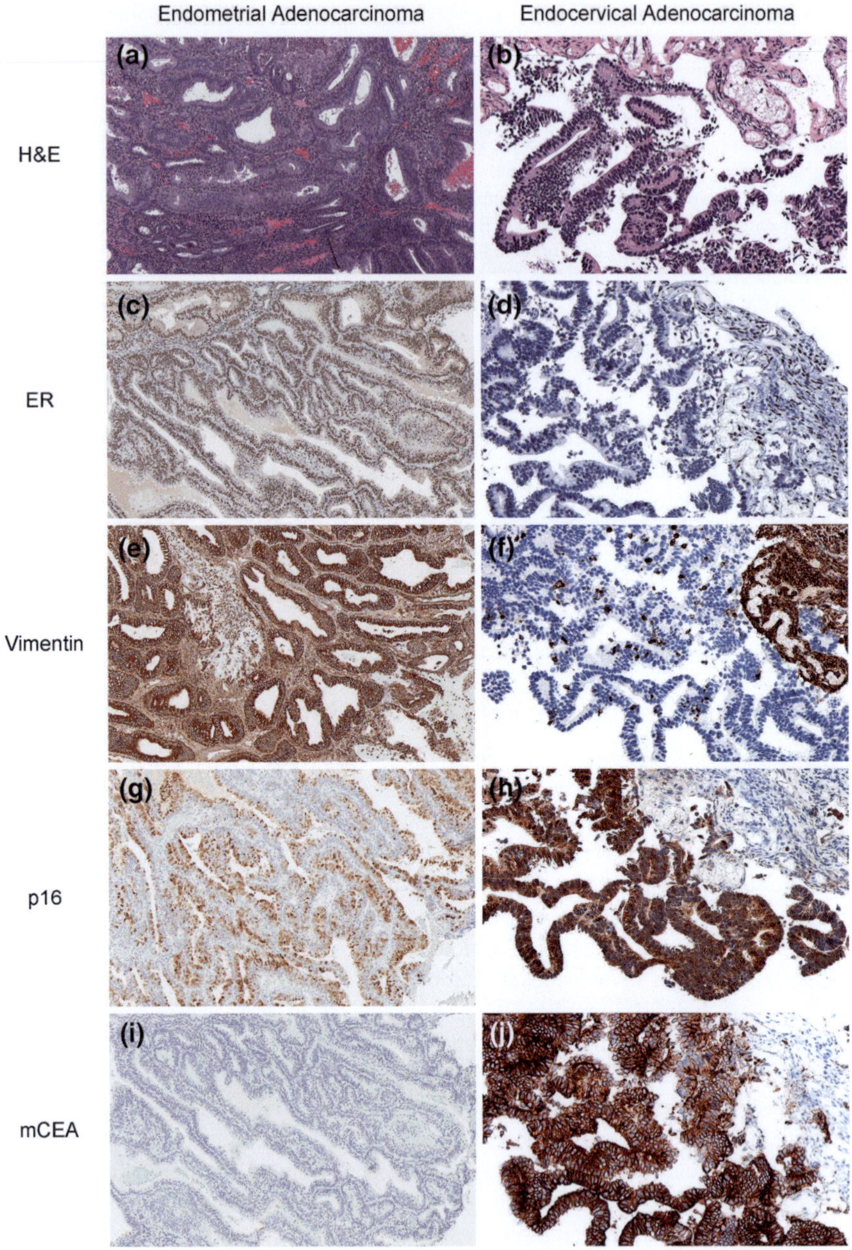

Fig. 3.3 Immunohistochemical panel to aid in the distinction of endometrial (**a**, **c**, **e**, **g**, **i**) and endocervical carcinomas (**b**, **d**, **f**, **h**, **j**). **a** and **b** H&E. **c** and **d** ER, **e** and **f** vimentin, **g** and **h** p16, **i** and **j** monoclonal CEA. Typical endometrial endometrioid adenocarcinoma is usually strongly and diffusely positive for vimentin and ER, has patchy expression of p16, and is negative for monoclonal CEA. Endocervical adenocarcinoma of the usual type is typically negative for ER and vimentin, and stains for monoclonal CEA. P16, a surrogate marker of HPV-driven tumorigenesis in this location, is diffusely expressed

The ER/vimentin/mCEA/p16 immunohistochemical panel must be interpreted carefully and in the context of tumor morphology, as up to 50% of endocervical, and as many as 70% of endometrial tumors may exhibit aberrant expression of at least one of the markers [40]. Tumor differentiation should be taken into account during interpretation [41]. For example, ER staining tends to be seen in endometrial tumors of both endometrioid or mucinous differentiation, but may also be retained in some endocervical adenocarcinomas [37]. On the other hand, tumors with endometrioid differentiation, regardless of endometrial or endocervical origin, may be positive for vimentin. Finally, mCEA works optimally in endocervical tumors with mucinous differentiation (of endocervical type) [41]. High-risk HPV is the pathogenetic agent in 67–91% of in situ and invasive endocervical adenocarcinomas [37]. Therefore, p16 is not diffusely expressed and HPV ISH is negative in a small percentage of endocervical adenocarcinomas of the usual type. The ER/vimentin/mCEA/p16 panel should be applied strictly to tumors with endometrioid or mucinous differentiation of the endocervical type. Data on the role of HPV in endocervical serous and clear carcinoma is scant and somewhat controversial [39, 42, 43]. Furthermore, these tumor histotypes, both endocervical and endometrial in origin, may overexpress p16 due to non-HPV related mechanisms. This can produce misleading p16 immunohistochemical patterns, and, in the cervix, discrepancies between p16 immunohistochemistry and HPV ISH results [39, 44]. HPV has not been reported in association with mesonephric adenocarcinoma, and HPV has only infrequently been associated with mucinous cervical adenocarcinoma (including the NOS, gastric type, signet ring cell) [43, 45–47]. Adenoid basal cell carcinoma [43, 48], small cell carcinoma [42, 43, 49], and adenosquamous carcinoma [43] are generally accepted as HPV-associated cervical carcinomas.

Rarely, independent primary endometrial and endocervical adenocarcinomas co-exist in the same patient. In this instance, the endometrial and endocervical tumors generally have a different histologic appearance and, in most cases, discordant immunohistochemical profiles [50].

Carcinomas arising in the lower uterine segment are generally thought to be endometrial carcinomas, although experience with these tumors is limited. One study has found that adenocarcinomas of the lower uterine segment generally have the same immunohistochemical profile as conventional endometrioid adenocarcinomas arising in the uterine fundus [51].

Tumors from the upper genital tract originating in the ovary, fallopian tube, or peritoneum may on occasion present in an endometrial biopsy and mimic an endometrial primary [52, 53]. The morphologic clues in this situation include detached fragments of tumor in a background of benign endometrium and/or tumor involvement limited to the endometrial glands. Tumor from the upper genital tract is thought to undergo intramucosal spread to the endometrium or the cervix. In the case of serous carcinoma, immunohistochemistry for WT-1 and ER may be most useful for identifying a possible extrauterine primary in endometrial biopsy specimens. Serous carcinomas of ovarian, fallopian tube, and peritoneal origin typically have strong and diffuse reactivity for WT-1 and ER. Endometrial serous carcinomas, on the other hand, tend to be WT-1 negative and only a proportion express ER

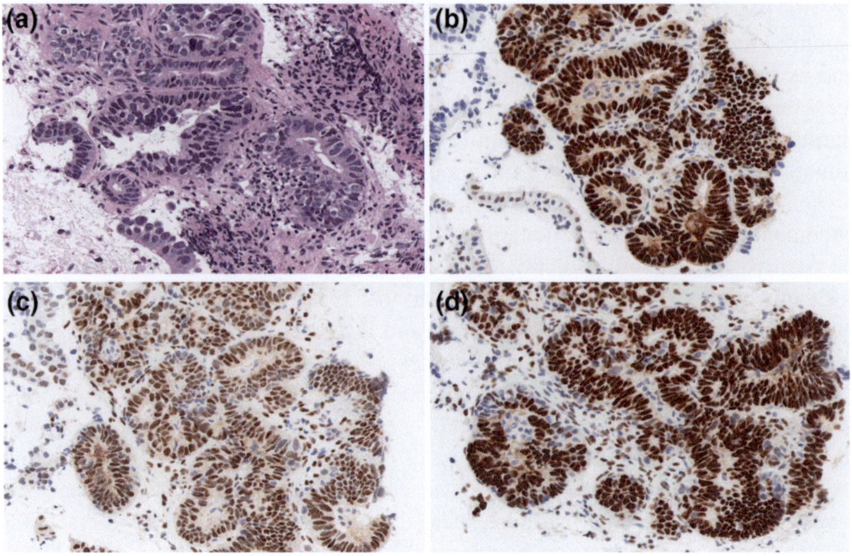

Fig. 3.4 Serous carcinoma involving endometrial glands in an endometrial biopsy (**a**). The tumor overexpresses p53 (**b**) and has diffuse expression of ER (**c**) and WT-1 (**d**). Given that many serous carcinomas of the endometrium are WT-1 negative, and that ER expression is either absent or reduced, the possibility of an upper genital tract primary, including from the ovary, fallopian tube, or peritoneum, with intramucosal spread to the endometrium should be considered

[54–60] (Fig. 3.4). Similarly, WT-1 and ER can be employed in establishing the origin of synchronous endometrial and upper genital tract tumors on resection specimens. Additionally, for all tumor histotypes, mismatch repair protein immunohistochemistry (discussed later in detail in part 4) for MLH1, MSH2, MSH6, and PMS2 may be helpful in this context [61].

Subtyping of Endometrial Carcinoma

The first attempts at endometrial carcinoma classification recognized two broad categories [62]. Bokhman type I tumors were well-to-moderately differentiated adenocarcinomas that arose in the background of endometrial hyperplasia, had superficial myometrial invasion, were responsive to progestin therapy, and had an excellent prognosis. Women with hyperestrogenism and/or disturbances in carbohydrate metabolism typically developed these tumors. Bokhman type II tumors, on the other hand, had no apparent precursor lesion, were poorly differentiated adenocarcinomas with deep myometrial invasion and metastasis to lymph nodes, and were associated with a poor prognosis. While this initial model was informative, our understanding of the complexity of endometrial carcinoma biology has since evolved significantly. Several key issues have arisen: (1) While most endometrial cancers can be reproducibly classified using morphologic criteria [63], tumors with ambiguous morphological features do exist [64]. Unlike mixed carcinomas in which prototypical tumor types are found adjacent to each other in one neoplasm, tumors with ambiguous morphology are characterised by a hybrid appearance, borrowing from more than one established tumor histotype, and cannot be definitively classified as either of those histotypes. (2) Reproducible classification of high-grade endometrial carcinomas, including grade 3 endometrioid, serous, clear cell, undifferentiated carcinomas, and mixed carcinomas, is poor, even among gynecologic pathology experts [65].(3) Endometrial cancers have complex molecular profiles with sometimes overlapping molecular abnormalities from one histotype to the next. For example, p53 mutations may be found in tumors with otherwise classic endometrioid or clear cell molecular profiles [66]. (4) Histologic features do not always correlate with tumor behavior. For example, a subgroup of low-grade and low-stage tumors is known to be clinically aggressive and recur or metastasize to lymph nodes. According to The Cancer Genome Atlas (TCGA) data for endometrium, 24% of grade 3 endometrioid tumors and 5% of grade 1 and 2 endometrioid tumors cluster into the poorest prognostic group along with non-endometrioid (predominantly serous) endometrial carcinomas [67]. On the other hand, tumors with mutations in the catalytic subunit of the DNA polymerase epsilon have been shown to have an excellent prognosis [67–70], and although about two-thirds of these tumors are endometrioid, the rest are mixed carcinomas or carcinomas with ambiguous features.

A relatively common problem in clinical practice arises in the differentiation of endometrioid from serous or clear cell histotypes. In either instance, assigning a non-endometrioid designation to the tumor, or tumor component, may subscribe the patient to more aggressive adjuvant therapy or more extensive surgery if the diagnosis is made on an endometrial biopsy. Thus, accurate histotype assignment is of clinical significance. While histologic diagnosis remains the mainstay of routine clinical practice, immunohistochemistry has recently emerged as an ancillary tool to help classify difficult cases and to improve interobserver variability. However, due to the biological complexities outlined above, the use of immunohistochemical panels rather than solitary immunomarkers is recommended, and the findings must be interpreted in the context of histologic features.

Endometrioid endometrial carcinoma may mimic clear cell carcinoma in areas of secretory change or areas of squamous metaplasia with cytoplasmic clearing [71, 72]. Although clear cell carcinoma typically has nuclear pleomorphism that exceeds that of typical endometrioid carcinoma, in endometrioid adenocarcinomas with more atypical nuclei, this may be a diagnostic dilemma. The most reliable markers that are of utility in making this distinction, include ER, hepatocyte nuclear factor 1 beta (HNF-1b), Napsin A, and racemase (Fig. 3.5). Most clear cell carcinomas do not express ER, and in cases that do, the staining is typically focal or weak [73–75]. On the other hand, ER is positive in a majority of grade 1 and 2 endometrioid adenocarcinomas, and in approximately 50% of grade 3 tumors [12]. Most clear cell carcinomas are positive for HNF-1b [73, 76], a nuclear marker. However, up to

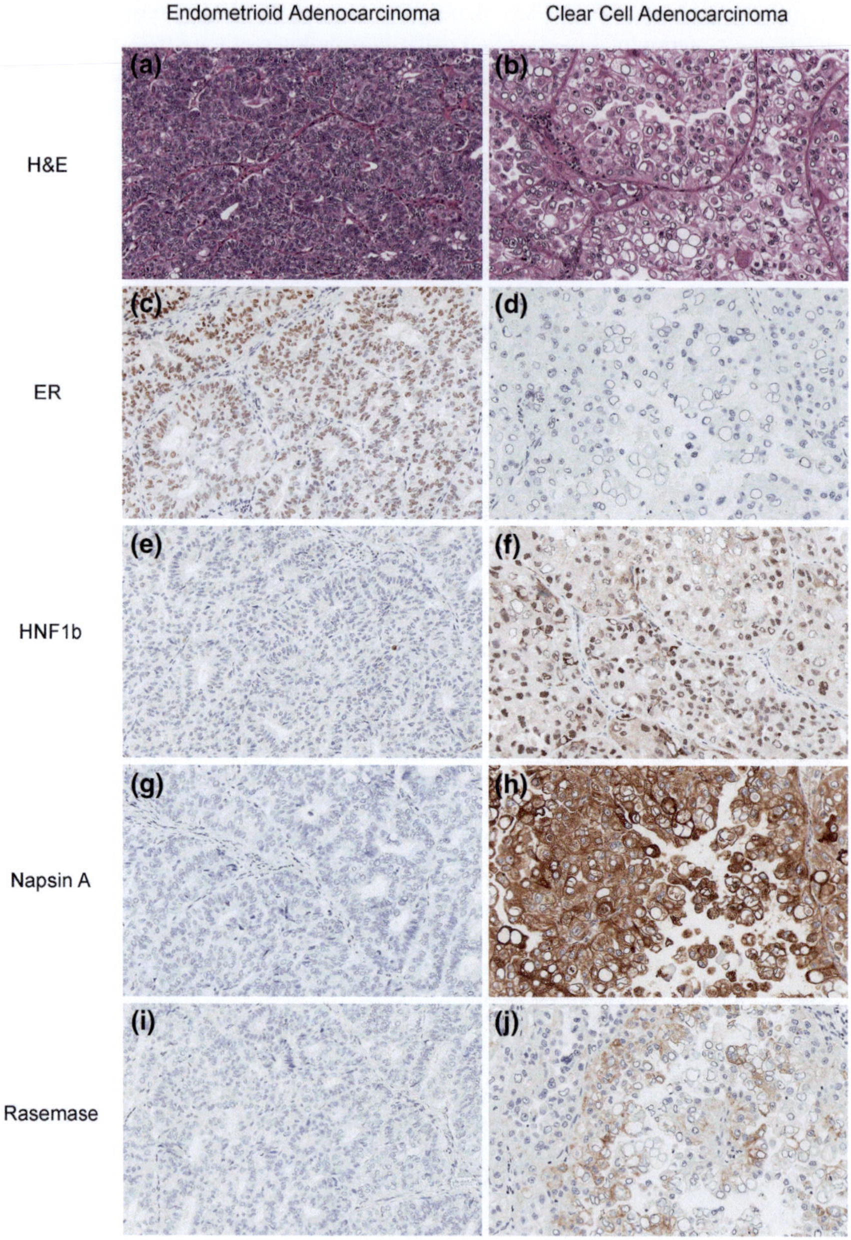

Fig. 3.5 Novel markers that may aid in distinction between endometrial endometrioid (**a**, **c**, **e**, **g**, **i**) and clear cell carcinoma (**b**, **d**, **f**, **h**, **j**). **a**, **b** H&E, **c**, **d** ER, **e**, **f** HNF1b, **g**, **h** Napsin A, **i**, **j** racemase. An immunophenotype favoring endometrioid adenocarcinoma includes a positive ER, and a negative or a focally positive HNF-1b, Napsin A, and racemase. An immunoprofile that favors clear cell carcinoma includes a negative ER, and positive HNF-1b, Napsin A, and racemase

50% of endometrioid adenocarcinomas may have weak focal expression of HNF-1b [73, 76, 77]. Napsin A, a cytoplasmic marker, has recently been reported to be expressed in 67–88% of clear cell and 0–5% of endometrioid endometrial carcinomas [78, 79]. Alpha-methylacyl-coenzyme-A racemase, or p504s, is a sensitive and specific cytoplasmic marker of prostate adenocarcinoma [80] and several other neoplasms [81, 82]. In endometrial tumors, racemase is expressed not only in 75% of clear cell, but also in 22% of endometrioid adenocarcinomas. In addition, in a third of clear cell carcinomas racemase expression is focal (5% of cells or less), which limits its practical utility in this situation. Nuclear BAF250a protein is lost in tumors with *ARID1A* gene mutations. Although 20–40% of clear cell carcinomas have BAF250a loss, the same immunohistochemical result is found in 39–54% of high-grade endometrioid adenocarcinomas [83–87]. Therefore, BAF250a is not particularly helpful in this differential diagnosis. Aberrant p53 staining, defined as either overexpression (>90% of cells with 3+ staining intensity) or complete absence of staining, and diffuse staining for p16 (as opposed to patchy p16 staining) favor clear cell carcinoma over endometrioid adenocarcinoma. However, these changes are present in less than a third of clear cell carcinomas and may be found in some high-grade endometrioid adenocarcinomas [12, 66, 75, 83, 85, 88], thus making these markers of limited utility in this differential.

Serous and endometrioid adenocarcinoma are typically reliably distinguished on the basis of nuclear pleomorphism and nuclear size variability, as well as loss of nuclear polarity, all features typically found in serous carcinoma. However, in high-grade endometrioid tumors, this distinction may be more difficult. In addition, architectural features including endometrioid tumors with papillae (with or without fibrovascular cores), predominantly gland-forming serous tumors, or serous or endometrioid carcinomas with a solid growth pattern, may make accurate classification on morphologic grounds alone problematic [72, 89, 90]. For the differential diagnosis of endometrioid versus serous carcinoma, useful markers include PTEN, IMP3, BAF250a, ER, p16, and p53 (Fig. 3.6). Although PTEN immunohistochemistry historically has been challenging, recent success and reproducible results have been demonstrated with the 6H2.1 antibody [91–93]. In order for a tumor to be considered as having PTEN loss (a predominantly cytoplasmic and focal nuclear marker), greater than 90% of cells in the tumor or in large geographic areas of tumor should be negative in the presence of a strong internal cytoplasmic control [94]. PTEN is lost in up to 75% of endometrioid adenocarcinomas [94], but is retained in a majority of serous carcinomas [66, 95–98]. IMP 3, a cytoplasmic marker, has been shown to be expressed in 63–98% of serous carcinomas, while negative in 97% of low grade and 80% of grade 3 endometrioid adenocarcinomas [59, 99]. BAF250a expression is lost in 39–54% of high-grade endometrioid adenocarcinomas and in 9–18% of serous carcinomas [83–87]. ER is lost in about 50% of serous endometrial carcinomas, but as mentioned earlier is expressed in most low grade and in 50% of grade 3 endometrioid adenocarcinomas [12, 31, 32, 98]. Ninety-two percentage of serous carcinomas have diffuse p16 expression, compared to only 7% of low-grade and 25% of high-grade endometrioid tumors [12]. Similarly, the rate of aberrant p53 expression (overexpression or complete absence

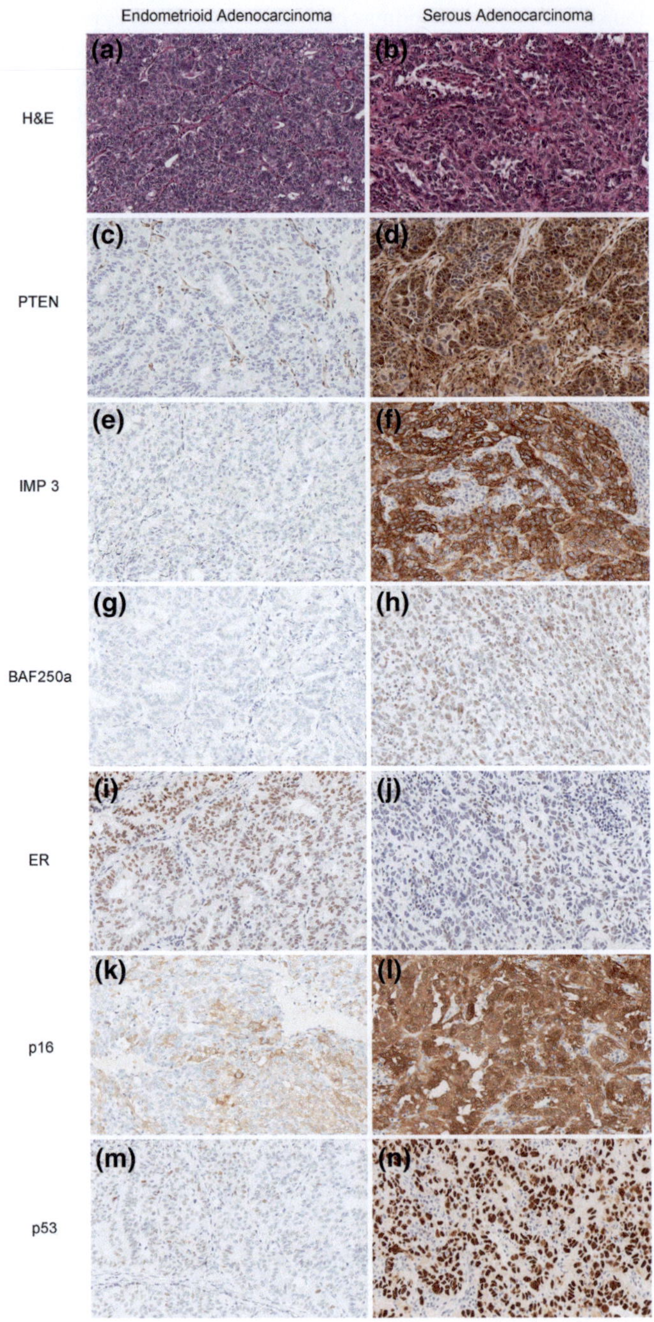
Endometrioid Adenocarcinoma
Serous Adenocarcinoma
H&E
PTEN
IMP 3
BAF250a
ER
p16
p53
(a)
(b)
(c)
(d)
(e)
(f)
(g)
(h)
(i)
(j)
(k)
(l)
(m)
(n)

◂**Fig. 3.6** Novel markers that may aid in distinction of endometrial endometrioid (**a**, **c**, **e**, **g**, **i**, **k**, **m**) and serous carcinoma (**b**, **d**, **f**, **h**, **j**, **l**, **n**). **a**, **b** H&E, **c**, **d** PTEN, **e**, **f** IMP 3, **g**, **h** BAF250a, **i**, **j** ER, **k**, **l** p16, **m**, **n** p53. An immunoprofile favoring endometrioid adenocarcinoma includes loss of PTEN, negative IMP3, loss of BAF250A, diffusely expressed ER, patchy p16, and wild type p53 expression. An immunoprofile favoring serous carcinoma includes retained PTEN, positive IMP3, retained BAF250a, negative or focally positive ER, diffuse p16, and aberrant p53 expression (overexpression or complete absence of expression)

of expression, as stated earlier) in serous carcinoma is 77–93%, compared to less than 20% in endometrioid adenocarcinoma (83, 100).

Endometrial Carcinoma and Lynch Syndrome

Lynch syndrome occurs due to a germ line mutation in a gene corresponding to a family of DNA mismatch repair (MMR) proteins, MLH1, MSH2, MSH6, and PMS2. The hallmark cancers of Lynch syndrome are colorectal adenocarcinoma and endometrial carcinoma, while less common cancer types include ovarian carcinoma, urothelial carcinomas of the ureter and renal pelvis, duodenal adenocarcinoma, and gastric adenocarcinoma. Loss of DNA MMR protein function typically results in high levels of DNA microsatellite instability (MSI). In 15–20% of all sporadic endometrial carcinomas, MLH1 immunohistochemical loss and MSI are secondary to *MLH1* gene promoter methylation with subsequent transcriptional silencing [101–105].

Early identification of Lynch syndrome in a patient with endometrial cancer is essential, not only to identify other family members with the syndrome, but also to proactively manage the patient's own increased risk of developing subsequent cancers. In particular, for women with Lynch syndrome, endometrial cancer is considered to be a "sentinel cancer" that precedes colorectal cancer by approximately one decade [106]. It is currently recommended that all newly diagnosed colorectal cancer patients undergo tissue testing for Lynch syndrome regardless of their family or personal history [107, 108], since clinical screening tools that are based on age and personal and family history of Lynch-associated tumors miss a significant proportion of patients [109]. Tumor tissue testing for Lynch syndrome involves MMR immunohistochemistry, MSI analysis and *MLH-1* methylation analysis. *MLH-1* methylation analysis is required for all tumors that exhibit MLH1 immunohistochemical loss, which may be due to *MLH-1* promoter methylation (in sporadic cases) or MLH-1 gene mutation (in Lynch syndrome). For optimal testing sensitivity, MMR immunohistochemistry and MSI analysis should be used in conjunction [110]; however, a number of different groups have demonstrated that immunohistochemistry alone has high sensitivity and specificity in identifying endometrial carcinomas with high levels of MSI [111–115]. The remainder of the discussion in this chapter will focus on practical issues concerning MMR immunohistochemistry.

Immunohistochemistry for MMR proteins is carried out using commercially available antibodies that work quite reliably [116]. Gene mutation of *MMR* genes or methylation of the *MLH1* gene promoter typically results in loss of immunohistochemical expression of the corresponding protein. Complete absence of nuclear expression should be observed in order for a tumor to be considered as having loss of an MMR marker. Strong nuclear staining in the surrounding endometrial stroma, myometrium, lymphocytes, or normal endometrium serves as an internal positive control. The MSH2 and MSH6 proteins and the MLH1 and PMS2 proteins act as functional pairs [117]. Therefore, when MLH1 protein expression is lost (due to mutation of the *MLH1* gene or methylation of *MLH1* gene promoter), there is typically secondary loss of PMS2 protein expression. Mutation of the PMS2 gene is typically associated with loss of PMS2 protein alone with retained MLH1 immunohistochemical expression. Similarly, mutation of the *MSH2* gene usually results in immunohistochemical loss of MSH2 and MSH6 proteins. On the other hand, mutation of *MSH6* gene results only in MSH6 protein loss, while MSH2 protein expression remains intact.

In terms of MMR immunohistochemistry reporting recommendations, it is important to note that for the vast majority of cases the percentage or intensity of staining is not relevant and that the interpretation result should be either positive or negative. Terminology such as "focally positive," "patchy staining," "weakly positive," "positive in *X%* of cells," or "equivocal staining" should be avoided. If the tumor is negative, it should be indicated that internal control stromal cells/normal mucosa are positive.

Several pitfalls in the interpretation of MMR immunohistochemistry exist. Most commonly, false negative results occur in the setting of an inadequate internal positive control (Fig. 3.7). On the other hand, immunohistochemical staining of the tumor may be focal or relatively weak, particularly in the case of MSH6. In most cases, this represents genuine nuclear staining. Both of these problems may be resolved by repeating the immunohistochemistry with prolongation of the antibody incubation time or by using a different tissue block. Another immunohistochemical issue involves cytoplasmic tumor staining, regardless of the presence or the absence of nuclear staining, especially when the tissue has previously been frozen for the purposes of intraoperative consultation. Cytoplasmic staining should be disregarded in the evaluation of MMR immunohistochemistry. Finally, endometrial stroma or tumor infiltrating lymphocytes may cause difficulties in MMR immunohistochemistry interpretation. Typically, however, these cells are relatively focal and appear within a background of immunohistochemically negative nests and sheets of tumor cells. Awareness of this pattern and correlation with the corresponding H&E features should resolve this particular diagnostic dilemma.

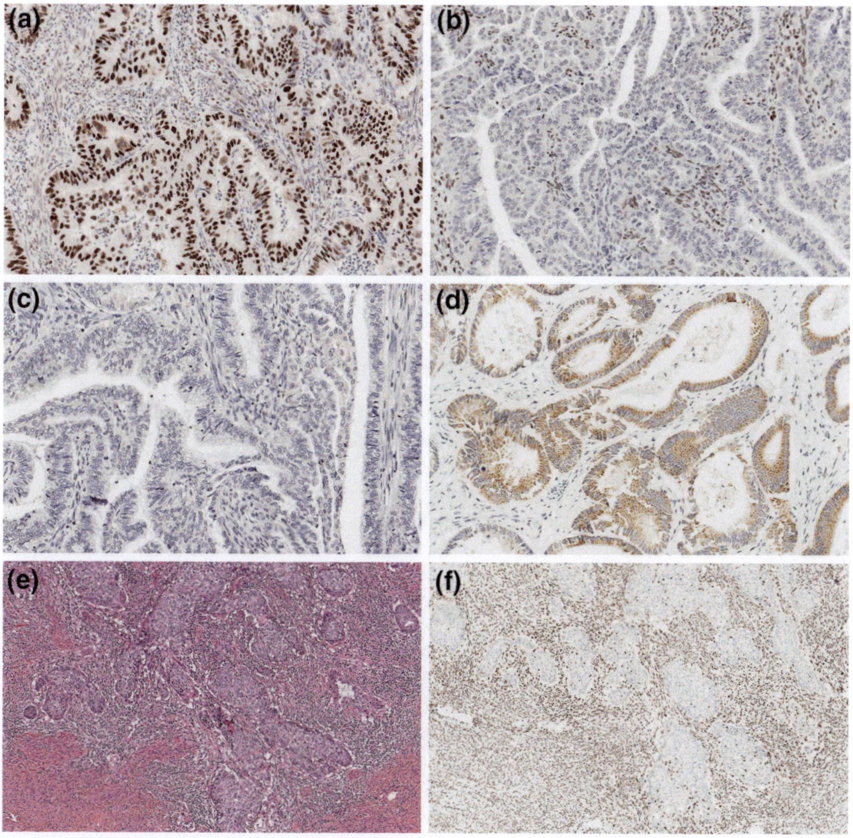

Fig. 3.7 Application of immunohistochemistry in testing for Lynch syndrome. **a** Expression of mismatch protein repair proteins (MLH-1, MSH-2, MSH-6, or PMS-2) is nuclear. **b** When interpretation of loss of mismatch repair protein expression is made, a good internal positive control should be found in the stroma. **c** If expression is absent in both the epithelium and the stroma, the immunohistochemical reaction did not work and should be repeated under different conditions or in a different block. **d** Cytoplasmic tumor staining should be disregarded. **e** Endometrial tumor with numerous tumor infiltrating lymphocytes. **f** Tumor infiltrating lymphocytes mimic tumor cells with retained MLH1 expression, which appear within otherwise immunonegative islands of tumor

Acknowledgements This work was supported by NIH 1P50CA098258 (SPORE in Uterine Cancer).

References

1. Mazur MT, Hsueh S, Gersell DJ. Metastases to the female genital tract. Analysis of 325 cases. Cancer. 1984;53(9):1978–84.
2. Kumar NB, Hart WR. Metastases to the uterine corpus from extragenital cancers. A clinicopathologic study of 63 cases. Cancer. 1982;50(10):2163–9.

3. Lim D, Oliva E. Nonendometrioid endometrial carcinomas. Semin Diagn Pathol. 2010;27(4): 241–60.
4. Karvouni E, Papakonstantinou K, Dimopoulou C, et al. Abnormal uterine bleeding as a presentation of metastatic breast disease in a patient with advanced breast cancer. Arch Gynecol Obstet. 2009;279(2):199–201.
5. Alvarez C, Ortiz-Rey JA, Estevez F, de la Fuente A. Metastatic lobular breast carcinoma to an endometrial polyp diagnosed by hysteroscopic biopsy. Obstet Gynecol. 2003;102(5 Pt 2):1149–51.
6. Tiseo M, Bersanelli M, Corradi D, et al. Endometrial metastasis of lung adenocarcinoma: a case report. Tumori. 2011;97(3):411–4.
7. Ahmad Z, Raza A, Patel MR. Endometrial metastasis of lung adenocarcinoma: a report of two cases. Am J Case Rep. 2015;16:296–9.
8. Tretheway D, Gebhardt JG, Dogra VS, Schiffhauer LM. Metastatic versus primary oncocytic papillary adenocarcinoma of the endometrium: a report of a case and review of the literature. Int J Gynecol Pathol. 2009;28(3):256–61.
9. Kefeli M, Gonullu G, Can B, Malatyalioglu E, Kandemir B. Metastasis of adenocarcinoma of the gall bladder to an endometrial polyp detected by endometrial curettage: case report and review of the literature. Int J Gynecol Pathol. 2009;28(4):343–6.
10. Schust DJ, Moore DH, Baird DB, Novotny DB. Primary adenocarcinoma of the gallbladder presenting as primary gynecologic malignancy: a report of two cases. Obstet Gynecol. 1994;83(5 Pt 2):831–4.
11. Caldarella A, Crocetti E, Bianchi S, et al. Female breast cancer status according to ER, PR and HER2 expression: a population based analysis. Pathol Oncol Res. 2011;17(3):753–8.
12. Reid-Nicholson M, Iyengar P, Hummer AJ, Linkov I, Asher M, Soslow RA. Immunophenotypic diversity of endometrial adenocarcinomas: implications for differential diagnosis. Mod Pathol. 2006;19(8):1091–100.
13. Okoye EI, Bruegl AS, Fellman B, Luthra R, Broaddus RR. Defective DNA mismatch repair influences expression of endometrial carcinoma biomarkers. Int J Gynecol Pathol. 2015.
14. Tornos C, Soslow R, Chen S, et al. Expression of WT1, CA 125, and GCDFP-15 as useful markers in the differential diagnosis of primary ovarian carcinomas versus metastatic breast cancer to the ovary. Am J Surg Pathol. 2005;29(11):1482–9.
15. Bhargava R, Beriwal S, Dabbs DJ. Mammaglobin vs GCDFP-15: an immunohistologic validation survey for sensitivity and specificity. Am J Clin Pathol. 2007;127(1):103–13.
16. Yang M, Nonaka D. A study of immunohistochemical differential expression in pulmonary and mammary carcinomas. Mod Pathol. 2010;23(5):654–61.
17. Hagemann IS, Pfeifer JD, Cao D. Mammaglobin expression in gynecologic adenocarcinomas. Hum Pathol. 2013;44(4):628–35.
18. Higgins JP, Kaygusuz G, Wang L, et al. Placental S100 (S100P) and GATA3: markers for transitional epithelium and urothelial carcinoma discovered by complementary DNA microarray. Am J Surg Pathol. 2007;31(5):673–80.
19. Miettinen M, McCue PA, Sarlomo-Rikala M, et al. GATA3: a multispecific but potentially useful marker in surgical pathology: a systematic analysis of 2500 epithelial and nonepithelial tumors. Am J Surg Pathol. 2014;38(1):13–22.
20. Engelsen IB, Stefansson IM, Akslen LA, Salvesen HB. GATA3 expression in estrogen receptor α-negative endometrial carcinomas identifies aggressive tumors with high proliferation and poor patient survival. Am J Obstet Gynecol. 2008;199(5):543.e1–7.
21. Brunner AH, Riss P, Heinze G, Meltzow E, Brustmann H. Immunoexpression of PAX 8 in endometrial cancer: relation to high-grade carcinoma and p53. Int J Gynecol Pathol. 2011;30 (6):569–75.
22. Ozcan A, Shen SS, Hamilton C, et al. PAX 8 expression in non-neoplastic tissues, primary tumors, and metastatic tumors: a comprehensive immunohistochemical study. Mod Pathol. 2011;24(6):751–64.

23. McGregor DK, Wu TT, Rashid A, Luthra R, Hamilton SR. Reduced expression of cytokeratin 20 in colorectal carcinomas with high levels of microsatellite instability. Am J Surg Pathol. 2004;28(6):712–8.
24. Wani Y, Notohara K, Saegusa M, Tsukayama C. Aberrant Cdx2 expression in endometrial lesions with squamous differentiation: important role of Cdx2 in squamous morula formation. Hum Pathol. 2008;39(7):1072–9.
25. Chiarelli S, Buritica C, Litta P, Ciani S, Guarch R, Nogales FF. An immunohistochemical study of morules in endometrioid lesions of the female genital tract: CD10 is a characteristic marker of morular metaplasia. Clin Cancer Res. 2006;12(14 Pt 1):4251–6.
26. Laury AR, Perets R, Piao H, et al. A comprehensive analysis of PAX8 expression in human epithelial tumors. Am J Surg Pathol. 2011;35(6):816–26.
27. Hornick JL, Lauwers GY, Odze RD. Immunohistochemistry can help distinguish metastatic pancreatic adenocarcinomas from bile duct adenomas and hamartomas of the liver. Am J Surg Pathol. 2005;29(3):381–9.
28. Yantiss RK, Woda BA, Fanger GR, et al. KOC (K homology domain containing protein overexpressed in cancer): a novel molecular marker that distinguishes between benign and malignant lesions of the pancreas. Am J Surg Pathol. 2005;29(2):188–95.
29. Siami K, Glenn McCluggage W, Ordonez NG, et al. Thyroid transcription factor-1 expression in endometrial and endocervical adenocarcinomas. Am J Surg Pathol. 2007;31 (11):1759–63.
30. Bishop JA, Sharma R, Illei PB. Napsin A and thyroid transcription factor-1 expression in carcinomas of the lung, breast, pancreas, colon, kidney, thyroid, and malignant mesothelioma. Hum Pathol. 2010;41(1):20–5.
31. Carcangiu ML, Chambers JT, Voynick IM, Pirro M, Schwartz PE. Immunohistochemical evaluation of estrogen and progesterone receptor content in 183 patients with endometrial carcinoma. Part I: clinical and histologic correlations. Am J Clin Pathol. 1990;94(3):247–54.
32. Chambers JT, Carcangiu ML, Voynick IM, Schwartz PE. Immunohistochemical evaluation of estrogen and progesterone receptor content in 183 patients with endometrial carcinoma. Part II: correlation between biochemical and immunohistochemical methods and survival. Am J Clin Pathol. 1990;94(3):255–60.
33. McCluggage WG, Sumathi VP, McBride HA, Patterson A. A panel of immunohistochemical stains, including carcinoembryonic antigen, vimentin, and estrogen receptor, aids the distinction between primary endometrial and endocervical adenocarcinomas. Int J Gynecol Pathol. 2002;21(1):11–5.
34. Dabbs DJ, Sturtz K, Zaino RJ. The immunohistochemical discrimination of endometrioid adenocarcinomas. Hum Pathol. 1996;27(2):172–7.
35. Castrillon DH, Lee KR, Nucci MR. Distinction between endometrial and endocervical adenocarcinoma: an immunohistochemical study. Int J Gynecol Pathol. 2002;21(1):4–10.
36. Staebler A, Sherman ME, Zaino RJ, Ronnett BM. Hormone receptor immunohistochemistry and human papillomavirus in situ hybridization are useful for distinguishing endocervical and endometrial adenocarcinomas. Am J Surg Pathol. 2002;26(8):998–1006.
37. Ansari-Lari MA, Staebler A, Zaino RJ, Shah KV, Ronnett BM. Distinction of endocervical and endometrial adenocarcinomas: immunohistochemical p16 expression correlated with human papillomavirus (HPV) DNA detection. Am J Surg Pathol. 2004;28(2):160–7.
38. Yemelyanova A, Ji H, Shih Ie M, Wang TL, Wu LS, Ronnett BM. Utility of p16 expression for distinction of uterine serous carcinomas from endometrial endometrioid and endocervical adenocarcinomas: immunohistochemical analysis of 201 cases. Am J Surg Pathol. 2009; 33(10):1504–14.
39. Kong CS, Beck AH, Longacre TA. A panel of 3 markers including p16, ProExC, or HPV ISH is optimal for distinguishing between primary endometrial and endocervical adenocarcinomas. Am J Surg Pathol. 2010;34(7):915–26.
40. Han CP, Lee MY, Kok LF, et al. Adding the p16(INK4a) marker to the traditional 3-marker (ER/Vim/CEA) panel engenders no supplemental benefit in distinguishing between primary

endocervical and endometrial adenocarcinomas in a tissue microarray study. Int J Gynecol Pathol. 2009;28(5):489–96.

41. Kamoi S, AlJuboury MI, Akin MR, Silverberg SG. Immunohistochemical staining in the distinction between primary endometrial and endocervical adenocarcinomas: another viewpoint. Int J Gynecol Pathol. 2002;21(3):217–23.
42. Nofech-Mozes S, Khalifa MM, Ismiil N, et al. Detection of HPV-DNA by a PCR-based method in formalin-fixed, paraffin-embedded tissue from rare endocervical carcinoma types. Appl Immunohistochem Mol Morphol. 2010;18(1):80–5.
43. Pirog EC, Kleter B, Olgac S, et al. Prevalence of human papillomavirus DNA in different histological subtypes of cervical adenocarcinoma. Am J Pathol. 2000;157(4):1055–62.
44. Park KJ, Kiyokawa T, Soslow RA, et al. Unusual endocervical adenocarcinomas: an immunohistochemical analysis with molecular detection of human papillomavirus. Am J Surg Pathol. 2011;35(5):633–46.
45. Toki T, Zhai YL, Park JS, Fujii S. Infrequent occurrence of high-risk human papillomavirus and of p53 mutation in minimal deviation adenocarcinoma of the cervix. Int J Gynecol Pathol. 1999;18(3):215–9.
46. Xu JY, Hashi A, Kondo T, et al. Absence of human papillomavirus infection in minimal deviation adenocarcinoma and lobular endocervical glandular hyperplasia. Int J Gynecol Pathol. 2005;24(3):296–302.
47. Fukushima M, Shimano S, Yamakawa Y, et al. The detection of human papillomavirus (HPV) in a case of minimal deviation adenocarcinoma of the uterine cervix (adenoma malignum) using in situ hybridization. Jpn J Clin Oncol. 1990;20(4):407–12.
48. Grayson W, Taylor LF, Cooper K. Adenoid basal carcinoma of the uterine cervix: detection of integrated human papillomavirus in a rare tumor of putative "reserve cell" origin. Int J Gynecol Pathol. 1997;16(4):307–12.
49. Horn LC, Lindner K, Szepankiewicz G, et al. p16, p14, p53, and cyclin D1 expression and HPV analysis in small cell carcinomas of the uterine cervix. Int J Gynecol Pathol. 2006;25 (2):182–6.
50. Jiang L, Malpica A, Deavers MT, et al. Endometrial endometrioid adenocarcinoma of the uterine corpus involving the cervix: some cases probably represent independent primaries. Int J Gynecol Pathol. 2010;29(2):146–56.
51. Westin SN, Lacour RA, Urbauer DL, et al. Carcinoma of the lower uterine segment: a newly described association with Lynch syndrome. J Clin Oncol. 2008;26(36):5965–71.
52. Kos Z, Broaddus RR, Djordjevic B. Fallopian tube high-grade serous carcinoma with intramucosal spread and presenting as a malignancy on pap smear. Int J Gynecol Pathol. 2014;33(4):443–8.
53. McCluggage WG, Hurrell DP, Kennedy K. Metastatic carcinomas in the cervix mimicking primary cervical adenocarcinoma and adenocarcinoma in situ: report of a series of cases. Am J Surg Pathol. 2010;34(5):735–41.
54. Hashi A, Yuminamochi T, Murata S, Iwamoto H, Honda T, Hoshi K. Wilms tumor gene immunoreactivity in primary serous carcinomas of the fallopian tube, ovary, endometrium, and peritoneum. Int J Gynecol Pathol. 2003;22(4):374–7.
55. Nofech-Mozes S, Khalifa MA, Ismiil N, et al. Immunophenotyping of serous carcinoma of the female genital tract. Mod Pathol. 2008;21(9):1147–55.
56. Al-Hussaini M, Stockman A, Foster H, McCluggage WG. WT-1 assists in distinguishing ovarian from uterine serous carcinoma and in distinguishing between serous and endometrioid ovarian carcinoma. Histopathology. 2004;44(2):109–15.
57. Euscher ED, Malpica A, Deavers MT, Silva EG. Differential expression of WT-1 in serous carcinomas in the peritoneum with or without associated serous carcinoma in endometrial polyps. Am J Surg Pathol. 2005;29(8):1074–8.
58. Hirschowitz L, Ganesan R, McCluggage WG. WT1, p53 and hormone receptor expression in uterine serous carcinoma. Histopathology. 2009;55(4):478–82.

59. Alkushi A, Kobel M, Kalloger SE, Gilks CB. High-grade endometrial carcinoma: serous and grade 3 endometrioid carcinomas have different immunophenotypes and outcomes. Int J Gynecol Pathol. 2010;29(4):343–50.
60. Goldstein NS, Uzieblo A. WT1 immunoreactivity in uterine papillary serous carcinomas is different from ovarian serous carcinomas. Am J Clin Pathol. 2002;117(4):541–5.
61. Soliman PT, Broaddus RR, Schmeler KM, et al. Women with synchronous primary cancers of the endometrium and ovary: do they have Lynch syndrome? J Clin Oncol. 2005; 23(36):9344–50.
62. Bokhman JV. Two pathogenetic types of endometrial carcinoma. Gynecol Oncol. 1983;15(1): 10–7.
63. Kurman RJ, Carcangiu ML, Herrington CS, Young RH, editors. WHO classification of tumors of female reproductive organs. Lyon: International Agency for Research on Cancer (IARC); 2014.
64. Soslow RA. Endometrial carcinomas with ambiguous features. Semin Diagn Pathol. 2010;27 (4):261–73.
65. Gilks CB, Oliva E, Soslow RA. Poor interobserver reproducibility in the diagnosis of high-grade endometrial carcinoma. Am J Surg Pathol. 2013;37(6):874–81.
66. Hoang LN, McConechy MK, Kobel M, et al. Histotype-genotype correlation in 36 high-grade endometrial carcinomas. Am J Surg Pathol. 2013;37(9):1421–32.
67. Kandoth C, Schultz N, Cherniack AD, et al. Integrated genomic characterization of endometrial carcinoma. Nature. 2013;497(7447):67–73.
68. Meng B, Hoang LN, McIntyre JB, et al. POLE exonuclease domain mutation predicts long progression-free survival in grade 3 endometrioid carcinoma of the endometrium. Gynecol Oncol. 2014;134(1):15–9.
69. Hussein YR, Weigelt B, Levine DA, et al. Clinicopathological analysis of endometrial carcinomas harboring somatic POLE exonuclease domain mutations. Mod Pathol. 2015;28(4): 505–14.
70. Church DN, Stelloo E, Nout RA, et al. Prognostic significance of POLE proofreading mutations in endometrial cancer. J Natl Cancer Inst. 2015;107(1):402.
71. Tobon H, Watkins GJ. Secretory adenocarcinoma of the endometrium. Int J Gynecol Pathol. 1985;4(4):328–35.
72. Clement PB, Young RH. Endometrioid carcinoma of the uterine corpus: a review of its pathology with emphasis on recent advances and problematic aspects. Adv Anat Pathol. 2002;9(3):145–84.
73. Hoang LN, Han G, McConechy M, et al. Immunohistochemical characterization of prototypical endometrial clear cell carcinoma–diagnostic utility of HNF-1beta and oestrogen receptor. Histopathology. 2014;64(4):585–96.
74. Mhawech-Fauceglia P, Yan L, Liu S, Pejovic T. $ER^+/PR^+/TFF3^+/IMP3^-$ immunoprofile distinguishes endometrioid from serous and clear cell carcinomas of the endometrium: a study of 401 cases. Histopathology. 2013;62(7):976–85.
75. Lax SF, Pizer ES, Ronnett BM, Kurman RJ. Clear cell carcinoma of the endometrium is characterized by a distinctive profile of p53, Ki-67, estrogen, and progesterone receptor expression. Hum Pathol. 1998;29(6):551–8.
76. Yamamoto S, Tsuda H, Aida S, Shimazaki H, Tamai S, Matsubara O. Immunohistochemical detection of hepatocyte nuclear factor 1beta in ovarian and endometrial clear-cell adenocarcinomas and nonneoplastic endometrium. Hum Pathol. 2007;38(7):1074–80.
77. Fadare O, Liang SX. Diagnostic utility of hepatocyte nuclear factor 1-beta immunoreactivity in endometrial carcinomas: lack of specificity for endometrial clear cell carcinoma. Appl Immunohistochem Mol Morphol. 2012;20(6):580–7.
78. Fadare O, Desouki MM, Gwin K, et al. Frequent expression of napsin A in clear cell carcinoma of the endometrium: potential diagnostic utility. Am J Surg Pathol. 2014;38(2): 189–96.
79. Iwamoto M, Nakatani Y, Fugo K, Kishimoto T, Kiyokawa T. Napsin A is frequently expressed in clear cell carcinoma of the ovary and endometrium. Hum Pathol. 2015;46(7):957–62.

80. Jiang Z, Woda BA, Rock KL, et al. P504S: a new molecular marker for the detection of prostate carcinoma. Am J Surg Pathol. 2001;25(11):1397–404.
81. Jiang Z, Fanger GR, Woda BA, et al. Expression of alpha-methylacyl-CoA racemase (P504s) in various malignant neoplasms and normal tissues: a study of 761 cases. Hum Pathol. 2003;34(8):792–6.
82. Zhou M, Chinnaiyan AM, Kleer CG, Lucas PC, Rubin MA. Alpha-Methylacyl-CoA racemase: a novel tumor marker over-expressed in several human cancers and their precursor lesions. Am J Surg Pathol. 2002;26(7):926–31.
83. Allo G, Bernardini MQ, Wu RC, et al. ARID1A loss correlates with mismatch repair deficiency and intact p53 expression in high-grade endometrial carcinomas. Mod Pathol. 2014;27(2):255–61.
84. Zhang ZM, Xiao S, Sun GY, et al. The clinicopathologic significance of the loss of BAF250a (ARID1A) expression in endometrial carcinoma. Int J Gynecol Cancer. 2014;24(3):534–40.
85. Fadare O, Gwin K, Desouki MM, et al. The clinicopathologic significance of p53 and BAF-250a (ARID1A) expression in clear cell carcinoma of the endometrium. Mod Pathol. 2013;26(8):1101–10.
86. Fadare O, Renshaw IL, Liang SX. Does the loss of ARID1A (BAF-250a) expression in endometrial clear cell carcinomas have any clinicopathologic significance?. A pilot assessment. J Cancer. 2012;3:129–36.
87. Wiegand KC, Lee AF, Al-Agha OM, et al. Loss of BAF250a (ARID1A) is frequent in high-grade endometrial carcinomas. J Pathol. 2011;224(3):328–33.
88. Vang R, Barner R, Wheeler DT, Strauss BL. Immunohistochemical staining for Ki-67 and p53 helps distinguish endometrial Arias-Stella reaction from high-grade carcinoma, including clear cell carcinoma. Int J Gynecol Pathol. 2004;23(3):223–33.
89. Murray SK, Young RH, Scully RE. Uterine endometrioid carcinoma with small nonvillous papillae: an analysis of 26 cases of a favorable-prognosis tumor to be distinguished from serous carcinoma. Int J Surg Pathol. 2000;8(4):279–89.
90. Ambros RA, Ballouk F, Malfetano JH, Ross JS. Significance of papillary (villoglandular) differentiation in endometrioid carcinoma of the uterus. Am J Surg Pathol. 1994;18(6):569–75.
91. Garg K, Broaddus RR, Soslow RA, Urbauer DL, Levine DA, Djordjevic B. Pathologic scoring of PTEN immunohistochemistry in endometrial carcinoma is highly reproducible. Int J Gynecol Pathol. 2012;31(1):48–56.
92. Pallares J, Bussaglia E, Martinez-Guitarte JL, et al. Immunohistochemical analysis of PTEN in endometrial carcinoma: a tissue microarray study with a comparison of four commercial antibodies in correlation with molecular abnormalities. Mod Pathol. 2005;18(5):719–27.
93. Maiques O, Santacana M, Valls J, et al. Optimal protocol for PTEN immunostaining; role of analytical and preanalytical variables in PTEN staining in normal and neoplastic endometrial, breast, and prostatic tissues. Hum Pathol. 2014;45(3):522–32.
94. Djordjevic B, Hennessy BT, Li J, et al. Clinical assessment of PTEN loss in endometrial carcinoma: immunohistochemistry outperforms gene sequencing. Mod Pathol. 2012;25(5):699–708.
95. Tashiro H, Blazes MS, Wu R, et al. Mutations in PTEN are frequent in endometrial carcinoma but rare in other common gynecological malignancies. Cancer Res. 1997;57(18):3935–40.
96. Risinger JI, Hayes K, Maxwell GL, et al. PTEN mutation in endometrial cancers is associated with favorable clinical and pathologic characteristics. Clin Cancer Res. 1998;4(12):3005–10.
97. Sun H, Enomoto T, Fujita M, et al. Mutational analysis of the PTEN gene in endometrial carcinoma and hyperplasia. Am J Clin Pathol. 2001;115(1):32–8.
98. Darvishian F, Hummer AJ, Thaler HT, et al. Serous endometrial cancers that mimic endometrioid adenocarcinomas: a clinicopathologic and immunohistochemical study of a group of problematic cases. Am J Surg Pathol. 2004;28(12):1568–78.

99. Zheng W, Yi X, Fadare O, et al. The oncofetal protein IMP3: a novel biomarker for endometrial serous carcinoma. Am J Surg Pathol. 2008;32(2):304–15.
100. Lax SF, Kendall B, Tashiro H, Slebos RJ, Hedrick L. The frequency of p53, K-ras mutations, and microsatellite instability differs in uterine endometrioid and serous carcinoma: evidence of distinct molecular genetic pathways. Cancer. 2000;88(4):814–24.
101. Kane MF, Loda M, Gaida GM, et al. Methylation of the hMLH1 promoter correlates with lack of expression of hMLH1 in sporadic colon tumors and mismatch repair-defective human tumor cell lines. Cancer Res. 1997;57(5):808–11.
102. Herman JG, Umar A, Polyak K, et al. Incidence and functional consequences of hMLH1 promoter hypermethylation in colorectal carcinoma. Proc Natl Acad Sci U S A. 1998;95 (12):6870–5.
103. Salvesen HB, MacDonald N, Ryan A, et al. Methylation of hMLH1 in a population-based series of endometrial carcinomas. Clin Cancer Res. 2000;6(9):3607–13.
104. Goodfellow PJ, Buttin BM, Herzog TJ, et al. Prevalence of defective DNA mismatch repair and MSH6 mutation in an unselected series of endometrial cancers. Proc Natl Acad Sci U S A. 2003;100(10):5908–13.
105. Broaddus RR, Lynch HT, Chen LM, et al. Pathologic features of endometrial carcinoma associated with HNPCC: a comparison with sporadic endometrial carcinoma. Cancer. 2006;106(1):87–94.
106. Lu KH, Dinh M, Kohlmann W, et al. Gynecologic cancer as a "sentinel cancer" for women with hereditary nonpolyposis colorectal cancer syndrome. Obstet Gynecol. 2005;105 (3):569–74.
107. Backes FJ, Hampel H, Backes KA, et al. Are prediction models for Lynch syndrome valid for probands with endometrial cancer? Fam Cancer. 2009;8(4):483–7.
108. SGO clinical practice statement: screening for Lynch syndrome in endometrial cancer. 2014. Available from: https://www.sgo.org/clinical-practice/guidelines/screening-for-lynch-syndrome-in-endometrial-cancer/.
109. Mercado RC, Hampel H, Kastrinos F, et al. Performance of PREMM (1,2,6), MMRpredict, and MMRpro in detecting Lynch syndrome among endometrial cancer cases. Genet Med. 2012;14 (7):670–80.
110. Bartley AN, Luthra R, Saraiya DS, Urbauer DL, Broaddus RR. Identification of cancer patients with Lynch syndrome: clinically significant discordances and problems in tissue-based mismatch repair testing. Cancer Prev Res (Phila). 2012;5(2):320–7.
111. Rosen DG, Cai KQ, Luthra R, Liu J. Immunohistochemical staining of hMLH1 and hMSH2 reflects microsatellite instability status in ovarian carcinoma. Mod Pathol. 2006;19(11):1414–20.
112. Cai KQ, Albarracin C, Rosen D, et al. Microsatellite instability and alteration of the expression of hMLH1 and hMSH2 in ovarian clear cell carcinoma. Hum Pathol. 2004; 35(5):552–9.
113. Modica I, Soslow RA, Black D, Tornos C, Kauff N, Shia J. Utility of immunohistochemistry in predicting microsatellite instability in endometrial carcinoma. Am J Surg Pathol. 2007;31 (5):744–51.
114. Ferguson SE, Aronson M, Pollett A, et al. Performance characteristics of screening strategies for Lynch syndrome in unselected women with newly diagnosed endometrial cancer who have undergone universal germline mutation testing. Cancer. 2014;120 (24), 3932–9.
115. Buchanan DD, Tan YY, Walsh MD, et al. Tumor mismatch repair immunohistochemistry and DNA MLH1 methylation testing of patients with endometrial cancer diagnosed at age younger than 60 years optimizes triage for population-level germline mismatch repair gene mutation testing. J Clin Oncol. 2014;32(2):90–100.
116. Djordjevic B, Barkoh BA, Luthra R, Broaddus RR. Relationship between PTEN, DNA mismatch repair, and tumor histotype in endometrial carcinoma: retained positive expression of PTEN preferentially identifies sporadic non-endometrioid carcinomas. Mod Pathol. 2013;26(10):1401–12.
117. Boland CR, Fishel R. Lynch syndrome: form, function, proteins, and basketball. Gastroenterology. 2005;129(2):751–5.

Chapter 4
Molecular Pathology of Endometrioid Adenocarcinoma

Katherine C. Kurnit, Bojana Djordjevic and Russell R. Broaddus

Introduction

The most common subtype of endometrial adenocarcinoma is endometrioid adenocarcinoma, with prevalence rates of around 80% [1, 2]. According to the Bokhman classification [3], these tumors are generally classified as Type I and tend to be associated with a better prognosis than Type II tumors [1, 2]. Endometrioid endometrial adenocarcinomas generally present at an earlier stage than non-endometrioid tumors and often have lower rates of recurrence [2]. Despite these less aggressive clinical characteristics, a subset of endometrioid carcinomas does behave more aggressively, and recent research has focused on characterizing the genotypic differences that may account for this. Molecular characterization of endometrioid adenocarcinoma can also provide potential therapeutic targets for

K.C. Kurnit
Department of Gynecologic Oncology and Reproductive Medicine,
Unit 1362, University of Texas M.D. Anderson Cancer Center,
1515 Holcombe Blvd., Houston, TX 77030, USA
e-mail: kkurnit@mdanderson.org

B. Djordjevic
Department of Anatomic Pathology, Sunnybrook Health Sciences Centre,
Department of Laboratory Medicine and Pathobiology, University of Toronto,
2075 Bayview Ave, room E4-27b, Toronto, ON M4N 3M5, Canada
e-mail: bojanadjordjevicmd@gmail.com

R.R. Broaddus (✉)
Department of Pathology, Unit 85,
University of Texas M.D. Anderson Cancer Center,
1515 Holcombe Blvd., Houston, TX 77030, USA
e-mail: rbroaddus@mdanderson.org

M.T. Deavers and D.M. Coffey (eds.), *Precision Molecular Pathology of Uterine Cancer*, Molecular Pathology Library,
DOI 10.1007/978-3-319-57985-6_4

matched targeted therapy trials, as current chemotherapy and radiation therapy approaches to the treatment of advanced/recurrent endometrioid-type endometrial cancer are not optimal.

PI3K/AKT Pathway

Activation of the PI3K/AKT signaling pathway is common in endometrial cancer, with pathway alterations reported to occur in over 80% of endometrioid endometrial cancers [4–6]. *PTEN* alteration is the most common, but other genes in this pathway have been found to be mutated in endometrial cancer as well, including *PIK3CA*, *PIK3R1*, and *PIK3R2* [4, 6, 7]. Additionally, mutations in multiple genes comprising this pathway have been shown to occur concomitantly [4, 8–10]. Survival outcomes have been mixed, but the literature suggests that PI3K pathway mutations may be associated with worse clinical outcomes [8, 11, 12]. Further, a study by Nout et al. showed a worse disease-free survival in endometrioid endometrial carcinomas when mutations within multiple signaling pathways, including the PI3K/AKT pathway, co-occur [8].

PTEN

The phosphatase and tensin homolog (*PTEN*) gene encodes a protein which functions as a tumor suppressor within the PI3K/AKT pathway [13, 14]. Inactivation of the *PTEN* gene is one of the most frequent mutations within this pathway and within endometrioid endometrial cancer in general, with described prevalence rates ranging from 15 to 80% [4, 13, 15–20].

PTEN mutations have been identified in both endometrial hyperplasia and in endometrial cancer and are thought to be an early event in tumorigenesis [21–23]. These mutations have been seen in both sporadic tumors and, to a lesser extent, in tumors associated with Lynch Syndrome [24]. *PTEN* mutations are more common in endometrioid endometrial cancer than in mixed or serous tumors [14, 16–18, 25]. Data regarding the relationship between *PTEN* mutations and microsatellite instability (MSI) status are mixed, with some studies showing higher rates of MSI-high in tumors with *PTEN* mutations, while others show no relationship [5, 25, 26].

However, Djordjevic et al. recently demonstrated that intact PTEN protein expression (and the presence of *PTEN* wild-type gene) was associated with microsatellite-stable (MSS) non-endometrioid endometrial carcinomas, while no such relationship existed in endometrioid endometrial tumors [27]. Approximately 90% of deleterious *PTEN* mutations are associated with immunohistochemical (IHC) loss of PTEN protein [14] (Fig. 4.1). Interestingly, in approximately 40% of endometrial carcinomas, IHC loss of PTEN protein expression is associated with no gene sequence abnormality [14]. This is likely due to the fact that PTEN protein and

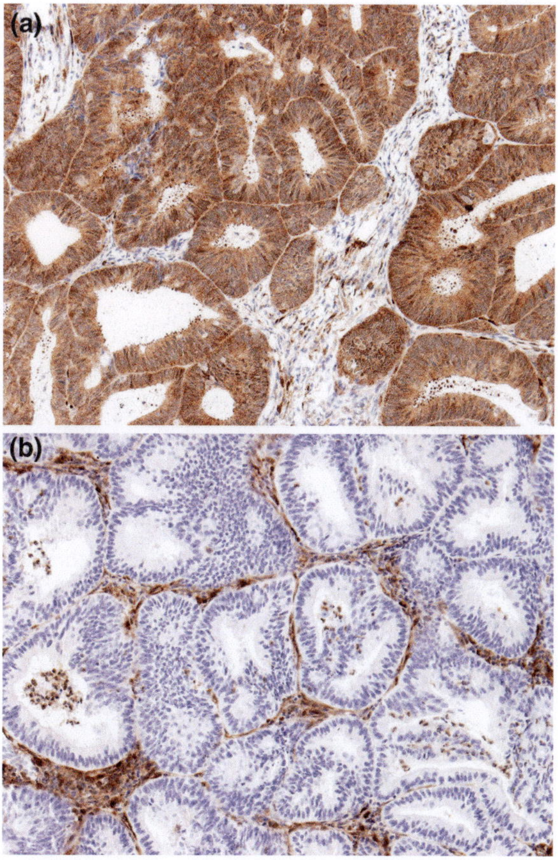

Fig. 4.1 PTEN immunohistochemistry. **a** Endometrial carcinoma with intact positive protein expression of PTEN. No *PTEN* gene mutation was detected by next-generation sequencing. **b** Endometrial carcinoma with *PTEN* gene mutation and associated loss of PTEN protein expression. Note intact expression of PTEN protein in adjacent stromal cells, which acts as an internal positive control

mRNA can be regulated by a variety of different mechanisms independent of gene mutation [28]. Therefore, for clinical purposes, immunohistochemistry may be a preferable method of detecting endometrial carcinomas with loss of PTEN function.

Multiple studies have attempted to characterize the relationship between *PTEN* endometrial cancer mutations and survival outcomes. In a single institution study of 221 endometrial cancer patients, Akiyama-Abe et al. performed IHC staining for PTEN and found loss of protein expression in 25% of tumors. In those with loss of PTEN expression, the authors found a significant association with endometrioid histology and decreased lymphatic–vascular invasion, as well as a significant improvement in overall survival [16]. Interestingly, they did not find any differences in rates of advanced stage at presentation or early grade tumors. Improved outcomes including survival and recurrence rates with *PTEN* mutations have similarly been shown in some, but not all, prior studies [25, 29, 30]. In contrast, a recent study of 187 endometrioid endometrial cancer patients by Westin et al. found that, in aggregate, there was no difference in progression-free survival of patients with IHC-determined loss of PTEN function compared with those tumors that retained PTEN function. However, on a sub-analysis of stratification by body mass index (BMI), loss of PTEN function in the presence of obesity (BMI ≥ 30) was associated with significantly improved progression-free survival, whereas non-obese patients (BMI <30) were found to have significantly worse progression-free survival in the setting of PTEN loss [31].

PIK3CA

The *PIK3CA* gene encodes the p110-alpha subunit of PI3K, which functions as the catalytic subunit of the protein complex [6, 32]. Mutation prevalence for endometrial cancer has been reported to be between 20 and 36% [4, 10, 11, 32–35], with mutations being more frequent in endometrioid than non-endometrioid tumors [4, 32]. Concurrent *PIK3CA* and *PTEN* mutations in endometrial carcinomas have been found in multiple studies [4, 10, 11]. There are also some data to support higher rates of MSI-high in endometrial tumors with *PIK3CA* mutations [36, 37], though not all studies have found this to be the case [5].

In general, endometrial tumors with *PIK3CA* mutation appear to be more aggressive than those without, with trends toward worse survival outcomes [12, 17, 36]. McIntyre et al. [36] found that *PIK3CA* mutations were associated with worse disease-specific survival in grade 3 endometrioid tumors, but this association did not persist on multivariate analysis and, interestingly, was not present for serous tumors harboring *PIK3CA* mutations. Catasus and colleagues similarly investigated 109 predominantly endometrioid endometrial carcinomas and found increased rates of myometrial invasion and lymphatic–vascular space invasion in association with *PIK3CA* mutations. Interestingly, they showed higher rates of grade 3 tumors as well as increased myometrial invasion or cervical involvement when mutations occurred in exon 20, compared with mutations on exon 9 which were more often associated with early grade tumors and invasion of less than half of the myometrium [11]. These data suggested that, in addition to *PIK3CA* mutations being important for survival outcomes, some *PIK3CA* mutations may be more relevant than others. This mutational diversity phenomenon, the overall tendency toward worse prognosis associated with *PIK3CA* mutations, and the complex nature of the PI3K/AKT pathway may account for some of the reasons why, despite the availability of multiple PI3K/AKT pathway inhibitors, clinical trials have failed to show consistent benefit with the use of PI3K/AKT targeted therapy in endometrial cancer [38].

PIK3R1 and *PIK3R2*

The *PIK3R1* and *PIK3R2* genes encode the p85-alpha and p85-beta regulatory subunits of PI3K [4, 6], which form a dimer that assists in stabilization of PTEN. A 2011 study by Cheung et al. further characterized the role of *PIK3R1* in endometrial tumors and described largely for the first time the presence of *PIK3R2* mutation in endometrial cancer [4, 39]. Mutation rates in endometrial carcinoma are 20–43% for *PIK3R1* [4, 40], and 5% for *PIK3R2* [4]. Findings from these studies suggest that *PIK3R1* and *PIK3R2* mutations may lead to activation of the PI3K/AKT pathway and thereby contribute to endometrial cancer tumorigenesis.

ARID1A

The *ARID1A* gene encodes a non-catalytic subunit of the SWI/SNF complex, which aids in chromatin remodeling [41, 42]. Bosse et al. [42] found that 27% of endometrioid endometrial cancers had *ARID1A* mutation and that these mutations were commonly associated with PI3K/AKT pathway mutations. *ARID1A* mutations appear to be more common with MSI-high tumors [37, 42–44], and it has been suggested that *ARID1A* may play a role in epigenetic silencing of *MLH1* [42]. An interesting study by Mao et al. analyzed *ARID1A* mutations in 246 cases ranging from normal endometrium to high-grade endometrial cancer. They found no mutations in normal tissue, areas of clonal but not complete loss within 16% of complex atypical hyperplasia cases, complete loss in 25% of low-grade endometrioid endometrial cancers, and complete loss in 44% of high-grade endometrioid tumors [45]. These results were notable, as they suggested a possible role in tumor progression for *ARID1A* mutations which had not previously been well described. As data are still limited regarding *ARID1A* mutations in endometrial cancer, little is available regarding survival outcomes. While Allo and colleagues found that *ARID1A* mutations do appear to be present within high-grade endometrioid tumors, they were unable to find a difference in progression-free survival within the endometrioid endometrial cancer group [43].

KRAS

The *KRAS* gene encodes the K-Ras protein, which functions along the RAS/MAPK pathway and helps regulate cell division [46]. Prevalence rates of *KRAS* mutation in endometrial cancers have been reported to be between 10 and 30% [4, 47, 48]. Several studies have found similar rates of *KRAS* mutation in endometrial hyperplasias and endometrial cancers, suggesting that *KRAS* mutation may represent an early event during tumorigenesis [47, 49].

KRAS mutations are more frequent among endometrioid and mixed endometrioid histologies, compared to non-endometrioid endometrial cancers [18, 50, 51]. Furthermore, *KRAS* mutation rates are higher in endometrioid tumors showing increasing amounts of mucinous differentiation [52], which may be clinically significant since mucinous differentiation has been associated with lymph node involvement [53]. Some studies have suggested that endometrial cancers with

KRAS mutation tend to be associated with lower endometrioid grade, though others have found no association with grade [50, 51, 54]. Like many other mutations in endometrioid endometrial cancer, *KRAS* mutations are more frequently found in MSI-high tumors than MSS tumors [44]. Interestingly, atypical endometrial hyperplasia with MSI-high exhibits wild-type *KRAS*, suggesting that defects in DNA mismatch repair precede *KRAS* mutation [24, 55].

There are limited data regarding clinical outcomes in endometrioid endometrial cancers with *KRAS* mutation. Birkeland et al. analyzed *KRAS* mutations from 264 primary and 22 metastatic endometrial carcinomas. They found *KRAS* mutations to be more prevalent among grade 1 and 2 tumors, in those with endometrioid histology, and in obese women. There was no association with prognosis, and there were no differences in mutation rates among the primary and metastatic tumors [56]. In contrast, Ito et al. showed that in a cohort of 221 endometrioid endometrial cancers, there was a higher prevalence of *KRAS* mutation among patients older than 60 years of age who had recurrence of their disease or died due to disease [54].

Several studies have also examined for a possible association between tamoxifen use and *KRAS* mutation within the endometrium [46, 57, 58]. A small retrospective study by Turbiner et al. found that women with endometrial cancer who were taking tamoxifen for breast cancer had a higher incidence of *KRAS* mutations. Within the tamoxifen cohort, 16 of the 18 tumors were endometrioid, one was of mixed histology, and one was a clear cell carcinoma [46]. Interestingly, a subsequent study by Tsujioka et al. similarly saw increased *KRAS* mutations in benign polyps within the endometrium of women taking tamoxifen, but found that after cessation of tamoxifen use the *KRAS* mutations were no longer identified [58].

Several studies have suggested that the presence of a *KRAS* mutation may correlate with poorer responses to several targeted therapies, especially those targeting the PI3K/AKT pathways such as mTOR inhibitors [6, 59]. A small in vitro study by Weigelt et al. found an increased resistance to mTOR inhibitors in endometrial cancer cell lines harboring *PIK3CA* and/or *PTEN* mutations with a coexisting *KRAS* mutation, though it did show that a subset of these cells still retained some sensitivity to other forms of PI3K pathway modulation [60]. A recent phase II trial of everolimus in 35 patients with recurrent endometrial cancer showed that none of the patients with a *KRAS* mutation and positive staining for pS6 (a marker of downstream activation of the PI3K/AKT/mTOR pathway) had a prolonged response to the mTOR inhibitor [61]. In contrast, an in vitro and in vivo study of the effects of metformin on endometrial cancer cell lines by Iglesias et al. found increased apoptosis in cells with *KRAS* mutation, as well as lower mean tumor weights. Interestingly, the presence of a *PTEN* mutation had no effect on tumor response to metformin in these cell lines. Metformin's mechanism of action as a potential cancer therapeutic is thought to involve a decrease of tumor growth, and based on these data, it appears that this effect is potentiated in *KRAS* mutant cells. The authors therefore suggested that this may be due to phosphorylation of the activated K-Ras protein by Protein Kinase C, which subsequently leads to its removal from the plasma membrane and, ultimately, to apoptosis of the tumor cell [62].

CTNNB1

The *CTNNB1* gene encodes the protein β-catenin, which functions as a member of the canonical Wnt pathway. In normal endometrium, β-catenin is expressed primarily at the cell membrane of glandular epithelial cells. *CTNNB1* mutation leads to less degradation of β-catenin protein, causing the protein to accumulate in the cytoplasm or translocate to the nucleus (Fig. 4.2), where it subsequently serves as a transcription factor for Myc, cyclin D1, and E-cadherin [63–65]. *CTNNB1* mutations have been discovered in up to 45% of endometrioid endometrial cancers [20, 65–69]. In 2013, The Cancer Genome Atlas (TCGA) reported on a genomic investigation of 373 endometrial carcinomas, which identified frequent mutations in the *CTNNB1* gene, specifically in the subset of endometrioid carcinomas [44]. Interestingly, in this analysis, 52% of the microsatellite-stable (MSS) tumors tested had a mutation in *CTNNB1*. In contrast, tumors with high microsatellite instability showed infrequent *CTNNB1* mutations [44].

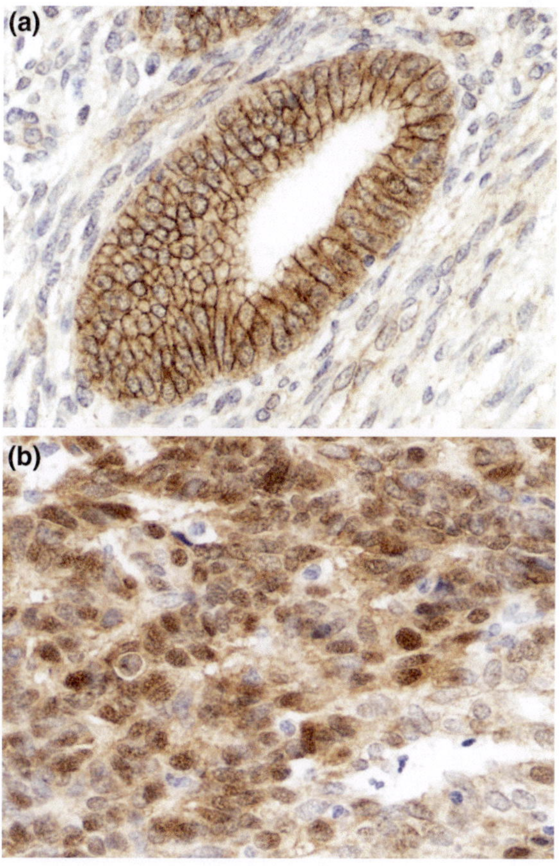

Fig. 4.2 β-catenin immunohistochemistry in normal endometrium (**a**) and endometrial carcinoma with *CTNNB1* gene mutation (**b**). In normal endometrial epithelium, β-catenin protein shows strong, membranous expression, with little-to-no cytoplasmic or nuclear expression. In endometrial carcinomas with *CTNNB1* (encodes β-catenin) mutation, β-catenin protein is inhibited from degradation, allowing translocation from the membrane to the cytoplasm and nucleus. Nuclear expression helps to drive activation of the WNT signaling pathway

Several earlier studies have suggested an association of *CTNNB1* mutations with lower grade and earlier stage endometrial cancers, as well as with endometrioid histology [63, 66, 70–72]. Moreno-Bueno et al. investigated 128 endometrial cancers, including 95 with endometrioid and 33 with non-endometrioid histology. *CTNNB1* mutations were detected in 14.9% of the endometrioid tumors, but in none of the non-endometrioid tumors [66]. Fukuchi et al. analyzed 76 endometrial tumors and found that of the 10 tumors with *CTNNB1* mutations, all except one were well- or moderately differentiated endometrioid carcinomas. Among these tumors, all except one were stage 1 or 2 at the time of diagnosis [63]. Similarly, findings of a predominance of grade 1 or 2 tumors have been reported by several other studies [70–72].

Recent findings suggest that endometrial cancers with beta-catenin mutations may represent a more aggressive subset of early endometrioid endometrial cancers [72–75]. Liu et al. performed consensus clustering of 271 of the endometrioid endometrial cancers used in TCGA, which revealed four distinct clusters of gene signatures. The group designated Cluster 2 represented a subset of low-grade, low-stage tumors with significantly higher frequencies of *CTNNB1* mutations and evidence for activation of the WNT/β-catenin signaling pathway. This group exhibited lower overall survival than even the higher grade and higher stage clusters, and was comprised of a younger, more obese subset of patients [73]. Similarly, Myers et al. performed a case-control analysis of 50 patients with low-grade, stage IA endometrioid endometrial carcinomas in order to further characterize those patients who had a recurrence of their early disease [74]. This study investigated the frequency of three commonly mutated genes in endometrial cancer, including *PIK3CA*, *CTNNB1*, and *KRAS*. They found that *CTNNB1* mutations were more frequent among the 12 patients with recurrent disease than among the 38 patients who did not recur and that there were no differences in rates of *PIK3CA* or *KRAS* mutations. In contrast to Liu et al., however, Myers et al. found the subset of patients with a recurrence to have a lower body mass index (BMI) than those without a recurrence of their disease.

TP53

The *TP53* gene encodes the p53 protein which assists in cell cycle arrest and apoptosis, and its mutation is frequent in numerous cancer types, including endometrial cancer [76, 77]. While prevalence rates are much higher in non-endometrioid than endometrioid endometrial carcinomas [18, 78], the majority of publications evaluating *TP53* mutations in endometrial cancer were done in predominantly endometrioid tumors, and rates of *TP53* mutation have still been reported to be 10–35% [44, 69, 77–83]. Lower grade endometrioid carcinomas may have higher frequencies of concurrent *TP53* and *PTEN* mutations compared with serous carcinomas and grade 3 endometrioid tumors, suggesting that the mechanism for p53-related tumorigenesis is different in endometrioid versus non-endometrioid tumors [44]. In support of this idea, Kaku et al. found a higher rate of *TP53* mutations in endometrial carcinomas without associated hyperplasia than in those with hyperplasia [84].

As discussed above, data from TCGA suggested that *TP53* mutations tended to cluster within the endometrial tumors showing serous histology and grade 3 endometrioid histology [44]. Other authors have found a similar association between grade 3 tumors and *TP53* mutation [78, 80, 85, 86]. Interestingly, a study by Kuhn et al. found prevalence rates of 30% within a sample of 20 undifferentiated endometrial tumors, 12 of which had both an endometrioid and undifferentiated component. When present, the *TP53* mutations were seen in both the undifferentiated and its corresponding endometrioid components, with the exception of one tumor which only showed a *TP53* mutation in the undifferentiated aspect of the tumor, suggesting a possible role of p53 in tumor progression (Kuhn). While several studies also suggest an association between *TP53* mutation and advanced stage, not all studies have found this to be the case [78, 82, 85, 87]. Similarly, no consensus findings of a relationship between *TP53* mutation and depth of invasion, lymphatic–vascular space invasion, or metastatic disease have been demonstrated [78, 82, 85, 87].

In general, clinical outcomes in patients with endometrioid endometrial cancer harboring *TP53* mutations appear to be worse than in those without *TP53* mutations. Lee et al. examined 131 patients with predominantly endometrioid endometrial cancer and found *TP53* mutation to be an independent prognostic indicator of poor overall survival and disease-free survival [82]. Other studies have shown a similar association with poor overall survival or disease-free survival, though many studies were unable to demonstrate a statistically significant difference in multivariate analysis [78, 80, 85, 88–93]. Reasons for the somewhat heterogeneous findings of these studies may include the wide range of numbers of patients, differences in histologic representation, and variation in methodologies for evaluation of *TP53* mutational status. Several studies have also looked at the effect of *TP53* mutations on outcomes in important subpopulations. For example, a study of 136 endometrial cancer patients by Oreskovic and colleagues found worse overall survival on multivariate analysis in those patients with grade 1 and grade 2, but not grade 3, tumors [94]. There is some evidence that the presence of *TP53* mutation can help impact therapeutic approaches to patients with endometrioid endometrial carcinoma. Saffari et al. found that, in a group of 53 endometrioid endometrial carcinoma patients, *TP53* mutation was associated with worse overall survival on multivariate analysis. In those women with *TP53* mutations who received adjuvant radiation therapy, survival outcomes were similar to wild-type patients with and without radiation treatment, and all three of these subgroups demonstrated better survival than patients with *TP53* mutation-containing tumors who did not receive adjuvant radiotherapy [93].

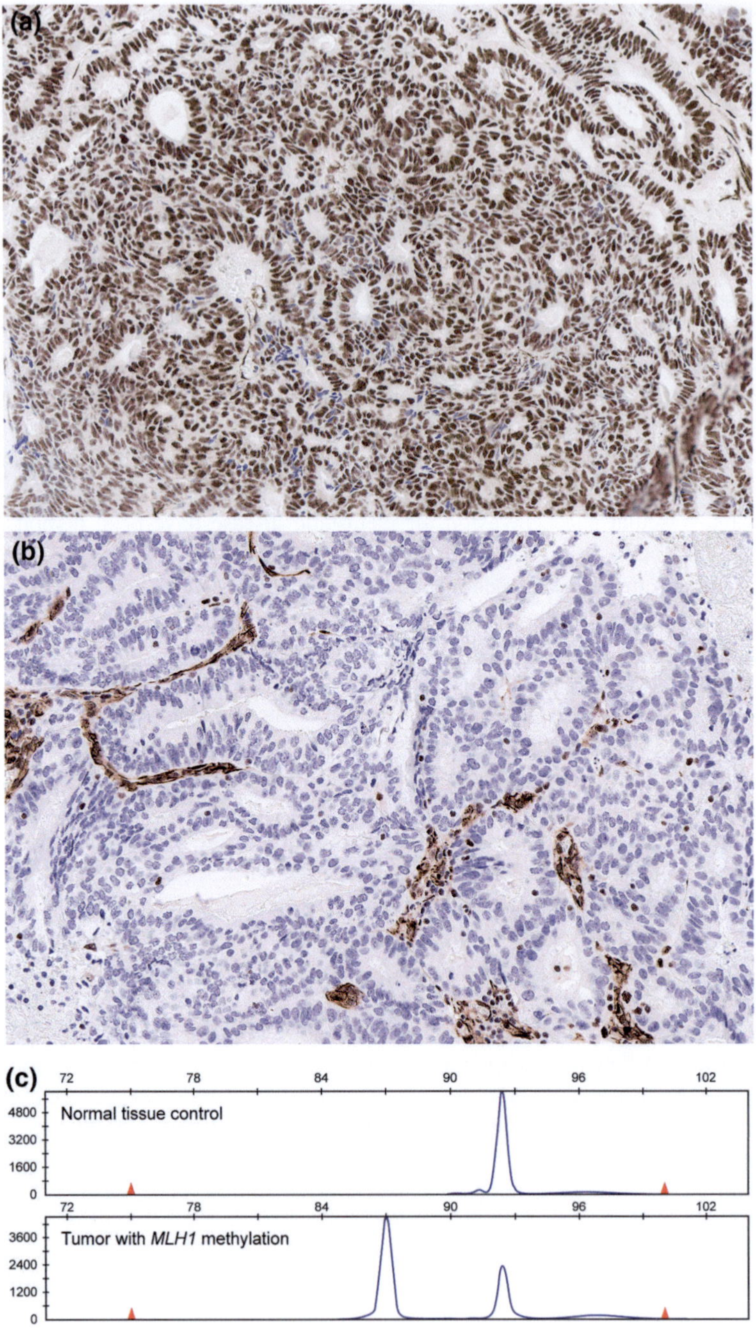
(a)
(b)
(c)
72
78
84
90
96
102
4800
3200
1600
0
Normal tissue control
3600
2400
1200
Tumor with MLH1 methylation

◂**Fig. 4.3** *MLH1* methylation associated with MLH1 protein loss by immunohistochemistry. **a** Endometrial carcinoma with retained nuclear expression of MLH1 protein. **b** Endometrial carcinoma with loss of MLH1 protein. Note retained positive expression of MLH1 in adjacent stromal cells. **c** PCR-based *MLH1* promoter methylation analysis. Tumor DNA is analyzed concurrently with DNA from normal tissue control from the same patient. Top tracing, normal tissue with no *MLH1* methylation; bottom tracing, tumor with presence of *MLH1* methylation

Microsatellite Instability

DNA mismatch repair (MMR) is controlled by a family of nuclear proteins, including MLH1, MSH2, MSH6, and PMS2. Defects in MMR can result from germline mutations in the genes encoding these proteins (Lynch Syndrome) or, in sporadic endometrial and colorectal carcinoma, from hypermethylation of the *MLH1* gene promoter. MMR defects are manifested as high levels of microsatellite instability (MSI-high, assessed clinically via a PCR-based assay) and by loss of mismatch repair protein expression in immunohistochemistry-based assays as demonstrated in Fig. 4.3 [95]. Prevalence of MSI-high in endometrial cancer has been reported to be around 15–40% [26, 50, 96–102], with 15–25% being the most common. In most published studies, no distinction is made between germline versus sporadic MMR loss, although it can be inferred that the vast majority of endometrial cancers with defective MMR are sporadic cancers with MLH1 protein loss due to *MLH1* gene methylation.

MMR loss and *MLH1* hypermethylation are thought to be early events during tumorigenesis in endometrial cancer, as hypermethylation patterns have been observed in endometrial hyperplasias [47, 103]. MSI-high is more common among endometrioid carcinomas compared to non-endometrioid tumors, including serous and clear cell carcinomas [27, 50, 101, 104, 105]. The relationship between tumor grade and MSI status is somewhat unclear, as some studies show an association with increasing grade in MSI-high tumors, while others show no association [104, 106–108]. Similarly, evaluating the relationship between MSI status and clinical stage has led to conflicting results, with several studies showing an association of MSI-high tumors with more advanced stage disease, others showing an association with earlier stages, and some studies showing no association with stage [101, 104, 106, 107, 109]. MSI-high tumors have been reported to have an increased risk of lymphatic–vascular space invasion [102, 104], but their relationship with depth of myometrial invasion is not clear [101, 104, 106]. MMR deficiency, particularly MLH1 protein loss and *MLH1* methylation, has been associated with a subset of undifferentiated endometrial carcinoma [110–113]. It is uncertain whether undifferentiated endometrial carcinoma should be considered a subtype of grade 3 endometrioid adenocarcinoma or a non-endometrioid carcinoma. Compared to grade 3 endometrioid adenocarcinoma, undifferentiated carcinomas typically have lower hormone receptor and cytokeratin expression [110] and may have a more aggressive disease course [111, 114, 115].

The impact of MSI-high on survival outcomes in endometrial cancer is similarly unclear, despite a number of different publications examining this issue. Details of several of the larger studies evaluating MMR status and survival outcomes are summarized in Table 4.1. Some authors have identified improved outcomes in MSI-high tumors [97, 98, 101, 102], others found worse outcomes [116, 117], and some have found no association [100, 105, 106, 118]. One large study by Zighelboim et al. analyzed 446 prospectively collected endometrioid endometrial carcinomas [100]. MSI status was determined by PCR, as was *MLH1* methylation status. No differences in overall survival or disease-free survival were observed between MSI-high and microsatellite-stable groups. Similarly, *MLH1* methylation status had no impact on overall or progression-free survival. One of the more recent larger analyses was performed by Ruiz and colleagues, who evaluated 212 endometrioid endometrial tumors. MSI status was evaluated by IHC. They evaluated OS and PFS both within early stage (I and II) and advanced stage (III and IV) and found no differences in survival measures within either subgroup [106]. The reasons for conflicting results between these various publications are unclear. As noted in Table 4.1, MMR deficiency has been measured in a variety of different ways in these studies, which could impact results. Endometrioid and non-endometrioid carcinomas have very different clinical courses and survival outcomes; an impact of MMR on survival may be missed in studies that include both these histologies. Lower grade, early-stage endometrioid carcinomas can recur five or more years following hysterectomy, so studies with shorter follow-up intervals may miss an association with MSI-high. It is also possible that these differences may be due at least in part to underlying differences in other concurrent gene mutations not fully evaluated in these studies.

POLE

As discussed previously, based on the molecular analysis of 373 endometrial carcinomas, TCGA [44] proposed a genomic categorization of endometrial cancer into four groups. "Ultramutated tumors" represent the first category in this classification and consist of tumors with very high mutations rates. All of these tumors harbor mutations in the *POLE* gene, which encodes the catalytic subunit of the DNA polymerase epsilon, which synthesizes the leading strand during DNA replication and also plays a role in the recognition and removal of mispaired nucleotides [119, 120]. Tumors with *POLE* mutations may have as many as a million base substitutions per tumor, particularly of the G:C>T:A form [121]. It has recently been shown that germline exonuclease domain mutations of *POLE* and *POLD1* genes confer a high risk of multiple colorectal adenomas and carcinomas [122]. In addition to endometrial and colorectal cancer, *POLE* mutations have also been reported in lung cancer and melanoma [123, 124]. Their inheritance is dominant, and they have a high penetrance with a variable phenotype.

Table 4.1 Selected studies evaluating survival outcomes in MMR deficient/MSI-high endometrial carcinomas

Study	Tumor histology	Tumor stage	Number of patients	MSI assessment method	Survival result
Maxwell et al., Obstet Gynecol [97]	Endometrioid	All stages	131	PCR (MSI-high when $\geq 2/3$ markers were abnormal)	MSI-high had improved OS
Cohn et al., Obstet Gynecol [102]	Endometrioid and non-endometrioid	All stages	294	IHC (MMR deficiency defined as loss of any of the 4 MMR proteins)	MMR loss had worse PFS, no difference in OS
Black et al., J Clin Oncol [101]	Endometrioid and non-endometrioid	All stages	473	PCR (MSI-high if $\geq 2/5$ markers with allelic shift)	MSI-high had improved RFS and OS
Zighelboim et al., J Clin Oncol [100]	Endometrioid	All stages	446	PCR (MSI-high if $\geq 2/5$ were abnormal; MSI-low if 1/5 abnormal)	MSI-high showed no difference in RFS and OS, also no difference when comparing methylation status
Cote et al., Int J Gynecol Pathol [118]	Endometrioid and non-endometrioid	All stages	76	PCR (MSI-high if $\geq 30\%$ of markers showed instability, MSI-low if $<30\%$)	MSI status not predictive of OS
Nelson et al., Gynecol Oncol [105]	Grade 3 or dedifferentiated endometrioid	All stages (then subanalyses)	102 (64 endometrioid)	IHC (MMR deficiency defined as loss of at least 1 MMR protein)	No difference when all or early stage only included; MMR loss associated with increased risk of disease-specific death in advanced stage endometrial cancer in univariate but not multivariate analysis
Ruiz et al., Gynecol Oncol [106]	Endometrioid	All stages (then subanalyses)	212	IHC (MMR deficiency defined as loss of at least 1 MMR protein)	In both early stage and advanced stage, no association seen between MSI and OS or PFS

The majority of *POLE* mutations in endometrial cancer are sporadic and have been reported to represent 5–7% [44, 121, 125] of endometrial cancers. In endometrial carcinoma, most *POLE* mutations tend to cluster in two hot spots, in exons 9 and 13 [126, 127]. Paradoxically, despite being "ultramutated," these tumors have been associated with a favorable prognosis [44, 126, 128]. This observation has recently been corroborated by a large study, which reported the *POLE* mutant tumors as having approximately one-third the risk of recurrence as that of *POLE* wild-type (predominantly endometrioid in this study) endometrial cancers, and an even lower risk of death [125]. It has been hypothesized that improved prognostic outcome in patients with these tumors may be attributable to the fact that the marked number of base substitutions leads to too many gene alterations, which hinder tumor cell growth and survival.

Endometrial *POLE* mutant tumors have characterized by pure endometrioid histology, mixed histology with endometrioid components, or ambiguous histology [121, 126, 128]. Several studies also reported small numbers of serous endometrial carcinoma with *POLE* mutations, but it is not certain whether the cases underwent a centralized review [121, 129–131]. The majority of endometrioid tumors are of high cytological grade; as many as 84% have been described to have tumor infiltrating lymphocytes [128].

Similar to *POLE* wild-type endometrioid tumors, *POLE* mutants frequently carry *PTEN* (94%), *PIK3CA* (71%), and *ARID1A* (76%) mutations; however, unlike most *POLE* wild-type tumors, the majority of *POLE* mutants are microsatellite stable (65–100%) [44, 121, 126, 128]. It has been suggested that in cases where microsatellite instability and *POLE* mutations coexist, the latter is likely a secondary event [132]. Furthermore, while all eight TCGA *POLE* mutant cases were found to have mutations in at least one mismatch repair gene, only two of these cases were microsatellite instability high, suggesting that some of the mutations are "functionally suboptimal" with respect to their classical mismatch repair gene mutant counterparts [44, 126, 133].

Approximately one-third (35%) of *POLE* mutant endometrial tumors also have *TP53* mutations [121, 126, 128]. Given the good prognostic outcome of the *POLE* mutant group, the clinical significance of these *TP53* mutations is likely different than that of the *TP53* mutations in serous carcinoma/copy number high (as per TCGA classification) tumors. The presence of *TP53* mutation in some *POLE* mutants with histological features other than those of clear-cut endometrioid adenocarcinoma is important to note, as the use of p53 immunohistochemistry may lead to misclassification of these tumors as serous carcinomas.

POLE mutations may be a useful biomarker in order to spare patients with high-grade endometrioid tumors from aggressive post-adjuvant treatments, as the tumors appear to have an indolent course. Currently, the only way to detect *POLE* mutations is by sequencing the *POLE* gene. Therefore, development of surrogate markers to enable their detection would be very important.

The Cancer Genome Atlas

The Cancer Genome Atlas (TCGA) is a National Cancer Institute-funded effort to comprehensively classify, at a genomic level, various types of cancer. Genomic characterization included next-generation sequencing of the whole exome, methylation profiles, miRNA profiling, gene expression analysis, and reverse phase protein lysate array. These data are publicly available for individual investigator analysis.

Endometrial cancer, both serous carcinoma and endometrioid carcinoma, has been characterized by TCGA [44]. These data reaffirmed high rates of PI3K/AKT pathway mutations within the endometrioid subtype and showed significant rates of *CTNNB1*, *KRAS*, and *POLE* mutation as well. Additionally, TCGA described a subset of endometrioid tumors which molecularly appeared to be more similar to type 2 tumors, and the authors therefore postulated that treatment approaches mirroring those used in uterine serous carcinomas may be beneficial in this group.

Re-analysis of the endometrioid group only (271 patients) revealed extraordinary heterogeneity in these tumors [73]. Four transcriptome clusters of endometrioid endometrial carcinoma were identified, as highlighted in Fig. 4.4. Clusters 1 and 2 each consisted mainly of patients with early-stage and grade 1 or 2 tumors. Clusters 3 and 4 primarily comprised patients with grade 3 tumors presenting with stage III or IV disease at the time of hysterectomy. At the transcriptome level, Cluster 1 is the "classic" endometrial cancer, with high expression of *ESR1* and *PGR* (genes encoding estrogen receptor and progesterone receptor). Remarkably, Cluster 2, which had a similar patient profile as Cluster 1, had significantly lower expression

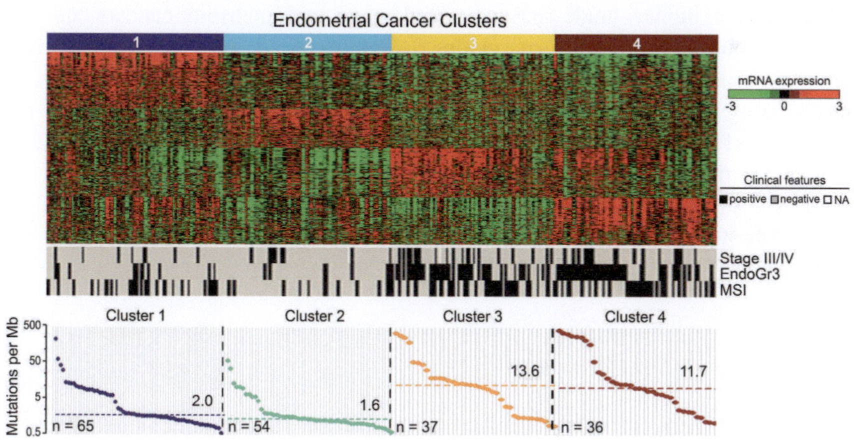

Fig. 4.4 Summary of The Cancer Genome Atlas (*TCGA*) analysis of 271 endometrioid-type endometrial carcinomas. Transcriptome Clusters 1 and 2 are primarily composed of patients with low-grade, early-stage disease, while Clusters 3 and 4 are dominated by patients with grade 3 endometrioid tumors, stages III or IV at the time of diagnosis. Clusters 3 and 4 also had significantly more mutations than tumors in Clusters 1 and 2

of these hormone receptors but higher expression of *WNT5A* and *WNT5B*, genes activated by WNT/β-catenin signaling. Cluster 2 patients were also significantly younger and more obese than patients in the other clusters, including Cluster 1. Unexpectedly, Cluster 2 patients had significantly worse survival than those in Cluster 1. Clusters 3 and 4 displayed similar transcriptome heterogeneity, with Cluster 3 characterized by higher expression of genes associated with cell cycle progression, such as *FOXM1*, *CCNB1*, and *CDC20*. This cluster had the worst survival of the 4 clusters. Cluster 4 had higher expression of genes associated with activation of the immune response, such as *STAT1*, *LCK*, *GIMAP5*, and *GIMAP7*. Although Cluster 4 was mainly composed of patients with high-grade, late-stage disease, these patients had better overall survival than the patients in Cluster 2. Cluster 3 patients had the worst overall survival.

The four clusters also had distinctive mutation spectra. *PTEN* and *PIK3CA* mutations were common in all four clusters. *KRAS* mutations were common in Clusters 1, 3, and 4, but infrequent in Cluster 2. *CTNNB1* mutations were most common in Cluster 2. Clusters 3 and 4 had the majority of the *TP53* mutations. Clusters 3 and 4 had the highest mutations per megabase, significantly higher than the mutational load in Clusters 1 and 2.

The TCGA data highlight the genetic and clinical diversity of the endometrioid histotype. These data also help to refute "dogma" that is commonly taught regarding endometrioid-type endometrial cancer. For example, conventional wisdom holds that young, obese women with endometrial cancer have good prognosis disease that is hormone driven. While certainly their prognosis is better than that for patients diagnosed with endometrial serous carcinoma, the TCGA data highlight above that a substantial subset of patients actually has endometrial cancers driven not by hormones but rather by activation of the WNT/β-catenin signaling pathway. Similarly, the higher grade and advanced stage endometrioid cancers are also heterogeneous. The subset of grade 3 endometrioid tumors with a more "immune-driven" genotype has better outcomes. The challenge to young investigators caring for endometrial cancer patients will be to productively incorporate this substantial TCGA data into rational clinical trials and, ultimately, into routine clinical practice.

Acknowledgement This work was supported by NIH 1P50CA098258 (SPORE in Uterine Cancer) (RRB) and NIH T32CA101642 (Research Training grant T32) (KCK).

References

1. Amant F, et al. Endometrial cancer. Lancet. 2005;366(9484):491–505.
2. Sherman ME. Theories of endometrial carcinogenesis: a multidisciplinary approach. Mod Pathol. 2000;13(3):295–308.
3. Bokhman JV. Two pathogenetic types of endometrial carcinoma. Gynecol Oncol. 1983;15 (1):10–7.

4. Cheung LW, et al. High frequency of PIK3R1 and PIK3R2 mutations in endometrial cancer elucidates a novel mechanism for regulation of PTEN protein stability. Cancer Discov. 2011;1(2):170–85.
5. Marchio C, et al. PIKing the type and pattern of PI3K pathway mutations in endometrioid endometrial carcinomas. Gynecol Oncol. 2015;137(2):321–8.
6. Slomovitz BM, Coleman RL. The PI3K/AKT/mTOR pathway as a therapeutic target in endometrial cancer. Clin Cancer Res. 2012;18(21):5856–64.
7. Berg A, et al. Molecular profiling of endometrial carcinoma precursor, primary and metastatic lesions suggests different targets for treatment in obese compared to non-obese patients. Oncotarget. 2015;6(2):1327–39.
8. Nout RA, et al. Improved risk assessment of endometrial cancer by combined analysis of MSI, PI3K-AKT, Wnt/beta-catenin and P53 pathway activation. Gynecol Oncol. 2012;126 (3):466–73.
9. Oda K, et al. PIK3CA cooperates with other phosphatidylinositol 3'-kinase pathway mutations to effect oncogenic transformation. Cancer Res. 2008;68(19):8127–36.
10. Oda K, et al. High frequency of coexistent mutations of PIK3CA and PTEN genes in endometrial carcinoma. Cancer Res. 2005;65(23):10669–73.
11. Catasus L, et al. PIK3CA mutations in the kinase domain (exon 20) of uterine endometrial adenocarcinomas are associated with adverse prognostic parameters. Mod Pathol. 2008;21(2):131–9.
12. Salvesen HB, et al. Integrated genomic profiling of endometrial carcinoma associates aggressive tumors with indicators of PI3 kinase activation. Proc Natl Acad Sci U S A. 2009;106(12):4834–9.
13. Lin MC, et al. Involution of latent endometrial precancers by hormonal and nonhormonal mechanisms. Cancer. 2009;115(10):2111–8.
14. Djordjevic B, et al. Clinical assessment of PTEN loss in endometrial carcinoma: immunohistochemistry outperforms gene sequencing. Mod Pathol. 2012;25(5):699–708.
15. Boruban MC, et al. From endometrial hyperplasia to endometrial cancer: insight into the biology and possible medical preventive measures. Eur J Cancer Prev. 2008;17(2):133–8.
16. Akiyama-Abe A, et al. Loss of PTEN expression is an independent predictor of favourable survival in endometrial carcinomas. Br J Cancer. 2013;109(6):1703–10.
17. Garcia-Dios DA, et al. High-throughput interrogation of PIK3CA, PTEN, KRAS, FBXW7 and TP53 mutations in primary endometrial carcinoma. Gynecol Oncol. 2013;128(2): 327–34.
18. Coenegrachts L, et al. Mutation profile and clinical outcome of mixed endometrioid-serous endometrial carcinomas are different from that of pure endometrioid or serous carcinomas. Virchows Arch. 2015;466(4):415–22.
19. Koul A, et al. Distinct sets of gene alterations in endometrial carcinoma implicate alternate modes of tumorigenesis. Cancer. 2002;94(9):2369–79.
20. Byron SA, et al. FGFR2 point mutations in 466 endometrioid endometrial tumors: relationship with MSI, KRAS, PIK3CA, CTNNB1 mutations and clinicopathological features. PLoS ONE. 2012;7(2):e30801.
21. Joshi A, et al. Activated mutant p110alpha causes endometrial carcinoma in the setting of biallelic Pten deletion. Am J Pathol. 2015;185(4):1104–13.
22. Hayes MP, et al. PIK3CA and PTEN mutations in uterine endometrioid carcinoma and complex atypical hyperplasia. Clin Cancer Res. 2006;12(20 Pt 1):5932–5.
23. Albertini AF, Devouassoux-Shisheboran M, Genestie C. Pathology of endometrioid carcinoma. Bull Cancer. 2012;99(1):7–12.
24. Huang M, et al. Molecular pathogenesis of endometrial cancers in patients with Lynch syndrome. Cancer. 2013;119(16):3027–33.
25. Risinger JI, et al. PTEN mutation in endometrial cancers is associated with favorable clinical and pathologic characteristics. Clin Cancer Res. 1998;4(12):3005–10.
26. Bilbao C, et al. The relationship between microsatellite instability and PTEN gene mutations in endometrial cancer. Int J Cancer. 2006;119(3):563–70.

27. Djordjevic B, et al. Relationship between PTEN, DNA mismatch repair, and tumor histotype in endometrial carcinoma: retained positive expression of PTEN preferentially identifies sporadic non-endometrioid carcinomas. Mod Pathol. 2013;26(10):1401–12.
28. Zhang S, Yu D. PI(3)king apart PTEN's role in cancer. Clin Cancer Res. 2010;16(17): 4325–30.
29. Mackay HJ, et al. Prognostic value of microsatellite instability (MSI) and PTEN expression in women with endometrial cancer: results from studies of the NCIC Clinical Trials Group (NCIC CTG). Eur J Cancer. 2010;46(8):1365–73.
30. Kanamori Y, et al. PTEN expression is associated with prognosis for patients with advanced endometrial carcinoma undergoing postoperative chemotherapy. Int J Cancer. 2002; 100(6):686–9.
31. Westin SN, et al. PTEN loss is a context-dependent outcome determinant in obese and non-obese endometrioid endometrial cancer patients. Mol Oncol. 2015;9(8):1694–703.
32. Rudd ML, et al. A unique spectrum of somatic PIK3CA (p110alpha) mutations within primary endometrial carcinomas. Clin Cancer Res. 2011;17(6):1331–40.
33. Catasus L, et al. Concomitant PI3K-AKT and p53 alterations in endometrial carcinomas are associated with poor prognosis. Mod Pathol. 2009;22(4):522–9.
34. Velasco A, et al. PIK3CA gene mutations in endometrial carcinoma: correlation with PTEN and K-RAS alterations. Hum Pathol. 2006;37(11):1465–72.
35. Janku F, et al. PIK3CA mutations in patients with advanced cancers treated with PI3K/AKT/mTOR axis inhibitors. Mol Cancer Ther. 2011;10(3):558–65.
36. McIntyre JB, et al. PIK3CA missense mutation is associated with unfavorable outcome in grade 3 endometrioid carcinoma but not in serous endometrial carcinoma. Gynecol Oncol. 2014;132(1):188–93.
37. Huang HN, et al. Ovarian and endometrial endometrioid adenocarcinomas have distinct profiles of microsatellite instability, PTEN expression, and ARID1A expression. Histopathology. 2015;66(4):517–28.
38. Myers AP. New strategies in endometrial cancer: targeting the PI3K/mTOR pathway–the devil is in the details. Clin Cancer Res. 2013;19(19):5264–74.
39. Herrero-Gonzalez S, Di Cristofano A. New routes to old places: PIK3R1 and PIK3R2 join PIK3CA and PTEN as endometrial cancer genes. Cancer Discov. 2011;1(2):106–7.
40. Urick ME, et al. PIK3R1 (p85alpha) is somatically mutated at high frequency in primary endometrial cancer. Cancer Res. 2011;71(12):4061–7.
41. Wu RC, Wang TL, Shihle M. The emerging roles of ARID1A in tumor suppression. Cancer Biol Ther. 2014;15(6):655–64.
42. Bosse T, et al. Loss of ARID1A expression and its relationship with PI3K-Akt pathway alterations, TP53 and microsatellite instability in endometrial cancer. Mod Pathol. 2013; 26(11):1525–35.
43. Allo G, et al. ARID1A loss correlates with mismatch repair deficiency and intact p53 expression in high-grade endometrial carcinomas. Mod Pathol. 2014;27(2):255–61.
44. Cancer Genome Atlas Research Network, et al. Integrated genomic characterization of endometrial carcinoma. Nature. 2013;497(7447):67–73.
45. Mao TL, et al. Loss of ARID1A expression correlates with stages of tumor progression in uterine endometrioid carcinoma. Am J Surg Pathol. 2013;37(9):1342–8.
46. Turbiner J, et al. Clinicopathological and molecular analysis of endometrial carcinoma associated with tamoxifen. Mod Pathol. 2008;21(8):925–36.
47. Zauber P, et al. Strong correlation between molecular changes in endometrial carcinomas and concomitant hyperplasia. Int J Gynecol Cancer. 2015;25(5):863–8.
48. Lagarda H, et al. K-ras mutations in endometrial carcinomas with microsatellite instability. J Pathol. 2001;193(2):193–9.
49. Samarnthai N, Hall K, Yeh IT. Molecular profiling of endometrial malignancies. Obstet Gynecol Int. 2010;2010:162363.
50. Peterson LM, et al. Molecular characterization of endometrial cancer: a correlative study assessing microsatellite instability, MLH1 hypermethylation, DNA mismatch repair protein

expression, and PTEN, PIK3CA, KRAS, and BRAF mutation analysis. Int J Gynecol Pathol. 2012;31(3):195–205.
51. Lax SF, et al. The frequency of p53, K-ras mutations, and microsatellite instability differs in uterine endometrioid and serous carcinoma: evidence of distinct molecular genetic pathways. Cancer. 2000;88(4):814–24.
52. Xiong J, et al. Endometrial carcinomas with significant mucinous differentiation associated with higher frequency of k-ras mutations: a morphologic and molecular correlation study. Int J Gynecol Cancer. 2013;23(7):1231–6.
53. Musa F, et al. Mucinous histology is a risk factor for nodal metastases in endometrial cancer. Gynecol Oncol. 2012;125(3):541–5.
54. Ito K, et al. K-ras point mutations in endometrial carcinoma: effect on outcome is dependent on age of patient. Gynecol Oncol. 1996;63(2):238–46.
55. Cohn DE, et al. Genotypic and phenotypic progression in endometrial tumorigenesis: determining when defects in DNA mismatch repair and KRAS2 occur. Genes Chromosom Cancer. 2001;32(4):295–301.
56. Birkeland E, et al. KRAS gene amplification and overexpression but not mutation associates with aggressive and metastatic endometrial cancer. Br J Cancer. 2012;107(12):1997–2004.
57. Hachisuga T, et al. K-ras mutation in the endometrium of tamoxifen-treated breast cancer patients, with a comparison of tamoxifen and toremifene. Br J Cancer. 2005;92(6):1098–103.
58. Tsujioka H, et al. Monitoring of endometrial K-ras mutation in tamoxifen-treated patients with breast cancer. Int J Gynecol Cancer. 2009;19(6):1052–6.
59. Shoji K, et al. Genotype-dependent efficacy of a dual PI3K/mTOR inhibitor, NVP-BEZ235, and an mTOR inhibitor, RAD001, in endometrial carcinomas. PLoS ONE. 2012;7(5):e37431.
60. Weigelt B, et al. PI3K pathway dependencies in endometrioid endometrial cancer cell lines. Clin Cancer Res. 2013;19(13):3533–44.
61. Meyer LA, et al. The search continues: looking for predictive biomarkers for response to mammalian target of rapamycin inhibition in endometrial cancer. Int J Gynecol Cancer. 2014;24(4):713–7.
62. Iglesias DA, et al. Another surprise from Metformin: novel mechanism of action via K-Ras influences endometrial cancer response to therapy. Mol Cancer Ther. 2013;12(12):2847–56.
63. Fukuchi T, et al. Beta-catenin mutation in carcinoma of the uterine endometrium. Cancer Res. 1998;58(16):3526–8.
64. Markowska A, et al. Signalling pathways in endometrial cancer. Contemp Oncol (Pozn). 2014;18(3):143–8.
65. McConechy MK, et al. Ovarian and endometrial endometrioid carcinomas have distinct CTNNB1 and PTEN mutation profiles. Mod Pathol. 2014;27(1):128–34.
66. Moreno-Bueno G, et al. Abnormalities of the APC/beta-catenin pathway in endometrial cancer. Oncogene. 2002;21(52):7981–90.
67. O'Hara AJ, Bell DW. The genomics and genetics of endometrial cancer. Adv Genomics Genet. 2012;2012(2):33–47.
68. Yeramian A, et al. Endometrial carcinoma: molecular alterations involved in tumor development and progression. Oncogene. 2013;32(4):403–13.
69. McConechy MK, et al. Use of mutation profiles to refine the classification of endometrial carcinomas. J Pathol. 2012;228(1):20–30.
70. Saegusa M, et al. beta-Catenin mutations and aberrant nuclear expression during endometrial tumorigenesis. Br J Cancer. 2001;84(2):209–17.
71. Schlosshauer PW, et al. Mutational analysis of the CTNNB1 and APC genes in uterine endometrioid carcinoma. Mod Pathol. 2000;13(10):1066–71.
72. Athanassiadou P, et al. The prognostic value of PTEN, p53, and beta-catenin in endometrial carcinoma: a prospective immunocytochemical study. Int J Gynecol Cancer. 2007;17(3):697–704.

73. Liu Y, et al. Clinical significance of CTNNB1 mutation and Wnt pathway activation in endometrioid endometrial carcinoma. J Natl Cancer Inst. 2014;106(9).
74. Myers A, et al. beta-Catenin mutations in recurrent FIGO IA grade I endometrioid endometrial cancers. Gynecol Oncol. 2014;134(2):426–7.
75. Liu Y, Broaddus RR, Zhang W. Identifying aggressive forms of endometrioid-type endometrial cancer: new insights into molecular subtyping. Expert Rev Anticancer Ther. 2015;15(1):1–3.
76. Olivier M, Hollstein M, Hainaut P. TP53 mutations in human cancers: origins, consequences, and clinical use. Cold Spring Harb Perspect Biol. 2010;2(1):a001008.
77. Niederacher D, et al. Loss of heterozygosity of BRCA1, TP53 and TCRD markers analysed in sporadic endometrial cancer. Eur J Cancer. 1998;34(11):1770–6.
78. Graesslin O, et al. Fluorescence in situ hybridization and immunohistochemical analysis of p53 expression in endometrial cancer: prognostic value and relation to ploidy. Ann Surg Oncol. 2008;15(2):484–92.
79. Luo W, et al. Amifostine enhancement of the anti-cancer effects of paclitaxel in endometrial cancer is TP53-dependent. Int J Oncol. 2010;37(5):1187–94.
80. Kihana T, et al. Mutation and allelic loss of the p53 gene in endometrial carcinoma. Incidence and outcome in 92 surgical patients. Cancer. 1995;76(1):72–8.
81. Janiec-Jankowska A, et al. TP53 mutations in endometrial cancers: relation to PTEN gene defects. Int J Gynecol Cancer. 2010;20(2):196–202.
82. Lee EJ, et al. p53 alteration independently predicts poor outcomes in patients with endometrial cancer: a clinicopathologic study of 131 cases and literature review. Gynecol Oncol. 2010;116(3):533–8.
83. Stelloo E, et al. Refining prognosis and identifying targetable pathways for high-risk endometrial cancer; a TransPORTEC initiative. Mod Pathol. 2015;28(6):836–44.
84. Kaku T, et al. Endometrial carcinoma associated with hyperplasia–immunohistochemical study of angiogenesis and p53 expression. Gynecol Oncol. 1999;72(1):51–5.
85. Jeon YT, et al. Cyclooxygenase-2 and p53 expressions in endometrial cancer. Cancer Epidemiol Biomarkers Prev. 2004;13(9):1538–42.
86. Semczuk A, et al. Allelic loss at TP53 is not related to p53 protein overexpression in primary human endometrial carcinomas. Oncology. 2005;69(4):317–25.
87. Ozsaran AA, et al. p53 staining as a prognostic indicator in endometrial carcinoma. Eur J Gynaecol Oncol. 1999;20(2):156–9.
88. Erdem O, et al. Angiogenesis, p53, and bcl-2 expression as prognostic indicators in endometrial cancer: comparison with traditional clinicopathologic variables. Int J Gynecol Pathol. 2003;22(3):254–60.
89. Lundgren C, et al. Nuclear DNA content, proliferative activity, and p53 expression related to clinical and histopathologic features in endometrial carcinoma. Int J Gynecol Cancer. 2002;12(1):110–8.
90. Soong R, et al. Overexpression of p53 protein is an independent prognostic indicator in human endometrial carcinoma. Br J Cancer. 1996;74(4):562–7.
91. Engelsen IB, et al. Pathologic expression of p53 or p16 in preoperative curettage specimens identifies high-risk endometrial carcinomas. Am J Obstet Gynecol. 2006;195(4):979–86.
92. Kohler MF, et al. p53 overexpression in advanced-stage endometrial adenocarcinoma. Am J Obstet Gynecol. 1996;175(5):1246–52.
93. Saffari B, et al. Association of p53 mutations and a codon 72 single nucleotide polymorphism with lower overall survival and responsiveness to adjuvant radiotherapy in endometrioid endometrial carcinomas. Int J Gynecol Cancer. 2005;15(5):952–63.
94. Oreskovic S, et al. A significance of immunohistochemical determination of steroid receptors, cell proliferation factor Ki-67 and protein p53 in endometrial carcinoma. Gynecol Oncol. 2004;93(1):34–40.
95. Djordjevic B, Broaddus RR. Role of the clinical pathology laboratory in the evaluation of endometrial carcinomas for Lynch syndrome. Semin Diagn Pathol. 2014;31(3):195–204.

96. Kawaguchi M, et al. Analysis of candidate target genes for mononucleotide repeat mutation in microsatellite instability-high (MSI-H) endometrial cancer. Int J Oncol. 2009;35(5): 977–82.
97. Maxwell GL, et al. Favorable survival associated with microsatellite instability in endometrioid endometrial cancers. Obstet Gynecol. 2001;97(3):417–22.
98. Kato M, et al. DNA mismatch repair-related protein loss as a prognostic factor in endometrial cancers. J Gynecol Oncol. 2015;26(1):40–5.
99. Thoury A, et al. Evidence for different expression profiles for c-Met, EGFR, PTEN and the mTOR pathway in low and high grade endometrial carcinomas in a cohort of consecutive women. Occurrence of PIK3CA and K-Ras mutations and microsatellite instability. Histol Histopathol. 2014;29(11):1455–66.
100. Zighelboim I, et al. Microsatellite instability and epigenetic inactivation of MLH1 and outcome of patients with endometrial carcinomas of the endometrioid type. J Clin Oncol. 2007;25(15):2042–8.
101. Black D, et al. Clinicopathologic significance of defective DNA mismatch repair in endometrial carcinoma. J Clin Oncol. 2006;24(11):1745–53.
102. Cohn DE, et al. Improved survival with an intact DNA mismatch repair system in endometrial cancer. Obstet Gynecol. 2006;108(5):1208–15.
103. Esteller M, et al. hMLH1 promoter hypermethylation is an early event in human endometrial tumorigenesis. Am J Pathol. 1999;155(5):1767–72.
104. An HJ, et al. Microsatellite instability in endometrioid type endometrial adenocarcinoma is associated with poor prognostic indicators. Am J Surg Pathol. 2007;31(6):846–53.
105. Nelson GS, et al. MMR deficiency is common in high-grade endometrioid carcinomas and is associated with an unfavorable outcome. Gynecol Oncol. 2013;131(2):309–14.
106. Ruiz I, et al. Lack of association between deficient mismatch repair expression and outcome in endometrial carcinomas of the endometrioid type. Gynecol Oncol. 2014;134(1):20–3.
107. Joehlin-Price AS, et al. Mismatch repair protein expression in 1049 endometrial carcinomas, associations with body mass index, and other clinicopathologic variables. Gynecol Oncol. 2014;133(1):43–7.
108. Konopka B, et al. Molecular genetic defects in endometrial carcinomas: microsatellite instability, PTEN and beta-catenin (CTNNB1) genes mutations. J Cancer Res Clin Oncol. 2007;133(6):361–71.
109. Alvarez T, et al. Molecular profile of grade 3 endometrioid endometrial carcinoma: is it a type I or type II endometrial carcinoma? Am J Surg Pathol. 2012;36(5):753–61.
110. Broaddus RR, et al. Pathologic features of endometrial carcinoma associated with HNPCC: a comparison with sporadic endometrial carcinoma. Cancer. 2006;106(1):87–94.
111. Tafe LJ, et al. Endometrial and ovarian carcinomas with undifferentiated components: clinically aggressive and frequently underrecognized neoplasms. Mod Pathol. 2010;23 (6):781–9.
112. Garg K, et al. Selection of endometrial carcinomas for DNA mismatch repair protein immunohistochemistry using patient age and tumor morphology enhances detection of mismatch repair abnormalities. Am J Surg Pathol. 2009;33(6):925–33.
113. Garg K, et al. Endometrial carcinomas in women aged 40 years and younger: tumors associated with loss of DNA mismatch repair proteins comprise a distinct clinicopathologic subset. Am J Surg Pathol. 2009;33(12):1869–77.
114. Kuhn E, et al. Molecular characterization of undifferentiated carcinoma associated with endometrioid carcinoma. Am J Surg Pathol. 2014;38(5):660–5.
115. Altrabulsi B, et al. Undifferentiated carcinoma of the endometrium. Am J Surg Pathol. 2005;29(10):1316–21.
116. Kanopiene D, et al. Impact of microsatellite instability on survival of endometrial cancer patients. Medicina (Kaunas). 2014;50(4):216–21.
117. Bilbao-Sieyro C, et al. Microsatellite instability and ploidy status define three categories with distinctive prognostic impact in endometrioid endometrial cancer. Oncotarget. 2014;5(15): 6206–17.

118. Cote ML, et al. A pilot study of microsatellite instability and endometrial cancer survival in white and African American women. Int J Gynecol Pathol. 2012;31(1):66–72.
119. Nick McElhinny SA, et al. Division of labor at the eukaryotic replication fork. Mol Cell. 2008;30(2):137–44.
120. Pursell ZF, et al. Yeast DNA polymerase epsilon participates in leading-strand DNA replication. Science. 2007;317(5834):127–30.
121. Church DN, et al. DNA polymerase epsilon and delta exonuclease domain mutations in endometrial cancer. Hum Mol Genet. 2013;22(14):2820–8.
122. Palles C, et al. Germline mutations affecting the proofreading domains of POLE and POLD1 predispose to colorectal adenomas and carcinomas. Nat Genet. 2013;45(2):136–44.
123. Govindan R, et al. Genomic landscape of non-small cell lung cancer in smokers and never-smokers. Cell. 2012;150(6):1121–34.
124. Pleasance ED, et al. A comprehensive catalogue of somatic mutations from a human cancer genome. Nature. 2010;463(7278):191–6.
125. Church DN, et al. Prognostic significance of POLE proofreading mutations in endometrial cancer. J Natl Cancer Inst. 2015;107(1):402.
126. Meng B, et al. POLE exonuclease domain mutation predicts long progression-free survival in grade 3 endometrioid carcinoma of the endometrium. Gynecol Oncol. 2014;134(1):15–9.
127. Forbes SA, et al. COSMIC: mining complete cancer genomes in the catalogue of somatic mutations in cancer. Nucleic Acids Res. 2011;39(Database issue):945–50.
128. Hussein YR, et al. Clinicopathological analysis of endometrial carcinomas harboring somatic POLE exonuclease domain mutations. Mod Pathol. 2015;28(4):505–14.
129. Le Gallo M, et al. Exome sequencing of serous endometrial tumors identifies recurrent somatic mutations in chromatin-remodeling and ubiquitin ligase complex genes. Nat Genet. 2012;44(12):1310–5.
130. Zhao S, et al. Landscape of somatic single-nucleotide and copy-number mutations in uterine serous carcinoma. Proc Natl Acad Sci U S A. 2013;110(8):2916–21.
131. Kuhn E, et al. Identification of molecular pathway aberrations in uterine serous carcinoma by genome-wide analyses. J Natl Cancer Inst. 2012;104(19):1503–13.
132. Kim TM, Laird PW, Park PJ. The landscape of microsatellite instability in colorectal and endometrial cancer genomes. Cell. 2013;155(4):858–68.
133. Heitzer E, Tomlinson I. Replicative DNA polymerase mutations in cancer. Curr Opin Genet Dev. 2014;24:107–13.

Chapter 5
The Molecular Pathology of Serous Endometrial Cancer

Mary Ellen Urick, Meghan L. Rudd and Daphne W. Bell

Introduction

Serous endometrial cancers (SECs) represent 2–10% of all endometrial tumors and are the most common of the so-called type II or non-endometrioid ECs [1–7]. They are poorly differentiated tumors with a high propensity to metastasize [8, 9]. Despite comprising only a small faction of all EC diagnoses, SECs are responsible for a large proportion (up to 39%) of EC-related deaths [4, 7]. Accordingly, when compared to women with non-serous ECs, women with SECs exhibit significantly lower survival rates, even when corrected for stage, and an increased frequency of tumor recurrence [4, 5, 10]. Relapse in SEC patients typically occurs within two years of surgery, and relapse rates as high as 50–80.5% have been reported [5, 6, 11–13]. SECs are often found as an admixture with other histological subtypes, such as endometrioid adenocarcinoma and clear cell adenocarcinoma, and can also be a component of some uterine carcinosarcomas [9, 11, 14–18]. Improved survival is not observed in patients with mixed ECs containing a SEC component [1, 17].

Although there are a limited number of known risk factors for SEC, one well-documented risk factor is increasing age; SEC typically occurs in older, postmenopausal women with mean ages at diagnosis ranging from 53 to 75 years [1, 4, 9, 11, 14, 15, 19–24]. Tamoxifen treatment is also a risk factor for the subsequent development of SEC [24]. In this regard, the increased risk of SEC

M.E. Urick · M.L. Rudd · D.W. Bell (✉)
Cancer Genetics and Comparative Genomics Branch,
National Human Genome Research Institute, National Institutes of Health,
50 South Drive, Bethesda, MD 20892, USA
e-mail: belldaph@mail.nih.gov

M.E. Urick
e-mail: maryellen.urick@nih.gov

M.L. Rudd
e-mail: ruddmeg@mail.nih.gov

M.T. Deavers and D.M. Coffey (eds.), *Precision Molecular Pathology of Uterine Cancer*, Molecular Pathology Library,
DOI 10.1007/978-3-319-57985-6_5

noted among *BRCA1* mutation carriers by some [25, 26] has been largely attributed to prior tamoxifen treatment rather than germline genetic predisposition to SEC [27]. A prior history of pelvic radiation may represent another risk factor for SEC [1, 28–32]. Finally, although type II ECs have traditionally been thought of as estrogen-independent tumors, a recent large meta-analysis of epidemiological data suggests that increased body mass index, which may increase levels of unopposed estrogen, may cause an increased risk for developing type II ECs [33, 34].

At the molecular level, SECs have a distinct constellation of genomic aberrations as compared with most endometrioid ECs (reviewed in [35]). Recent advances in DNA sequencing, or so-called next-generation sequencing technologies, have shed new insights into the molecular pathogenesis of human cancers, including SECs. Herein, we review the most prominent features of the genomic landscape of SECs (Table 5.1), with an emphasis on somatically mutated driver genes and, where appropriate, we discuss how these features might be leveraged in the clinical setting (Fig. 5.1; Tables 5.2 and 5.3).

Introduction to the Molecular Pathology of SEC

The first genetic alterations observed in SECs were p53/*TP53* aberrations [36–41]. Diligent clinicopathological studies, combined with molecular analyses of *TP53*, have led to the development of a step-wise model of tumor evolution for SEC. In this model, cells with the so-called p53 signature evolve to endometrial glandular dysplasia (EmGD), followed by endometrial intraepithelial carcinoma (EIC), and ultimately SEC [17, 39, 40, 42–46].

Since the initial discovery of *TP53* mutations and p53 positivity in SEC, efforts to uncover additional genomic alterations that contribute to the disease have been the focus of a number of studies (reviewed in [35]). Rapid advancements in the understanding of the genomic landscape of SECs and new insights into their molecular pathology came with innovations in DNA sequencing technology [47–50]. Within the past three years, next-generation sequencing of 107 SEC tumor and 15 cell line exomes across multiple studies has systematically mapped SEC mutational landscapes, validating previous findings that had implicated *TP53* and phosphatidylinositol 3-kinase (PI3K) pathway aberrations in SECs [39, 40, 46, 51–53], and extending upon this knowledge by assembling a comprehensive catalogue of somatically mutated genes present in ~22,000 protein encoding genes [47–50]. The subsequent application of statistical methods to determine whether genes are mutated at significantly higher rates than the background mutation rate has nominated a subset of mutated genes as putative novel pathogenic "driver" genes for SEC [47–50]. In addition to mutations, genome-wide copy number aberrations, RNA expression, and DNA methylation have also been systematically analyzed in some studies [47, 48, 50], including the integrated genomic analysis of serous and endometrioid ECs by The Cancer Genome Atlas (TCGA)[47].

Table 5.1 Significant molecular aberrations identified in serous and serous-like ECs by whole exome sequencing studies [47–50]

Gene	Aberration	Aberration frequency in serous n = 42 and serous-like tumors n = 60 in TCGA dataset [47] (aberrant/total)	Aberration frequency in serous samples (aberrant/total)	Reference(s)
Mutations				
TP53	Mutation	88% (37/42) 92% (55/60)	100% (12/12)	[213]
			93% (25/27)	[38]
			90% (19/21)	[56]
			82% (62/76)	[48]
			71% (37/52)	[49]
			68% (25/37)	[214]
			60% (31/52)	[50]
			50% (2/4)	[81]
			20% (1/5)	[215]
PIK3CA	Mutation	45% (19/42) 47% (28/60)	56% (5/9)	[216]
			50% (2/4)	[81]
			40% (2/5)	[215]
			31% (16/52)	[49]
			27% (10/37)	[214]
			24% (18/76)	[48]
			23% (12/52)	[50]
			22% (10/46)	[217]
			20% (3/15)	[218]
			15% (5/34)	[54]
			8% (1/12)	[213]
FBXW7	Mutation	33% (14/42) 22% (13/60)	29% (15/52)	[49]
			20% (15/76)	[48]
			17% (9/52)	[50]
			8% (1/12)	[213]
PPP2R1A	Mutation	26% (11/42) 22% (13/60)	43% (16/37)	[214]
			41% (20/49)	[219]
			32% (8/25)	[220]
			25% (13/52)	[49]
			18% (14/76)	[48]
			17% (4/23)	[221]
			17% (2/12)	[213]
			15% (8/52)	[50]
CHD4	Mutation	17% (7/42) 13% (13/60)	19% (10/52)	[50]
			17% (9/52)	[49]
			10% (1/10)[a]	[48]

(continued)

Table 5.1 (continued)

Gene	Aberration	Aberration frequency in serous n = 42 and serous-like tumors n = 60 in TCGA dataset [47] (aberrant/total)	Aberration frequency in serous samples (aberrant/total)	Reference(s)
CSMD3	Mutation	12% (5/42) 10% (6/60)	8% (1/12)[a]	[49]
SPOP	Mutation	7% (3/42) 5% (3/60)	10% (1/10)[a]	[48]
			8% (4/52)	[49]
			4% (2/52)	[50]
PIK3R1	Mutation	2% (1/42) 13% (8/60)	13% (2/15)	[218]
			8% (4/46)	[52]
TAF1	Mutation	5% (2/42) 5% (3/60)	13% (7/52)	[50]
PTEN	Mutation	2% (1/42) 10% (6/60)	13% (6/46)	[51]
			11% (1/9)	[216]
			6% (3/52)	[50]
			3% (1/37)	[214]
Copy number alterations				
PIK3CA	Amplification	29% (12/42) 28% (17/60)	67% (4/6)	[222]
			52% (13/25)	[50]
			26% (6/23)	[48]
ERBB2	Amplification	29% (12/42) 25% (15/60)	57% (13/23)	[223]
			44% (11/25)	[50]
			29% (17/58)	[101]
			28% (7/25)	[114]
			21% (6/28)	[97]
			17% (2/12)	[105]
			17% (2/12)	[102]
			17% (18/105)	[224]
	CNV loss	NA	20% (5/25)	[50]
CCNE1	Amplification	31% (13/42) 23% (14/60)	48% (12/25)	[50]
			45% (20/44)	[133]
			26% (6/23)	[48]
	CNV loss	NA	8% (2/25)	[50]
MYC	Amplification	21% (9/42) 23% (14/60)	40% (10/25)	[50]
SOX17	Amplification	20% (12/60)	NA	NA
FGFR3	Amplification	8% (5/60)	NA	NA
	Loss	2% (1/60)	NA	NA

Aberrant genes are ranked by frequency among SECs in TCGA dataset.[a] indicates that the frequency represents data that did not reach significance in an individual study

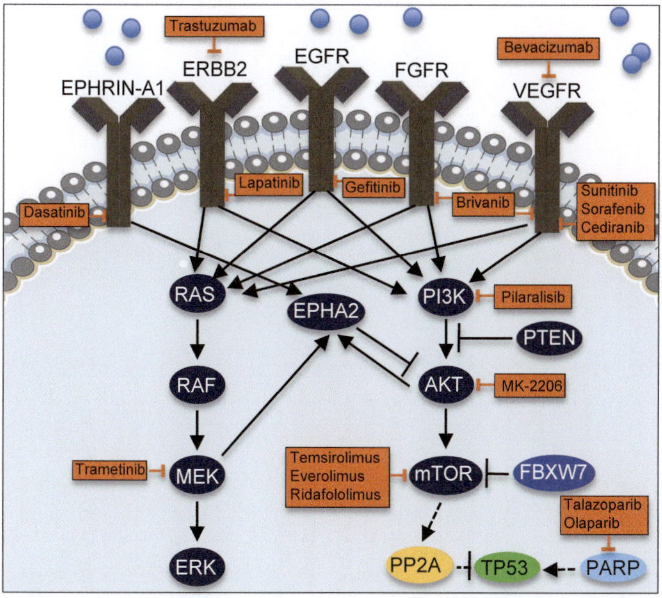

Fig. 5.1 Schematic representation of pathways affected by targeted therapies currently in clinical trials specifically recruiting EC patients (Table 5.2) and targeted therapies that have noted clinical responses in SEC patients in phase II trials (Table 5.3). Note that this figure is not intended to be a comprehensive representation of all molecular pathways relevant to SEC

The simultaneous assessment of serous, endometrioid, and mixed histology tumors by TCGA has permitted a direct comparison of the genomic landscapes of these traditional histological subtypes. This analysis revealed that a subset of high-grade endometrioid ECs and a subset of mixed histology ECs molecularly resemble SECs; these tumors, together with SECs, are thus referred to as the "serous-like" EC subgroup, which represents one of the four molecular subgroups defined by TCGA. The three remaining molecular subgroups are predominated by endometrioid ECs and are referred to as ultramutated/POLE-mutated, hypermutated/microsatellite instability positive (MSI+), and copy number low/microsatellite stable (MSS) [47]. Serous and serous-like ECs in TCGA's study are characterized by widespread copy number alterations and are thus referred to as copy number high, whereas endometrioid tumors tend to be copy number quiet (low). Additionally, serous and serous-like ECs have a relatively low mutational load in comparison with endometrioid ECs. The relatively low mutational load of serous and serous-like ECs may explain why fewer pathogenic driver genes have been nominated within these tumors than within endometrioid ECs.

Whole exome studies conducted to date have implicated *TP53*, *PIK3CA*, *FBXW7*, *PPP2R1A*, *CHD4, SPOP*, and *TAF1* as major driver genes for serous and serous-like ECs [47–50]. Additional genes that were not designated as statistically significantly mutated genes in whole exome studies can nonetheless be considered

Table 5.2 Clinical trials testing targeted therapies that are currently enrolling or scheduled to enroll for which SEC patients may be eligible (clinical trials.gov accessed June 2015)

Targeted therapy	Biomarker description	Clinical trial official title	Clinical trials.gov identifier	Phase	Trial status as of June 2015
Phosphatidylinositol 3-kinase (PI3K)/AKT/mTOR Pathway Inhibitors					
PI3K or dual PI3K/mTOR inhibitors					
Buparlisib (BKM120)	None specified	Phase Ib study of the combination of BKM120 and cisplatin or carboplatin in patients with advanced solid tumors	NCT02439489	Ph Ib	Recruiting
mTOR inhibitors					
Afinitor® (everolimus)	None specified	Phase II single-arm trial with combination of everolimus and letrozole in treatment of platinum resistant relapse or refractory or persistent ovarian cancer/endometrial cancer (CRAD001CUS242T)	NCT02188550	Ph II	Recruiting
Metformin	Ki-67, TUNEL assay, phosphor-AMPK, phosphor-IGF-1R, phosphor-IRS1, phospho-Akt, phospho-S6, phosphor-mTOR, pACC	A clinical trial to evaluate endometrial cancer biomarker changes following exposure to the insulin sensitizer metformin	NCT02042495	Ph II	Not yet open for participant recruitment
MLN0128 (INK-128)	Mutational analysis indicated for endometrial cancers; genes not specified	A phase 1 study of MLN0128 and bevacizumab in patients with recurrent glioblastoma and other solid tumors	NCT02142803	Ph I	Recruiting
AKT inhibitors					
ARQ092	None specified	A phase 1 dose escalation study of ARQ 092 in adult subjects with advanced solid tumors and recurrent malignant lymphoma	NCT01473095	Ph I	Recruiting

(continued)

Table 5.2 (continued)

Targeted therapy	Biomarker description	Clinical trial official title	Clinical trials.gov identifier	Phase	Trial status as of June 2015
AZD5363	*PIK3CA* mutation, *AKT1* mutation, or "dysregulatory aberration on the PIK/AKT pathway"	A phase I, open-label, multicenter study to assess the safety, tolerability, pharmacokinetics, and preliminary antitumor activity of ascending doses of AZD5363 under adaptable dosing schedules in patients with advanced solid malignancies	NCT01226316	Ph I	Recruiting
MEK Inhibitors					
Mekinist™ (trametinib)	KRAS status and baseline genomic biomarkers in the phosphatidylinositol 3 kinase (PI3K)/AKT pathway	A randomized phase II study with a safety lead-in to assess the antitumor efficacy of the MEK inhibitor trametinib alone or in combination with GSK2141795, an AKT inhibitor, in patients with recurrent or persistent endometrial cancer	NCT01935973	Ph II	Recruiting
Mekinist™ (trametinib)	Biomarkers not specified	A translational companion protocol to GOG229O: A randomized phase II study with a safety lead-in to assess the antitumor efficacy of the MEK inhibitor trametinib alone or in combination With GSK2141795, an AKT inhibitor, in patients with recurrent or persistent endometrial cancer	NCT02093546	Ph II	Recruiting
Inhibitors targeting HER2, HER3, or EGFR					
Herceptin® (trastuzumab)	Over-expression of HER2/NEU as detected by FISH or IHC	Randomized ph II evaluation of carboplatin/paclitaxel with and without trastuzumab (herceptin) in HER2/Neu+ patients with advanced/recurrent uterine serous papillary carcinoma	NCT01367002	Ph II	Recruiting

(continued)

Table 5.2 (continued)

Targeted therapy	Biomarker description	Clinical trial official title	Clinical trials.gov identifier	Phase	Trial status as of June 2015
Tykerb® (lapatinib)	*ErbB2* gene amplification by FISH	A phase I study of lapatinib (tykerb) plus ixabepilone (ixempra) as second-line treatment for patients with HER-2 over-expressed recurrent or persistent endometrial carcinoma or carcinosarcoma	NCT01454479	Ph I	Enrolling by invitation only
Neratinib (PB272)	*HER2*, *HER3*, and *EGFR* mutations; *EGFR* amplification	An open-label, multicenter, multinational, phase 2 study exploring the efficacy and safety of neratinib therapy in patients with solid tumors with activating HER2, HER3, or EGFR mutations or with EGFR gene amplification	NCT01953926	Ph II	Recruiting
Vascular Endothelial Growth Factor (VEGF) Targeted Therapies					
Avastin® (bevacizumab)	None specified	A randomized phase ii trial of carboplatin-paclitaxel compared to carboplatin-paclitaxel-bevacizumab in advanced (stage III–IV) or recurrent endometrial cancer	NCT01770171	Ph II	Recruiting
Poly (ADP-ribose) Polymerase (PARP) Inhibitors					
Talazoparib (BMN 673)	PTEN, MSI, and MRE11 aberrations	A single-arm phase II trial of BMN 673 for inoperable, advanced endometrial cancer with retrospective PTEN, MSI, and MRE11 analysis	NCT02127151	Ph II	Not yet open for patient recruitment
Lynparza™ (olaparib)	Aberrations in PI3K/AKT/mTOR and HR defect pathway	A phase ib study of the oral PARP inhibitor olaparib with the oral mTORC1/2 inhibitor AZD2014 or the oral AKT inhibitor AZD5363 for recurrent endometrial, triple negative breast, and ovarian, primary peritoneal, or fallopian tube cancer	NCT02208375	Ph Ib	Recruiting

(continued)

Table 5.2 (continued)

Targeted therapy	Biomarker description	Clinical trial official title	Clinical trials.gov identifier	Phase	Trial status as of June 2015
Veliparib (ABT-888)	None specified	An early phase 1 study of ABT-888 in combination with carboplatin and paclitaxel in patients with hepatic or renal dysfunction and solid tumors	NCT01366144	Ph I	Recruiting
BCR-ABL, Src, EphA2 Inhibitors					
Sprycel® (dasatinib)	EphA2 expression	Pilot and translational study of dasatinib (NSC#732517) paclitaxel and carboplatin in women with advanced stage and recurrent endometrial cancer	NCT01440998	Ph I	Recruiting

Biomarkers specified in the trial description are provided in the second column. Note that SEC patients may also be eligible to enroll in basket trials such as NCI-MATCH (NCT02465060), NCI-MPACT (NCT01827384), and the WINTHER trial (NCT01856296), which test multiple targeted agents and are not listed in this table.

Table 5.3 Results of phase II clinical trial of targeted therapies for the treatment of SEC

Targeted therapy	SEC patients (total patients)	Outcomes reported for SEC patients	Did patients receive prior chemotherapy?	Did the trial meet overall efficacy and safety criteria?
Phosphatidylinositol 3-kinase (PI3K)/AKT/mTOR Pathway Inhibitors				
PI3K or dual PI3K/mTOR inhibitors				
Pilaralisib	24 (67)	1 PFS > 6, 1 CR & PFS > 6 months	Yes	No
mTOR inhibitors				
Toriscl® (temsirolimus)	15 (54)	chemo naïve: 2 PR, 3 SD prior chemo: 5 SD	6 chemo naïve 9 treated	Yes—chemo naïve No—chemo treated
Torisel® (temsirolimus)	12 (50)	2 responses (PR or CR unknown)	Unknown	No
Afinitor® (everolimus)	11 (44)	1 PR 6 months, 2 SD 6 months	Yes	Yes
Ridaforolimus	10 (45)	1 PR, 1 SD	Yes	Yes
Ridaforolimus	5 (31)	4 SD	Unknown	No
AKT inhibitors				
MK-2206	14 (14)	2 PFS > 6 months, 2 still on treatment	Unknown	Ongoing
MEK inhibitors				
Selumetinib (AZD6244)	9 (52)	Not specified	Yes	No
Inhibitors Targeting HER2, HER3, or EGFR				
Iressa® (gefitinib)	6 (26)	1 CR	Yes	No
Multikinase/angiogenesis inhibitors				
Avastin® (bevacizumab)	14 (52)	1 CR, 3 PR, 36% PFS 6 months	Yes	Yes
Eylea® (VEGF Trap)	11 (44)	0 responders	Yes	No
Sutent® (sunitinib)	6 (33)	2 PFS $\geq$ 1 year	Yes	Yes
Dovitinib (TKI258)	7 (53)	Not specified	Yes	No
Brivanib (BMS-582664)	10 (43)	1 PFS > 6 months, 1 CR, 3 PR	Yes	Yes
Nexavar® (sorafenib)	3 (56)	1 PR	Unknown	Yes

(continued)

Table 5.3 (continued)

Targeted therapy	SEC patients (total patients)	Outcomes reported for SEC patients	Did patients receive prior chemotherapy?	Did the trial meet overall efficacy and safety criteria?
Ofev® (nintedanib)	13 (32)	median PFS 3.15 months	Yes	No
Cediranib (AZD2171)	11 (48)	1 PR	Unknown	Yes
ALK inhibitors				
Dalantercept	15 (28)	3 PFS > 6 months	Yes	No

Abbreviations: *CR* complete response, *PR* partial response, *SD* stable disease, *PFS* progression-free survival

contributing factors in SEC tumorigenesis based on prior knowledge of both their mutation spectrum in SEC and their biological function. For example, deleterious mutations in several known cancer genes are present in SEC exomes, including mutations in *PIK3R1* and *PTEN*, which are key players in the PI3K pathway [51, 52, 54]. Moreover, the frequent occurrence of copy number alterations in SECs and serous-like ECs highlights a number of additional driver genes including amplification of the *HER2/ERBB2*, *MYC*, and *CCNE1* oncogenes (Table 5.1). In the following subsections, we highlight the current state of knowledge of the proposed driver aberrations of SEC as well as the potential clinical relevance of these alterations.

TP53 Aberrations in SEC

Somatic *TP53* mutations are the most frequent molecular abnormalities observed in SECs, occurring in 20–100% of cases (Table 5.1). *TP53*/p53 aberrations are early events in SEC tumorigenesis as evidenced by their presence in benign-appearing glands adjacent to SEC (the so-called p53 signature), in EmGD and in EIC. The differential frequencies of *TP53* mutations observed among these lesions, as well as the presence of identical mutations in concurrent lesions, have contributed to the development of a model of tumor progression for SEC [40, 46, 55, 56].

The consequences of *TP53* mutations in human cancer are variable, and can be differentially classified as loss-of-function, dominant-negative, or gain-of-function [57–61]. In TCGA's analysis of EC in which mutations in *TP53* were predominantly found in serous and serous-like tumors, an in silico evaluation using the PARADIGM-SHIFT algorithm [62] predicted that missense mutations in *TP53* have distinct functional effects to insertions/deletions and splice site mutations [47]. Indeed, close to one-third of *TP53* mutations in the TCGA EC dataset were reported to be gain-of-function mutants [63], at least in certain cellular contexts. As noted elsewhere [61], understanding the functional effects of individual *TP53* mutations is important when designing strategies to leverage such mutations as actionable targets for cancer therapy, which includes the development of strategies to restore wild-type p53 function, degrade mutant p53, target downstream effectors of mutant p53, and develop synthetic lethal approaches [61, 64]. Notably, preclinical studies in small numbers of p53-mutant EC cell lines have indicated that REGgamma may be a potential therapeutic target for p53-mutated (R248Q) ECs [65]. Moreover, the sensitivity of *TP53*-deficient EC cells to paclitaxel is increased by exposure to the multityrosine kinase inhibitor and angiogenesis inhibitor BIBF1120 or amifostine [66, 67].

Murine models of EC corroborate the importance of *TP53*/p53 abnormalities in the pathogenesis of human SEC. Conditional deletion of *Trp53* in the murine genitourinary tract leads to the development of endometrial tumors including SEC, clear cell carcinoma, and carcinosarcoma in older animals (65–79 weeks) [68]. Consistent with the model of tumor progression proposed for human SEC, EmGD and EIC are not only observed adjacent to some papillary adenocarcinomas in tumor-bearing mice with conditional deletion of *Trp53*, but are also observed in younger, tumor-free, mice [68]. Interestingly, serous and clear cell tumors that arise within this murine model frequently exhibit upregulation of the AKT-mTOR signal transduction pathway, which occurs at the EIC to carcinoma transition [68]. Another murine model for the development of non-endometrioid ECs is provided by the conditional deletion of *Cdh1* and *Trp53* in the uterus [69], which suggests functional cooperation between *Cdh1* and *Trp53* in the development of type II EC. Of note, the combined ablation of *Cdh1* and *Trp53* results in the upregulation of genes associated with inflammation, suggesting a tumor microenvironment associated with chronic inflammation. Finally, the conditional deletion of *Trp53* and *Pot1A*, which regulates telomere length, provides a model for type II endometrial tumor progression, since animals develop in situ lesions akin to EIC, poorly differentiated ECs with nuclear atypia some of which exhibited focal regions of papillary differentiation, and metastatic disease [70]. Taken together, studies of human endometrial tumors and mouse models of EC solidify the importance of p53 dysregulation as an early event in SEC.

PI3K Pathway Aberrations in SEC

The PI3K signal transduction pathway is activated in response to the stimulation of growth factor receptors (including those encoded by *ERBB2/HER2*) and regulates a variety of cellular processes including cell survival, proliferation, growth, migration, and metabolism (reviewed in [71]). PI3K is a heterodimeric protein that consists of a catalytic subunit and a regulatory subunit, each of which has multiple isoforms (reviewed in [72]). *PIK3CA* and *PIK3R1*, which encode the p110α catalytic subunit and the p85α regulatory subunit, respectively, often acquire pathogenic somatic mutations in human cancers (reviewed in [73]). Likewise, the *PTEN* tumor suppressor gene, which negatively regulates PI3K signaling, is also highly mutated in human cancer (reviewed in [73]). We and others have uncovered frequent somatic mutations in the PIK3CA-PIK3R1-PTEN axis; incidences of somatic mutations in SEC range from 8–56% for *PIK3CA*, 8–13% for *PIK3R1*, and 2–13% for *PTEN* (Table 5.1).

Early work from our own laboratory showed that ECs, including SECs, have a unique pattern of *PIK3CA* mutations compared with other tumor types, which has implications for the design of mutation panels intended for clinical use in cancer patient stratification for targeted therapies. Approximately half of all *PIK3CA* mutations in EC occur in the adaptor-binding domain (ABD) and protein kinase-C homology 2 (C2) domain (exons 1–7) of p110α (Fig. 5.2), whereas these domains are infrequently mutated in other cancers [74]. Interestingly, biochemical studies of a subset of cancer-associated mutations in p110α have shown that not all mutations are functionally equivalent [75–77]. Likewise, not all mutations in *PIK3CA* may be equal in predicting clinical response to targeted therapies directed against the PI3K pathway. In this regard, one study that prospectively treated cancer patients (including nine EC patients) with *PIK3CA*-mutated tumors with PI3K/AKT/mTOR inhibitors found that the *PIK3CA* H1047R mutation was associated with significantly ($p = 0.018$) higher response rates to treatments with PI3K pathway inhibitors compared to other *PIK3CA* mutations [78]. It will be critical in future clinical trials of EC patients to determine which *PIK3CA* aberrations, if any, correlate with response to targeted therapies.

PIK3R1 encodes the p85α regulatory subunit of PI3K, which functions to stabilize and inhibit the p110α catalytic subunit encoded by *PIK3CA* [79]. Somatic mutations in *PIK3R1* have been reported in 8–13% of SECs (Table 5.1), and the majority of mutations in SEC occur in the inter-Src homology 2 (iSH2) domain (Fig. 5.2), which mediates binding to p110α [47, 52]. At the biochemical level, *PIK3R1* mutations within the iSH2 domain disrupt inhibition of p110α to allow downstream activation of the PI3K [52] and MAPK pathways [80]. In contrast, truncation mutations in the RhoGAP domain of p85α result in PTEN dysregulation via proteasome degradation [81]. Apart from comprehensive whole exome sequencing studies, the gene encoding a second isoform of the PI3K regulatory subunit, *PIK3R2*, has only been sequenced in four SECs and a mutation was found in one (25%) [81]. *PIK3R2* mutations were not identified by TCGA, but the gene was reportedly amplified in 20% of serous-like cases [47].

In studies that have simultaneously sequenced all three genes, somatic mutations in the PIK3CA-PIK3R1-PTEN axis have been found in 40% (17/46) of SECs and in 58% (35/60) of TCGA's serous-like subgroup [47, 51, 52]. Amplification of *PIK3CA* has also been reported in 26–67% of SECs and serous-like tumors (Table 5.1). Collectively, these genomic observations emphasize the importance of PI3K pathway dysregulation in the molecular pathology of SEC and implicate the PI3K pathway as a potential therapeutic target for SEC.

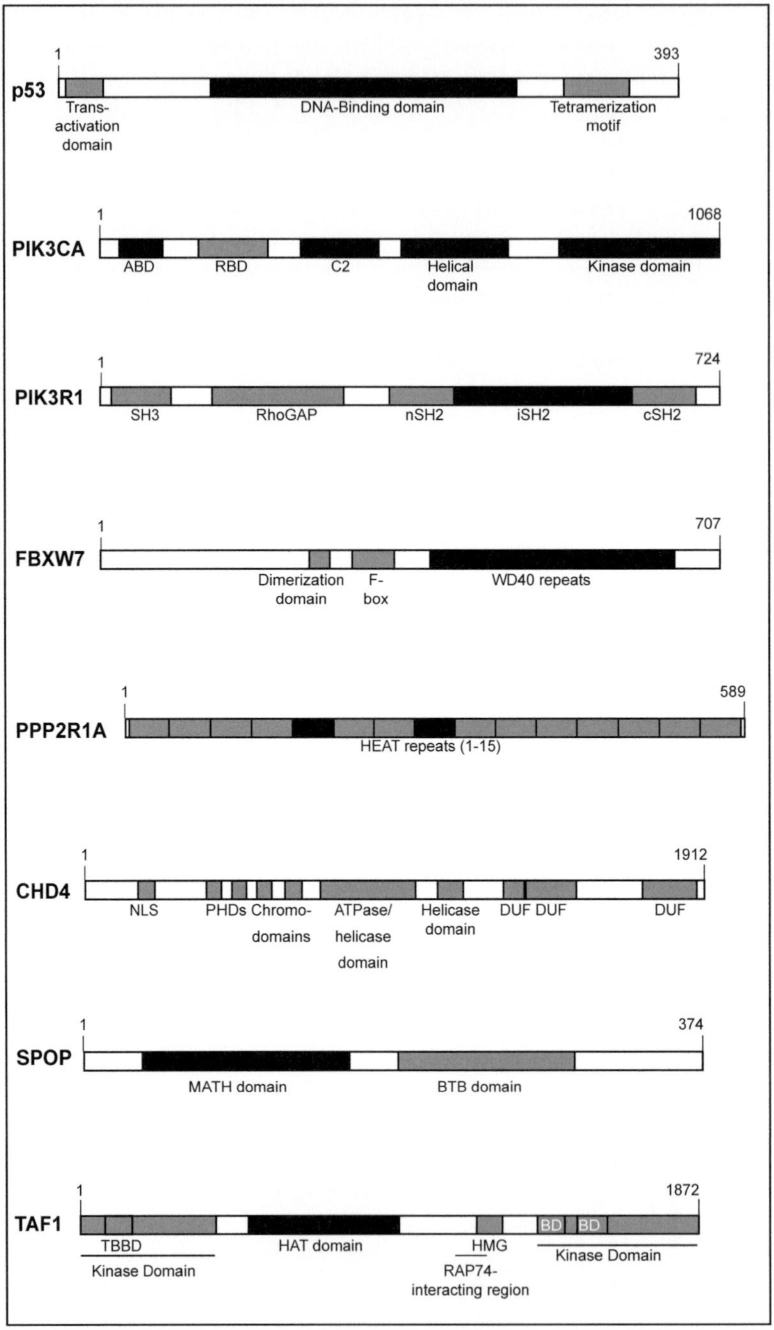
1
393
p53
Trans-
activation
domain
DNA-Binding domain
Tetramerization
motif
1
1068
PIK3CA
ABD
RBD
C2
Helical
domain
Kinase domain
1
724
PIK3R1
SH3
RhoGAP
nSH2
iSH2
cSH2
1
707
FBXW7
Dimerization
domain
F-
box
WD40 repeats
1
589
PPP2R1A
HEAT repeats (1-15)
1
1912
CHD4
NLS
PHDs
Chromo-
domains
ATPase/
helicase
domain
Helicase
domain
DUF DUF
DUF
1
374
SPOP
MATH domain
BTB domain
1
1872
TAF1
TBBD
Kinase Domain
HAT domain
HMG
RAP74-
interacting region
BD
BD
Kinase Domain

◂**Fig. 5.2** Schematic representation of known functional domains of a subset of genes frequently mutated in SECs. *Dark shading* denotes domains that exhibit clustering of somatic mutations in SECs. Abbreviations: *ABD* adaptor-binding domain, *RBD* Ras-binding domain, *C2* protein kinase-C homology 2, *SH* Src Homology, *RhoGAP* Rho GTPase-activating proteins, *WD repeat* tryptophan–aspartic acid repeat, *HEAT repeats* Huntington-Elongation-A subunit-TOR repeats, *NLS* Nuclear localization signal, *PHD* Plant homeodomain-type zinc finger, *DUF* Domain of unknown function, *MATH domain* Meprin And TRAF Homology domain, *BTB domain* Broad complex, Tramtrack and Bric-a-brac domain, *TBBD* TATA-box-binding protein-binding domain, *HAT* Histone Acetyltransferase, *RAP74* RNA Polymerase II Associated protein, 74 kDa, *HMG* High-mobility group

PI3K Pathway Aberrations as Therapeutic Targets in SEC

Clinical trials evaluating the safety and efficacy of PI3K inhibitors, mTOR inhibitors, dual PI3K/mTOR inhibitors, and AKT inhibitors in EC are underway (Table 5.2). Combined, these agents have produced 38.8% (7/18) of the responses observed in SEC patients in phase II clinical trials of targeted therapies (Table 5.3). Here, we describe phase II clinical trial results to date for PI3K pathway inhibitors in SEC patients.

The pan-PI3K inhibitor pilaralisib (SAR245408, XL147; Sanofi) has been evaluated in a phase II trial in patients ($n = 67$) with advanced or recurrent EC (NCT01013324) [82]. Although efficacy criteria were not met for the overall study, a favorable safety profile was reported [82]. Among 24 SEC patients included in this trial, all of whom had received at least one prior chemotherapy-based regimen, one patient had a complete response (objective response rate determined by RECIST 1.1) with progression-free survival >6 months, another exhibited a partial response with progression-free survival at >6 months, one exhibited stable disease with progression-free survival >6 months, and three patients exhibited progressive disease. Although the trial included an extensive assessment of molecular aberrations in *PTEN*, *PIK3CA*, *PIK3R1/2*, *AKT1/2*, *NRAS*, *KRAS*, *TP53*, *ARID1A*, *CTNNB1*, *ERBB2*, and *CCNE1*, and genetic aberrations of one or more markers were observed in responsive patients, there was no statistically significant correlation between the molecular status of markers and clinical outcome as a whole.

A phase II trial (NCT01307631) of MK-2206 (Merck & Co., Inc.), an allosteric inhibitor of AKT [83], in which patients with recurrent or advanced EC were stratified by *PIK3CA* mutation status, found that all patients with six-month progression-free survival harbored SEC [84]. These observations resulted in a phase II cohort expansion study of MK-2206 for patients with recurrent SEC, with up to two lines of prior chemotherapy, which is currently active (NCT01312753). Interim results of the expansion study noted that of 14 patients accrued, two patients met the six-month progression-free survival endpoint, two patients were still receiving treatment, and the remaining 10 patients did not meet efficacy endpoints [84]. A companion molecular analysis was planned but has not yet been reported.

AKT inhibitors are also being tested in combination with MEK inhibitors in patients with EC (Table 5.2); there is known cross talk and compensatory roles of the RAS/RAF/MEK/ERK pathways and the PI3K pathway [85]. The small-molecule MEK1/2 inhibitor, selumetinib (AZD6244; AstraZeneca), has been tested as a single agent in a phase II trial of patients with recurrent or persistent EC that included an exploratory objective of determining associations between biomarkers (mutation, immunohistochemical expression) and response (NCT01011933). Although selumetinib was reportedly well tolerated and 12% of patients experienced six-month event-free survival, this fell short of meeting pre-defined efficacy criteria of 15% six-month event-free survival. All patients received at least one prior chemotherapy regimen. Nine patients enrolled and treated had SEC (17.3% of 52 total), but study results were not reported by histology so it is unclear whether any SEC patients responded [86].

Three different mTOR inhibitors have been tested in phase II clinical trials for women with EC: Afinitor® (everolimus; Novartis), ridaforolimus (AP23573, MK-8669, deforolimus; Ariad Pharmaceutical), and Torisel® (temsirolimus; Pfizer) (Table 5.3). Biomarkers studied within these trials include PTEN expression (NCT00072176, NCT00770185), expression of hormone receptors as well as mTOR pathway members (NCT00729586), mutations in *PTEN*, *PIK3CA*, *KRAS*, *CTNNB1*, and microsatellite instability status (NCT02093598). To date, none of these biomarkers have been shown to be effective in predicting response to mTOR inhibition.

In an attempt to aggregate sufficient numbers of patients to identify biomarkers of mTOR inhibitor sensitivity, the results from three separate clinical trials that evaluated mTOR inhibitors in a total of 94 women with EC were combined [87]. Two of the trials tested intravenous temsirolimus (one included chemotherapy naïve patients and the other included patients who had received one prior chemotherapy), and the third trial tested ridaforolimus in patients who could have received prior adjuvant chemotherapy. Two of twelve treated patients with SEC in the three trials combined achieved a response [87]. No significant association was found between PTEN loss [measured by immunohistochemistry (IHC)], stathmin expression (measured by IHC), mutations in *PIK3CA*, *KRAS*, *MET*, *NRAS*, *AKT1*, or *EGFR*, and response or progression. A separate analysis of results from the temsirolimus trials described in the analysis above also failed to find a molecular biomarker of response, but found that prior chemotherapy was a significant predictor of progression; a greater frequency of increased tumor growth was observed in women treated with chemotherapy prior to temsirolimus as compared to the chemotherapy naïve population [88].

In the phase II ENDORAD trial of everolimus as second- or third-line treatment of advanced EC, 11 patients with chemotherapy refractory SEC (out of a total of 44 patients) were enrolled and treated with single-agent everolimus. One patient with SEC exhibited partial response (non-progressive disease rate) at 3 and 6 months, while two others had stable disease at 3 and 6 months. In addition to these promising results in SEC patients, the trial as a whole met efficacy and safety target criteria and therefore supported further development of this type of targeted therapy [89]. As of June 2015, everolimus was also being tested in a phase II trial in combination with the aromatase inhibitor letrozole in women with recurrent or persistent EC (NCT02188550). No biomarkers were specified for this trial.

Phase II trials of ridaforolimus in EC have also been promising. One 59-year-old woman with papillary SEC was highlighted in results from a phase II trial of ridaforolimus for remarkably decreased lung metastasis size [90]. Overall, this study successfully recruited and treated 10 patients with SEC; one patient achieved partial response (described previously with decreased lung metastasis size) and one achieved stable disease. However, no biomarkers were specified or reported in this study [90]. A separate phase II trial of oral ridaforolimus in women with recurrent or metastatic EC recruited five women with SEC; four responded with stable disease and one exhibited progressive disease [91]. No correlation between PTEN loss (measured by IHC), *PIK3CA* mutation, or *AKT* mutation with partial response or disease stabilization was found [91]. This study reported prolonged stabilization of disease and supported additional studies that combine ridaforolimus with hormone therapies and chemotherapies [91].

A phase II trial of single-agent temsirolimus therapy for patients with recurrent or metastatic EC successfully enrolled and treated six patients with chemotherapy naïve and nine patients with chemotherapy treated SEC [92] and resulted in encouraging responses. Partial response was observed in 33.3% (2/6) and stable disease was observed in 50% (3/6) of chemotherapy naïve patients. In patients previously treated with chemotherapy, stable disease was observed in 55.5% (5/9); no partial responses were reported in this group. This trial found that *PTEN* mutation, phosphorylated AKT, MTOR, and S6 were not biomarkers for temsirolimus response [92]. Another phase II trial of temsirolimus in women with stage II or IV disease or persistent or recurrent disease after treatment for earlier stage disease successfully enrolled 12 patients with SEC and treated them with single-agent temsirolimus. Two of these patients responded, although it was unclear whether they achieved partial or complete responses and whether or not they received prior chemotherapy [93].

Combination therapies with temsirolimus are also being tested in phase II clinical trials recruiting SEC patients. These are testing temsirolimus in combination with hormonal therapy (NCT00729586), with the VEGF inhibitor Avastin® (bevacizumab; Genentech) (NCT01010126), or with temsirolimus [94].

HER2 (ERBB2) Aberrations in SEC

The epidermal growth factor receptor (EGFR) family consists of EGFR (HER1, ERBB1), HER2 (NEU, ERBB2), HER3 (ERBB3), and HER4 transmembrane receptors. This family of receptors lies upstream of signaling pathways including the PI3K and RAS/RAF pathways that are often dysregulated in oncogenesis (reviewed in [95, 96]). Although *HER2* mutations are rare in SECs [47, 49], *HER2* gene amplification is common and has been reported in 17–57% of SECs and serous-like tumors (Table 5.1). Similarly, HER2 over-expression occurs at a significantly higher frequency in SECs compared to the other histological subtypes of EC [97]. The reported frequencies of HER2 over-expression in SECs are highly variable and range from 17 to 80% [97–108]. HER2 over-expression is associated with advanced stage [109] and is an independent prognostic factor correlated with poor outcome in patients with SEC [106, 110], suggesting HER2 may be advantageous to target therapeutically.

HER2 as a Therapeutic Target in SEC

Therapies targeting HER2 and other members of the EGFR family are currently being tested in clinical trials (Table 5.2) or have been tested in phase II trials (Table 5.3). Clinical trials of HER2-targeted therapies often require HER2 "positivity" as an inclusion criteria or endpoint measurement. However, it should be noted that a standardized definition of HER2 "positivity," and standardized tests for HER2 protein levels and gene amplification have not been established for SEC patients. In an attempt to begin to establish standards for HER2 testing in EC, one study compared the American Society of Clinical Oncology and the College of American Pathologists (ASCO/CAP) and US Food and Drug Administration (FDA) scoring criteria that are used for measurements of HER positivity in breast cancer in 85 SECs and found a superior concordance between HER2 fluorescence in situ hybridization (FISH) [PathVysion Kit (Abbott Molecular)] and IHC [Herceptest (Dako Denmark A/S)] results using the ASCO/CAP scoring criteria [111]. Concordance between HER2 FISH and IHC has been confirmed in other studies of SEC [102, 112, 113], and both FISH and IHC are currently being utilized to measure HER2 expression in phase II trials recruiting patients with SEC (Table 5.3). Here, we summarize the most advanced clinical trial results of HER2-targeted therapies in SEC to date.

Clinical investigations into the efficacy of Herceptin® (trastuzumab; Genentech), a humanized monoclonal antibody directed against HER2, for the treatment of SEC are underway. Although trastuzumab gained FDA approval for the treatment of breast cancer patients with HER-positive tumors, early results in SEC are mixed. Encouragingly, two SEC patients in one report who achieved a complete response and stable disease after trastuzumab treatment exhibited HER2 over-expression in the associated tumors, as defined by strong (3+) IHC staining [107]. In contrast, a phase II trial of trastuzumab in HER2-positive (as measured by IHC or FISH) EC patients with advanced or recurrent disease, with or without prior therapy, observed no objective responses [114]. However, there has been some debate as to whether this trial was adequately powered to detect responsiveness [115]. Moreover, at the molecular level, it has been suggested that higher levels of the p95HER2 variant observed in SECs compared with breast cancers might confer primary resistance to trastuzumab in SEC [116].

Lapatinib is a reversible small-molecule dual inhibitor of both HER1 and HER2 [117] that, unlike trastuzumab, binds the intracellular domain of HER2 (which is preserved in p95HER2) [118]. In preclinical studies utilizing xenograft models of SEC, no attenuation of tumor growth was observed with single-agent trastuzumab whereas a significant reduction in tumor growth of HER2-amplified tumor xenografts was observed with the combination of lapatinib and trastuzumab [112]. However, a phase II trial of lapatinib in persistent or recurrent EC indicated limited activity, but very few tumors were either HER2-positive by IHC or EGFR-mutated; one patient with a novel EGFR mutation showed a partial response and prolonged progression-free survival [119].

Gilotrif® (afatinib; Boehringer Ingelheim Pharmaceuticals, Inc.) is a small-molecule irreversible inhibitor of EGFR and HER2 [120]. Preclinical results show that SEC cell lines with *HER2* amplification were not only sensitive to afatinib, but these cell lines were more sensitive than cell lines not harboring *HER2* amplification; furthermore, mice treated with afatinib displayed decreased growth of tumors established from SEC cell lines [121]. Of note, a 63-year-old woman with metastatic papillary SEC with *HER2*-positive pulmonary nodes (as measured by FISH) upon recurrence following two rounds of chemotherapy indicated a complete response to afatinib that lasted almost a year after being taken off the drug [122].

FBXW7 Aberrations in SEC

The FBXW7 tumor suppressor is an integral component of the SCF-FBXW7-E3 ubiquitin ligase complex, which regulates the turnover of numerous protein substrates including several that have been implicated in tumorigenesis such as cyclin E, MYC, NOTCH, MCL1, and mTOR (reviewed in [123]) (Fig. 5.3). *FBXW7* is somatically mutated in a wide range of solid tumors and hematological malignancies and functions as a haploinsufficient tumor suppressor gene [124, 125]. *FBXW7* mutations are common in SEC and serous-like tumors, with frequencies of 8–33% (Table 5.1). Copy number losses encompassing *FBXW7*, possibly resulting in haploinsufficiency, have also been noted in 13–52% SEC [48, 50]. Somatic mutations in *FBXW7* appear to be relatively early events in serous endometrial tumorigenesis based on their presence in concurrent cases of EIC and SEC [48], and in a case of superficial serous carcinoma [126].

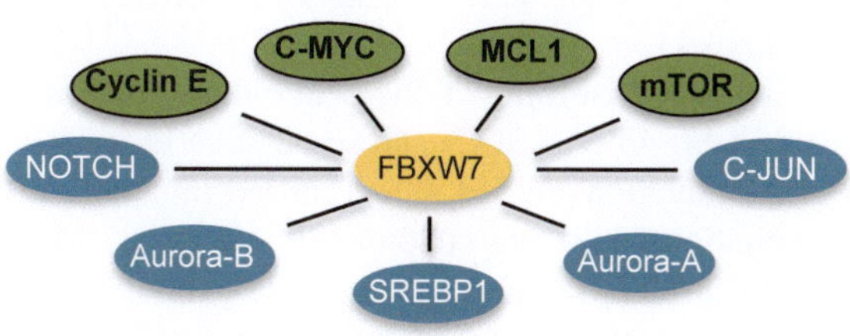

Fig. 5.3 Schematic representation of FBWX7 and a subset of known substrates that are targeted by the FBXW7 ubiquitin ligase complex for proteosomal degradation. Substrate proteins that are known to be dysregulated in EC are indicated in bold font

Most *FBXW7* mutations in serous and serous-like ECs are missense mutations within the WD repeat domain, which mediates FBXW7-substrate interactions (Fig. 5.2). Within this domain, codons 465, 479, 505, and 689 are major mutational hot spots in SEC. Codons 465, 479, and 505 are also mutation hot spots in other tumor types, and mutations at these residues can impair FBXW7-substrate interactions [124, 127–130], and are associated with elevated levels of SCF^{FBXW7} substrates [125, 131, 132]. In SEC, *FBXW7* mutations have been implicated in the dysregulation of cyclin E based on observations that *FBXW7* mutations and *CCNE1* amplification, which is also a frequent and early event in SEC [133], exhibit mutual exclusivity in SEC [48]. However, the overall effect of *FBXW7* mutations on the turnover of other SCF^{FBXW7} protein substrates, including mTOR, has not yet been addressed.

Given the abundance of *FBXW7* mutations across multiple tumor types, strategies that have been proposed to leverage mutant FBXW7 as a druggable target in solid tumors include synthetic lethal approaches, targeting oncoproteins that are upregulated by mutant FBXW7, and the use of small-molecule agonists to facilitate binding of mutant FBXW7 to protein substrates [125, 134]. In this regard, it is notable that FBXW7-deficient cancer cell lines exhibit increased sensitivity to HDAC inhibition [135–137]. Moreover, in T-ALL and ovarian cancer cells, *FBXW7* mutations correlate with high MCL1 levels, resistance to antitubulin chemotherapeutics including paclitaxel and vincristine, resistance to the BCL-2 inhibitor ABT-727, and sensitivity to sorafenib, a small-molecule multikinase inhibitor [127, 130]. The potential clinical relevance of *FBXW7* mutations in SEC awaits preclinical investigations. Of note, inhibitors of mTOR, a substrate of FBXW7, are currently being tested in clinical trials on EC but it is unclear at this time whether *FBXW7* mutations will serve as biomarkers of response.

PPP2R1A Mutations in SEC

The PP2A serine-threonine phosphatase is a trimeric holoenzyme composed of a catalytic subunit (the C subunit), a scaffolding subunit (the Aα or Aβ isoforms), and a variable regulatory subunit (a member of the B, B′, B″, B‴ family subunits). There is a large body of evidence ascribing tumor suppressor activity to PP2A in various cellular contexts [138, 139].

PPP2R1A encodes the α-isoform of the scaffolding subunit of PP2A and is somatically mutated in 17–43% of SECs and serous-like ECs (Table 5.1). The vast majority of *PPP2R1A* mutations in SECs, and indeed in certain other gynecologic cancers, occur at mutational hot spot codons 179, 182, 183, 256, and 257 within HEAT domains 5 and 8 (exons 5 and 6) (Fig. 5.2). Although the cellular consequences of somatic tumor-associated mutations in *PPP2R1A* have yet to be determined, in vitro biochemical studies have shown that several tumor-associated mutations in PPP2R1A ($PPP2R1A^{Pro179Ala,\ Arg182Ala/Glu,\ Arg183Ala/Glu,\ Trp257Ala}$) have a reduced ability to bind one or more regulatory “B” subunits of PP2A [140].

Interestingly, in addition to being present as somatic mutations in SECs, the PPP2R1A^{Pro179Leu} and PPP2R1A^{Arg182Trp} variants also occur as rare de novo germline variants in individuals with autosomal dominant mental retardation, suggesting they are pathogenic and function in a dominant or dominant-negative manner in this clinical context [141].

Whether mutant forms of PPP2R1A represent druggable targets in SEC remains to be seen. However, it is noteworthy that Gilenya® (Fingolimod, FTY720, Novartis) is a drug that activates PP2A and has received FDA approval for the treatment of relapsing multiple sclerosis [142]. Thus, it has been proposed that preclinical studies to assess the efficacy of fingolimod in animal models of PPP2R1A-mutated cancers may be warranted [143].

CHD4 Mutations in SEC

Chromodomain-helicase-DNA-binding protein 4 (CHD4; also known as Mi-2β) is a core subunit of the nucleosome remodeling and histone deacetylase (NuRD) complex (reviewed in [144]). Within this complex, CHD4 is one of the two catalytic subunits (the other being CHD3) that provide ATPase enzymatic activity to mobilize nucleosomes [145, 146] and facilitate chromatin remodeling associated with transcriptional regulation [147, 148], cell proliferation [149], maintenance of DNA integrity [150], and DNA repair [151]. Depletion of CHD4 has been shown to enhance cell line sensitivity to DNA damaging agents [150–154], result in resistance to cisplatin in *BRCA*-mutated ovarian cancer cells [152], inhibit DNA double-strand break repair [150, 151, 154], increase accumulated DNA damage [150, 155], decrease cell proliferation [149, 151] and chromatin decondensation [156], and result in altered cell cycle [149] following exposure to DNA damaging agents [150, 151, 154]. Specifically with respect to altered DNA repair, siRNA-mediated depletion of CHD4 impairs the recruitment of a number of DNA repair proteins including HDAC1, MTA2, BRCA1, RNF168, BRIT1, and RPA to sites of DNA damage, following exposure to DNA damaging agents [150, 153, 154, 157]. In addition, CHD4 also has NuRD-independent functions in the transcriptional activation of CD4, Th2 cytokine, and *KLF1* and *BCL11A* genes [158–160].

Whole exome sequencing studies have implicated *CHD4* mutations in the development of SEC [47, 49, 50]. Somatic mutations have been reported in 10–19% of SECs and serous-like tumors (Table 5.1), and *CHD4* has also been reported in amplifications in SEC [47, 50]. The majority of *CHD4* mutations in SECs are missense mutations that localize to the ATPase domain and the helicase domain (Fig. 5.2) [47, 49, 50], which are required for DNA binding and catalytic activity [161, 162]. Point mutations in these domains might therefore affect DNA binding or may disrupt regulatory intramolecular interactions with the PHD and chromodomains, thus resulting in increased enzymatic activity [162, 163]. Mutations in CHD4 may also affect interactions with other members of the NuRD complex, or other proteins known to interact with CHD4, with a non-exhaustive list of these other proteins to include ATM [154, 157], ATR [164], BRIT1 [153], BRG1 [165], Gata3 [159], HEB [160], NAB1/2 [166], p300 [160], RFP [160], and RNF8 [156]. Future research will be needed to determine the significance of *CHD4* somatic mutations in SEC with respect to both protein function and potential therapeutic relevance.

SPOP Mutations in SEC

Speckle-type BTB/POZ protein (SPOP) is a Cul3-Ub E3 ligase-adaptor protein, which binds to a number of substrate proteins, targeting them for ubiquitination and subsequent proteolysis [167, 168]. Known substrates of SPOP include AR [169], BMI1 [168], BRMS1 [170], Daxx [171, 172], DDIT3/CHOP [173], Gli2/3 [174, 175], DEK [176], ERα [177, 178], macroH2A [168, 179], PIPKIIβ [180], Pdx1 [181], SRC-3/AIB1 [182], and TRIM24 [176] (Fig. 5.4). SPOP normally localizes to the nucleus but has been shown to accumulate in the cytoplasm under hypoxic conditions [183]. Within the context of hypoxia, cytoplasmic targets of SPOP that have been identified are PTEN, DUSP7, Daxx, and Gli2 [183].

We initially identified *SPOP* as a significantly mutated gene within SEC exomes, and subsequent exome sequencing studies have validated this finding. Across studies, SPOP mutations have been noted in 4–10% of SECs and in 5% of serous-like ECs (Table 5.1). All somatic SPOP mutations identified within SEC and serous-like tumors occur within the MATH (Meprin and TRAF homology) domain [47–50] (Fig. 5.2), which directly binds protein substrates [184]. This pattern recapitulates the localization of *SPOP* mutations in prostate cancer, which are also almost exclusively found in the MATH domain [185–188]. Interestingly, the spectrum of mutations within the MATH domain differs somewhat between endometrial and prostate cancers [49, 185–188]. Whether this reflects different mechanisms of mutagenesis, different functional consequences, or both is not yet known. Thus far, the functional analysis of SPOP mutants is at an early stage, but it has been reported that a subset of SPOP mutants found in EC exhibit decreased ERα binding, degradation and ubiquitination, and, in some instances, increased cell

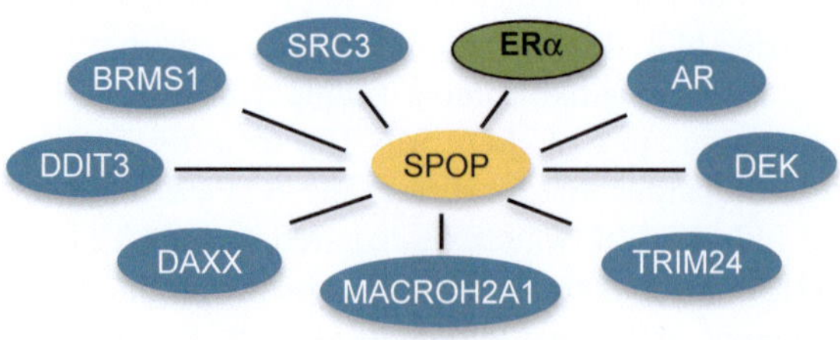

Fig. 5.4 Schematic representation of SPOP and a subset of known substrates that are targeted by the SPOP ubiquitin ligase complex for proteosomal degradation. Substrate proteins that are known to be dysregulated in EC are highlighted in *bold* font

growth of the Ishikawa cell line [178]. Future research will be needed to determine whether there are other key substrates of SPOP that are deregulated by somatic MATH domain mutations in SEC.

TAF1 Mutations in SEC

TBD-associated factor 1 (TAF1) is an X-linked gene that is part of the transcription factor IID (TFIID) complex, which is a core complex that is integral to the initiation of gene transcription and is comprised of TATA-box-binding protein (TBD) and at least 13 TAFs (reviewed in [189]). *TAF1* is the largest subunit of TFIID and has a number of reported functions within the complex (reviewed in [190]), including serving as a major structural component [191, 192], localizing the complex through co-activator, promoter [193], and histone binding [194], regulation of the activity other TFIID subunits [195–197], as well as providing enzymatic activity. TAF1 is a complex protein that has been reported to exhibit kinase [196, 198], ubiquitin-activating/conjugating [199, 200], and acetyltransferase activities [196, 201].

TAF1 was nominated as a significantly mutated gene in SEC as a result of whole exome sequencing [50]. In addition to being mutated in 5–13% of SEC and serous-like tumors (Table 5.1), *TAF1* mutations have also been associated with diffuse large B cell lymphoma [202], medulloblastoma [203], and lung cancers [204, 205]. A pan-cancer analysis also nominated *TAF1* as a significantly mutated gene [205]. In SEC, the majority of somatic mutations reported in *TAF1* are missense mutations that occur within the putative histone acetyltransferase (HAT) domain and a region between the HAT domain and the bromodomains [47, 50] (Fig. 5.2). In the absence of functional studies of these mutations, we can only speculate at this time on their possible effects. In this regard, it is conceivable that mutations in the HAT domain might alter TAF1 acetyltransferase activity possibly by releasing the regulatory contact between TAF1 and TAF7 [195], or they might affect the ability of the TAF1 HAT domain to bind DNA [206]. It may prove challenging to pinpoint the exact effects of somatic mutations in *TAF1*, given the diverse functional roles of the TAF1 protein within the TFIID complex. Although it is premature to speculate on the clinical significance, if any, of TAF1 mutants in SEC, it is noteworthy that UMB-32, a lead compound in a chemical library screen for bromodomain inhibitors, targets TAF1 and a related protein TAF1L [207].

Novel Clinical Trial Designs

Identification of predictive biomarkers of response to targeted therapies in SEC patients could catalyze the clinical translation of what is known of the molecular pathology of SEC. Although there have been anecdotal reports of responses to targeted therapies in SEC, clinically relevant biomarkers have not yet been uncovered. This might reflect the evolution of the tumor genome between the time of tissue resection and the administration of therapy, limitations in the numbers of SEC patients included in clinical trials, the statistical power of study design, or the evaluation of a limited number of molecular alterations. In this regard, clinical studies such as NCI's National Clinical Trials Network (NCTN)—Exceptional Responders Initiative (NCT02243592) may prove informative in revealing biomarkers of drug responsiveness for SEC patients. Within this study, whole exome and/or targeted deep sequencing and potentially other molecular approaches will be used to search for biomarkers of response in patients who have previously achieved "a complete or partial response lasting at least 6 months after receiving a treatment for which <10% of patients are expected to have a complete or partial response for this duration" (reviewed in [208]). Moving forward, basket trial design [209] may also prove to be informative for comparatively rare cancer types such as SEC for which it can be difficult to accrue sufficient numbers of patients for traditional or umbrella clinical trial designs. Currently, at least three basket trials have the potential to enroll SEC patients: the National Cancer Institute's Molecular Analysis for Therapy Choice [NCI-MATCH; (NCT02465060)], the National Cancer Institute's Molecular Profiling-Based Assignment of Cancer Therapy [NCI-MPACT; (NCT01827384)], and the Worldwide Innovative Networking Consortium's WINTHER (NCT01856296) clinical trials [210–212].

Summary and Conclusion

In this chapter, we have provided an overview of the current state of knowledge regarding the molecular pathology of SEC. In the current understanding, the major pathogenic drivers are TP53, the PI3K pathway, HER2 (ERBB2), FBXW7, MYC, CCNE1, PPP2R1A, CHD4, SPOP, and TAF. Precisely how this knowledge will translate into clinical practice remains to be seen, but against the backdrop of genomic and functional studies, ongoing clinical trials of targeted therapies, and novel clinical trial designs, we hope that advancements in the understanding of the molecular pathology of SEC will eventually translate into identification of clinically relevant biomarkers and, most importantly, increased quality of life and survival times for SEC patients.

References

1. Carcangiu ML, Chambers JT. Uterine papillary serous carcinoma: a study on 108 cases with emphasis on the prognostic significance of associated endometrioid carcinoma, absence of invasion, and concomitant ovarian carcinoma. Gynecol Oncol. 1992;47(3):298–305.
2. Christopherson WM, Alberhasky RC, Connelly PJ. Carcinoma of the endometrium. II. Papillary adenocarcinoma: a clinical pathological study, 46 cases. Am J Clin Pathol. 1982;77(5):534–40.

3. Clement PB, Young RH. Non-endometrioid carcinomas of the uterine corpus: a review of their pathology with emphasis on recent advances and problematic aspects. Adv Anat Pathol. 2004;11(3):117–42.
4. Hamilton CA, Cheung MK, Osann K, Chen L, Teng NN, Longacre TA, et al. Uterine papillary serous and clear cell carcinomas predict for poorer survival compared to grade 3 endometrioid corpus cancers. Br J Cancer. 2006;94(5):642–6.
5. Sutton GP, Brill L, Michael H, Stehman FB, Ehrlich CE. Malignant papillary lesions of the endometrium. Gynecol Oncol. 1987;27(3):294–304.
6. Cirisano FD Jr, Robboy SJ, Dodge RK, Bentley RC, Krigman HR, Synan IS, et al. The outcome of stage I–II clinically and surgically staged papillary serous and clear cell endometrial cancers when compared with endometrioid carcinoma. Gynecol Oncol. 2000;77(1):55–65.
7. Ueda SM, Kapp DS, Cheung MK, Shin JY, Osann K, Husain A, et al. Trends in demographic and clinical characteristics in women diagnosed with corpus cancer and their potential impact on the increasing number of deaths. Am J Obstet Gynecol. 2008;198(2):218 e1-6.
8. Bokhman JV. Two pathogenetic types of endometrial carcinoma. Gynecol Oncol. 1983;15(1):10–7.
9. Goff BA, Kato D, Schmidt RA, Ek M, Ferry JA, Muntz HG, et al. Uterine papillary serous carcinoma: patterns of metastatic spread. Gynecol Oncol. 1994;54(3):264–8.
10. Alkushi A, Kobel M, Kalloger SE, Gilks CB. High-grade endometrial carcinoma: serous and grade 3 endometrioid carcinomas have different immunophenotypes and outcomes. Int J Gynecol Pathol. 2010;29(4):343–50.
11. Hendrickson M, Ross J, Eifel P, Martinez A, Kempson R. Uterine papillary serous carcinoma: a highly malignant form of endometrial adenocarcinoma. Am J Surg Pathol. 1982;6(2):93–108.
12. Rosenberg P, Blom R, Hogberg T, Simonsen E. Death rate and recurrence pattern among 841 clinical stage-I endometrial cancer-patients with special reference to uterine papillary serous carcinoma. Gynecol Oncol. 1993;51(3):311–5.
13. Scarfone G, Secomandi R, Parazzini F, Vigano R, Mangili G, Frigerio L, et al. Clear cell and papillary serous endometrial carcinomas: survival in a series of 128 cases. Arch Gynecol Obstet. 2013;287(2):351–6.
14. Gehrig PA, Groben PA, Fowler WC, Walton LA, Van le L. Noninvasive papillary serous carcinoma of the endometrium. Obstet Gynecol. 2001;97(1):153–7.
15. Grice J, Ek M, Greer B, Koh WJ, Muntz HG, Cain J, et al. Uterine papillary serous carcinoma: evaluation of long-term survival in surgically staged patients. Gynecol Oncol. 1998;69(1):69–73.
16. Lee KR, Belinson JL. Recurrence in noninvasive endometrial carcinoma. Relationship to uterine papillary serous carcinoma. Am J Surg Pathol. 1991;15(10):965–73.
17. Sherman ME, Bitterman P, Rosenshein NB, Delgado G, Kurman RJ. Uterine serous carcinoma. A morphologically diverse neoplasm with unifying clinicopathologic features. Am J Surg Pathol. 1992;16(6):600–10.
18. Williams KE, Waters ED, Woolas RP, Hammond IG, McCartney AJ. Mixed serous-endometrioid carcinoma of the uterus: pathologic and cytopathologic analysis of a high-risk endometrial carcinoma. Int J Gynecol Cancer. 1994;4(1):7–18.
19. Idrees R, Din NU, Fatima S, Kayani N. Serous carcinoma arising in endometrial polyps: clinicopathologic study of 4 cases. Ann Diagn Pathol. 2013;17(3):256–8.
20. Yasuda M, Katoh T, Hori S, Suzuki K, Ohno K, Maruyama M, et al. Endometrial intraepithelial carcinoma in association with polyp: review of eight cases. Diagn Pathol. 2013;8:25.
21. Lauchlan SC. Tubal (serous) carcinoma of the endometrium. Arch Pathol Lab Med. 1981;105(11):615–8.

22. Kato DT, Ferry JA, Goodman A, Sullinger J, Scully RE, Goff BA, et al. Uterine papillary serous carcinoma (UPSC): a clinicopathologic study of 30 cases. Gynecol Oncol. 1995;59 (3):384–9.
23. Benito V, Lubrano A, Arencibia O, Alvarez EE, Leon L, Medina N, et al. Pure papillary serous tumors of the endometrium: a clinicopathological analysis of 61 cases from a single institution. Int J Gynecol Cancer. 2009;19(8):1364–9.
24. McCluggage WG, Sumathi VP, McManus DT. Uterine serous carcinoma and endometrial intraepithelial carcinoma arising in endometrial polyps: report of 5 cases, including 2 associated with tamoxifen therapy. Hum Pathol. 2003;34(9):939–43.
25. Lavie O, Ben-Arie A, Segev Y, Faro J, Barak F, Haya N, et al. BRCA germline mutations in women with uterine serous carcinoma—still a debate. Int J Gynecol Cancer. 2010;20 (9):1531–4.
26. Lavie O, Hornreich G, Ben Arie A, Renbaum P, Levy-Lahad E, Beller U. BRCA1 germline mutations in women with uterine serous papillary carcinoma. Obstet Gynecol. 2000;96 (1):28–32.
27. Segev Y, Iqbal J, Lubinski J, Gronwald J, Lynch HT, Moller P, et al. The incidence of endometrial cancer in women with BRCA1 and BRCA2 mutations: an international prospective cohort study. Gynecol Oncol. 2013;130(1):127–31.
28. Behtash N, Tehranian A, Ardalan FA, Hanjani P. Uterine papillary serous carcinoma after pelvic radiation therapy for cancer of the cervix. J Obstet Gynaecol. 2002;22(1):96–7.
29. Gallion HH, van Nagell JR Jr., Donaldson ES, Powell DE. Endometrial cancer following radiation therapy for cervical cancer. Gynecol Oncol. 1987;27(1):76–83.
30. Park MH, Cho SH, Kang HJ, Kim SR, Hwang YY. Uterine papillary serous carcinoma following radiation therapy for carcinoma of cervix: a case report. Int J Gynecol Cancer. 2000;10(3):253–6.
31. Parkash V, Carcangiu ML. Uterine papillary serous carcinoma after radiation therapy for carcinoma of the cervix. Cancer. 1992;69(2):496–501.
32. Pothuri B, Ramondetta L, Martino M, Alektiar K, Eifel PJ, Deavers MT, et al. Development of endometrial cancer after radiation treatment for cervical carcinoma. Obstet Gynecol. 2003;101(5 Pt 1):941–5.
33. McCullough ML, Patel AV, Patel R, Rodriguez C, Feigelson HS, Bandera EV, et al. Body mass and endometrial cancer risk by hormone replacement therapy and cancer subtype. Cancer Epidemiol, Biomarkers Prev. 2008;17(1):73–9.
34. Setiawan VW, Yang HP, Pike MC, McCann SE, Yu H, Xiang YB, et al. Type I and II endometrial cancers: have they different risk factors? J Clin Oncol. 2013;31(20):2607–18.
35. O'Hara AJ, Bell DW. The genomics and genetics of endometrial cancer. Adv Genomics Genet. 2012;2012(2):33–47.
36. Ambros RA, Sheehan CE, Kallakury BV, Ross JS, Malfetano J, Paunovich E, et al. MDM2 and p 53 protein expression in the histologic subtypes of endometrial carcinoma. Mod Pathol. 1996;9(12):1165–9.
37. Kovalev S, Marchenko ND, Gugliotta BG, Chalas E, Chumas J, Moll UM. Loss of p53 function in uterine papillary serous carcinoma. Hum Pathol. 1998;29(6):613–9.
38. Lax SF, Kendall B, Tashiro H, Slebos RJ, Hedrick L. The frequency of p53, K-ras mutations, and microsatellite instability differs in uterine endometrioid and serous carcinoma: evidence of distinct molecular genetic pathways. Cancer. 2000;88(4):814–24.
39. Moll UM, Chalas E, Auguste M, Meaney D, Chumas J. Uterine papillary serous carcinoma evolves via a p53-driven pathway. Hum Pathol. 1996;27(12):1295–300.
40. Sherman ME, Bur ME, Kurman RJ. p53 in endometrial cancer and its putative precursors: evidence for diverse pathways of tumorigenesis. Hum Pathol. 1995;26(11):1268–74.
41. Tashiro H, Isacson C, Levine R, Kurman RJ, Cho KR, Hedrick L. p53 gene mutations are common in uterine serous carcinoma and occur early in their pathogenesis. Am J Pathol. 1997;150(1):177–85.

42. Ambros RA, Sherman ME, Zahn CM, Bitterman P, Kurman RJ. Endometrial intraepithelial carcinoma: a distinctive lesion specifically associated with tumors displaying serous differentiation. Hum Pathol. 1995;26(11):1260–7.
43. Liang SX, Chambers SK, Cheng L, Zhang S, Zhou Y, Zheng W. Endometrial glandular dysplasia: a putative precursor lesion of uterine papillary serous carcinoma. Part II: molecular features. Int J Surg Pathol. 2004;12(4):319–31.
44. Zheng W, Liang SX, Yu H, Rutherford T, Chambers SK, Schwartz PE. Endometrial glandular dysplasia: a newly defined precursor lesion of uterine papillary serous carcinoma. Part I: morphologic features. Int J Surg Pathol. 2004;12(3):207–23.
45. Wheeler DT, Bell KA, Kurman RJ, Sherman ME. Minimal uterine serous carcinoma: diagnosis and clinicopathologic correlation. Am J Surg Pathol. 2000;24(6):797–806.
46. Zheng W, Xiang L, Fadare O, Kong B. A proposed model for endometrial serous carcinogenesis. Am J Surg Pathol. 2011;35(1):e1–14.
47. Cancer Genome Atlas Research Network, Kandoth C, Schultz N, Cherniack AD, Akbani R, Liu Y, et al. Integrated genomic characterization of endometrial carcinoma. Nature. 2013;497(7447):67–73.
48. Kuhn E, Wu RC, Guan B, Wu G, Zhang J, Wang Y, et al. Identification of molecular pathway aberrations in uterine serous carcinoma by genome-wide analyses. J Natl Cancer Inst. 2012;104(19):1503–13.
49. Le Gallo M, O'Hara AJ, Rudd ML, Urick ME, Hansen NF, O'Neil NJ, et al. Exome sequencing of serous endometrial tumors identifies recurrent somatic mutations in chromatin-remodeling and ubiquitin ligase complex genes. Nat Genet. 2012;44(12):1310–5.
50. Zhao S, Choi M, Overton JD, Bellone S, Roque DM, Cocco E, et al. Landscape of somatic single-nucleotide and copy-number mutations in uterine serous carcinoma. Proc Natl Acad Sci USA. 2013;110(8):2916–21.
51. Rudd ML, Price JC, Fogoros S, Godwin AK, Sgroi DC, Merino MJ, et al. A unique spectrum of somatic PIK3CA (p110alpha) mutations within primary endometrial carcinomas. Clin Cancer Res. 2011;17(6):1331–40.
52. Urick ME, Rudd ML, Godwin AK, Sgroi D, Merino M, Bell DW. PIK3R1 (p85alpha) is somatically mutated at high frequency in primary endometrial cancer. Can Res. 2011;71(12):4061–7.
53. Wild PJ, Ikenberg K, Fuchs TJ, Rechsteiner M, Georgiev S, Fankhauser N, et al. p53 suppresses type II endometrial carcinomas in mice and governs endometrial tumour aggressiveness in humans. EMBO Mol Med. 2012;4(8):808–24.
54. Hayes MP, Douglas W, Ellenson LH. Molecular alterations of EGFR and PIK3CA in uterine serous carcinoma. Gynecol Oncol. 2009;113(3):370–3.
55. Jia L, Liu Y, Yi X, Miron A, Crum CP, Kong B, et al. Endometrial glandular dysplasia with frequent p53 gene mutation: a genetic evidence supporting its precancer nature for endometrial serous carcinoma. Clin Cancer Res. 2008;14(8):2263–9.
56. Tashiro H, Blazes MS, Wu R, Cho KR, Bose S, Wang SI, et al. Mutations in PTEN are frequent in endometrial carcinoma but rare in other common gynecological malignancies. Can Res. 1997;57(18):3935–40.
57. Brosh R, Rotter V. When mutants gain new powers: news from the mutant p53 field. Nat Rev Cancer. 2009;9(10):701–13.
58. Hanel W, Marchenko N, Xu S, Yu SX, Weng W, Moll U. Two hot spot mutant p53 mouse models display differential gain of function in tumorigenesis. Cell Death Differ. 2013;20(7):898–909.
59. Hong B, van den Heuvel AP, Prabhu VV, Zhang S, El-Deiry WS. Targeting tumor suppressor p53 for cancer therapy: strategies, challenges and opportunities. Curr Drug Targets. 2014;15(1):80–9.
60. Lang GA, Iwakuma T, Suh YA, Liu G, Rao VA, Parant JM, et al. Gain of function of a p53 hot spot mutation in a mouse model of Li-Fraumeni syndrome. Cell. 2004;119(6):861–72.

61. Muller PA, Vousden KH. Mutant p53 in cancer: new functions and therapeutic opportunities. Cancer Cell. 2014;25(3):304–17.
62. Ng S, Collisson EA, Sokolov A, Goldstein T, Gonzalez-Perez A, Lopez-Bigas N, et al. PARADIGM-SHIFT predicts the function of mutations in multiple cancers using pathway impact analysis. Bioinformatics. 2012;28(18):i640–6.
63. Brachova P, Mueting SR, Devor EJ, Leslie KK. Oncomorphic 53 mutations in gynecologic cancers lose the normal protein: protein interactions with the microrna microprocessing complex. J Cancer Therapy. 2014;5(6):506–16.
64. Beckta JM, Ahmad SF, Yang H, Valerie K. Revisiting p53 for cancer-specific chemo- and radiotherapy: ten years after. Cell Cycle. 2014;13(5):710–3.
65. Wang H, Bao W, Jiang F, Che Q, Chen Z, Wang F, et al. Mutant p53 (p53-R248Q) functions as an oncogene in promoting endometrial cancer by up-regulating REGgamma. Cancer Lett. 2015;360(2):269–79.
66. Luo W, Wu F, Elmaoued R, Beck BB, Fischer E, Meng X, et al. Amifostine enhancement of the anti-cancer effects of paclitaxel in endometrial cancer is TP53-dependent. Int J Oncol. 2010;37(5):1187–94.
67. Meng X, Dizon DS, Yang S, Wang X, Zhu D, Thiel KW, et al. Strategies for molecularly enhanced chemotherapy to achieve synthetic lethality in endometrial tumors with mutant p53. Obstet Gynecol Int. 2013;2013:828165.
68. Wild PJ, Ikenberg K, Fuchs TJ, Rechsteiner M, Georgiev S, Fankhauser N, et al. p53 suppresses type II endometrial carcinomas in mice and governs endometrial tumour aggressiveness in humans. EMBO Mol Med. 2012;4(8):808–24.
69. Stodden GR, Lindberg ME, King ML, Paquet M, MacLean JA, Mann JL, et al. Loss of Cdh1 and Trp53 in the uterus induces chronic inflammation with modification of tumor microenvironment. Oncogene. 2015;34(19):2471–82.
70. Akbay EA, Pena CG, Ruder D, Michel JA, Nakada Y, Pathak S, et al. Cooperation between p53 and the telomere-protecting shelterin component Pot1a in endometrial carcinogenesis. Oncogene. 2013;32(17):2211–9.
71. Yuan TL, Cantley LC. PI3K pathway alterations in cancer: variations on a theme. Oncogene. 2008;27(41):5497–510.
72. Vanhaesebroeck B, Guillermet-Guibert J, Graupera M, Bilanges B. The emerging mechanisms of isoform-specific PI3K signalling. Nat Rev Mol Cell Biol. 2010;11(5): 329–41.
73. Fruman DA, Rommel C. PI3K and cancer: lessons, challenges and opportunities. Nat Rev Drug Discov. 2014;13(2):140–56.
74. Samuels Y, Wang Z, Bardelli A, Silliman N, Ptak J, Szabo S, et al. High frequency of mutations of the PIK3CA gene in human cancers. Science. 2004;304(5670):554.
75. Gymnopoulos M, Elsliger MA, Vogt PK. Rare cancer-specific mutations in PIK3CA show gain of function. Proc Natl Acad Sci USA. 2007;104(13):5569–74.
76. Zhao L, Vogt PK. Helical domain and kinase domain mutations in p110alpha of phosphatidylinositol 3-kinase induce gain of function by different mechanisms. Proc Natl Acad Sci U S A. 2008;105(7):2652–7.
77. Zhao L, Vogt PK. Hot-spot mutations in p110alpha of phosphatidylinositol 3-kinase (pI3K): differential interactions with the regulatory subunit p85 and with RAS. Cell Cycle. 2010;9 (3):596–600.
78. Janku F, Wheler JJ, Naing A, Falchook GS, Hong DS, Stepanek VM, et al. PIK3CA mutation H1047R is associated with response to PI3K/AKT/mTOR signaling pathway inhibitors in early-phase clinical trials. Cancer Res. 2013;73(1):276–84.
79. Yu J, Zhang Y, McIlroy J, Rordorf-Nikolic T, Orr GA, Backer JM. Regulation of the p85/p110 phosphatidylinositol 3′-kinase: stabilization and inhibition of the p110alpha catalytic subunit by the p85 regulatory subunit. Mol Cell Biol. 1998;18(3):1379–87.
80. Cheung LW, Yu S, Zhang D, Li J, Ng PK, Panupinthu N, et al. Naturally occurring neomorphic PIK3R1 mutations activate the MAPK pathway, dictating therapeutic response to MAPK pathway inhibitors. Cancer Cell. 2014;26(4):479–94.

81. Cheung LW, Hennessy BT, Li J, Yu S, Myers AP, Djordjevic B, et al. High frequency of PIK3R1 and PIK3R2 mutations in endometrial cancer elucidates a novel mechanism for regulation of PTEN protein stability. Cancer Discov. 2011;1(2):170–85.
82. Matulonis U, Vergote I, Backes F, Martin LP, McMeekin S, Birrer M, et al. Phase II study of the PI3K inhibitor pilaralisib (SAR245408; XL147) in patients with advanced or recurrent endometrial carcinoma. Gynecol Oncol. 2015;136(2):246–53.
83. Bilodeau MT, Balitza AE, Hoffman JM, Manley PJ, Barnett SF, Defeo-Jones D, et al. Allosteric inhibitors of Akt1 and Akt2: a naphthyridinone with efficacy in an A2780 tumor xenograft model. Bioorg Med Chem Lett. 2008;18(11):3178–82.
84. Panagiotis Konstantinopoulos VM, William TB, Liu J, Horowitz NS, Birrer MJ, Doyle LA, Berlin ST, Whalen C, Van Hummelen P, Coleman RL, Aghajanian C, Mills GB, Matulonis U, Westin SN, Myers AP. Phase II, single stage, cohort expansion study of MK-2206 in recurrent endometrial serous cancer. Available from: http://meetinglibrary.asco.org/content/134284–144.
85. Mendoza MC, Er EE, Blenis J. The Ras-ERK and PI3K-mTOR pathways: cross-talk and compensation. Trends Biochem Sci. 2011;36(6):320–8.
86. Coleman RL, Sill MW, Thaker PH, Bender DP, Street D, McGuire WP, et al. A phase II evaluation of selumetinib (AZD6244, ARRY-142886), a selective MEK-1/2 inhibitor in the treatment of recurrent or persistent endometrial cancer: an NRG oncology/gynecologic oncology group study. Gynecol Oncol. 2015;138(1):30–5.
87. Mackay HJ, Eisenhauer EA, Kamel-Reid S, Tsao M, Clarke B, Karakasis K, et al. Molecular determinants of outcome with mammalian target of rapamycin inhibition in endometrial cancer. Cancer. 2014;120(4):603–10.
88. Goodwin RA, Jamal R, Tu D, Walsh W, Dancey J, Oza AM, et al. Clinical and toxicity predictors of response and progression to temsirolimus in women with recurrent or metastatic endometrial cancer. Gynecol Oncol. 2013;131(2):315–20.
89. Ray-Coquard I, Favier L, Weber B, Roemer-Becuwe C, Bougnoux P, Fabbro M, et al. Everolimus as second- or third-line treatment of advanced endometrial cancer: ENDORAD, a phase II trial of GINECO. Br J Cancer. 2013;108(9):1771–7.
90. Colombo N, McMeekin DS, Schwartz PE, Sessa C, Gehrig PA, Holloway R, et al. Ridaforolimus as a single agent in advanced endometrial cancer: results of a single-arm, phase 2 trial. Br J Cancer. 2013;108(5):1021–6.
91. Tsoref D, Welch S, Lau S, Biagi J, Tonkin K, Martin LA, et al. Phase II study of oral ridaforolimus in women with recurrent or metastatic endometrial cancer. Gynecol Oncol. 2014;135(2):184–9.
92. Oza AM, Elit L, Tsao MS, Kamel-Reid S, Biagi J, Provencher DM, et al. Phase II study of temsirolimus in women with recurrent or metastatic endometrial cancer: a trial of the NCIC Clinical Trials Group. J Clin Oncol. 2011;29(24):3278–85.
93. Fleming GF, Filiaci VL, Marzullo B, Zaino RJ, Davidson SA, Pearl M, et al. Temsirolimus with or without megestrol acetate and tamoxifen for endometrial cancer: a gynecologic oncology group study. Gynecol Oncol. 2014;132(3):585–92.
94. Alvarez EA, Brady WE, Walker JL, Rotmensch J, Zhou XC, Kendrick JE, et al. Phase II trial of combination bevacizumab and temsirolimus in the treatment of recurrent or persistent endometrial carcinoma: a gynecologic oncology group study. Gynecol Oncol. 2013;129 (1):22–7.
95. Prenzel N, Fischer OM, Streit S, Hart S, Ullrich A. The epidermal growth factor receptor family as a central element for cellular signal transduction and diversification. Endocr Relat Cancer. 2001;8(1):11–31.
96. Yarden Y. The EGFR family and its ligands in human cancer. signalling mechanisms and therapeutic opportunities. Eur J Cancer. 2001;37(Suppl 4):S3–8.
97. Grushko TA, Filiaci VL, Mundt AJ, Ridderstrale K, Olopade OI, Fleming GF, et al. An exploratory analysis of HER-2 amplification and overexpression in advanced endometrial carcinoma: a gynecologic oncology group study. Gynecol Oncol. 2008;108(1):3–9.

98. Caduff RF, Svoboda-Newman SM, Bartos RE, Ferguson AW, Frank TS. Comparative analysis of histologic homologues of endometrial and ovarian carcinoma. Am J Surg Pathol. 1998;22(3):319–26.
99. Diaz-Montes TP, Ji H, Smith Sehdev AE, Zahurak ML, Kurman RJ, Armstrong DK, et al. Clinical significance of Her-2/neu overexpression in uterine serous carcinoma. Gynecol Oncol. 2006;100(1):139–44.
100. Macwhinnie N, Monaghan H. The use of P53, PTEN, and C-erbB-2 to differentiate uterine serous papillary carcinoma from endometrioid endometrial carcinoma. Int J Gynecol Cancer. 2004;14(5):938–46.
101. Morrison C, Zanagnolo V, Ramirez N, Cohn DE, Kelbick N, Copeland L, et al. HER-2 is an independent prognostic factor in endometrial cancer: association with outcome in a large cohort of surgically staged patients. J Clin Oncol. 2006;24(15):2376–85.
102. Odicino FE, Bignotti E, Rossi E, Pasinetti B, Tassi RA, Donzelli C, et al. HER-2/neu overexpression and amplification in uterine serous papillary carcinoma: comparative analysis of immunohistochemistry, real-time reverse transcription-polymerase chain reaction, and fluorescence in situ hybridization. Int J Gynecol Cancer. 2008;18(1):14–21.
103. Prat J, Oliva E, Lerma E, Vaquero M, Matias-Guiu X. Uterine papillary serous adenocarcinoma. A 10-case study of p53 and c-erbB-2 expression and DNA content. Cancer. 1994;74(6):1778–83.
104. Santin AD, Bellone S, Van Stedum S, Bushen W, De Las Casas LE, Korourian S, et al. Determination of HER2/neu status in uterine serous papillary carcinoma: comparative analysis of immunohistochemistry and fluorescence in situ hybridization. Gynecol Oncol. 2005;98(1):24–30.
105. Slomovitz BM, Broaddus RR, Burke TW, Sneige N, Soliman PT, Wu W, et al. Her-2/neu overexpression and amplification in uterine papillary serous carcinoma. J Clin Oncol. 2004;22(15):3126–32.
106. Togami S, Sasajima Y, Oi T, Ishikawa M, Onda T, Ikeda S, et al. Clinicopathological and prognostic impact of human epidermal growth factor receptor type 2 (HER2) and hormone receptor expression in uterine papillary serous carcinoma. Cancer Sci. 2012;103(5):926–32.
107. Villella JA, Cohen S, Smith DH, Hibshoosh H, Hershman D. HER-2/neu overexpression in uterine papillary serous cancers and its possible therapeutic implications. Int J Gynecol Cancer. 2006;16(5):1897–902.
108. Santin AD, Bellone S, Gokden M, Palmieri M, Dunn D, Agha J, et al. Overexpression of HER-2/neu in uterine serous papillary cancer. Clin Cancer Res. 2002;8(5):1271–9.
109. Berchuck A, Rodriguez G, Kinney RB, Soper JT, Dodge RK, Clarke-Pearson DL, et al. Overexpression of HER-2/neu in endometrial cancer is associated with advanced stage disease. Am J Obstet Gynecol. 1991;164(1 Pt 1):15–21.
110. Santin AD, Bellone S, Siegel ER, Palmieri M, Thomas M, Cannon MJ, et al. Racial differences in the overexpression of epidermal growth factor type II receptor (HER2/neu): a major prognostic indicator in uterine serous papillary cancer. Am J Obstet Gynecol. 2005;192(3):813–8.
111. Buza N, English DP, Santin AD, Hui P. Toward standard HER2 testing of endometrial serous carcinoma: 4-year experience at a large academic center and recommendations for clinical practice. Mod Pathol. 2013;26(12):1605–12.
112. Groeneweg JW, Hernandez SF, Byron VF, DiGloria CM, Lopez H, Scialabba V, et al. Dual HER2 targeting impedes growth of HER2 gene-amplified uterine serous carcinoma xenografts. Clin Cancer Res. 2014;20(24):6517–28.
113. Singh P, Smith CL, Cheetham G, Dodd TJ, Davy ML. Serous carcinoma of the uterus-determination of HER-2/neu status using immunohistochemistry, chromogenic in situ hybridization, and quantitative polymerase chain reaction techniques: its significance and clinical correlation. Int J Gynecol Cancer. 2008;18(6):1344–51.

114. Fleming GF, Sill MW, Darcy KM, McMeekin DS, Thigpen JT, Adler LM, et al. Phase II trial of trastuzumab in women with advanced or recurrent, HER2-positive endometrial carcinoma: a Gynecologic Oncology Group study. Gynecol Oncol. 2010;116(1):15–20.
115. Santin AD. Phase II trial of trastuzumab in women with advanced or recurrent HER-positive endometrial carcinoma: a gynecologic oncology group study. Gynecol Oncol. 2010;118 (1):95–6.
116. Growdon WB, Groeneweg J, Byron V, DiGloria C, Borger DR, Tambouret R, et al. HER2 over-expressing high grade endometrial cancer expresses high levels of p95HER2 variant. Gynecol Oncol. 2015;137(1):160–6.
117. Xia W, Mullin RJ, Keith BR, Liu LH, Ma H, Rusnak DW, et al. Anti-tumor activity of GW572016: a dual tyrosine kinase inhibitor blocks EGF activation of EGFR/erbB2 and downstream Erk1/2 and AKT pathways. Oncogene. 2002;21(41):6255–63.
118. Scaltriti M, Rojo F, Ocana A, Anido J, Guzman M, Cortes J, et al. Expression of p95HER2, a truncated form of the HER2 receptor, and response to anti-HER2 therapies in breast cancer. J Natl Cancer Inst. 2007;99(8):628–38.
119. Leslie KK, Sill MW, Lankes HA, Fischer EG, Godwin AK, Gray H, et al. Lapatinib and potential prognostic value of EGFR mutations in a gynecologic oncology group phase II trial of persistent or recurrent endometrial cancer. Gynecol Oncol. 2012;127(2):345–50.
120. Li D, Ambrogio L, Shimamura T, Kubo S, Takahashi M, Chirieac LR, et al. BIBW2992, an irreversible EGFR/HER2 inhibitor highly effective in preclinical lung cancer models. Oncogene. 2008;27(34):4702–11.
121. Schwab CL, Bellone S, English DP, Roque DM, Lopez S, Cocco E, et al. Afatinib demonstrates remarkable activity against HER2-amplified uterine serous endometrial cancer in vitro and in vivo. Br J Cancer. 2014;111(9):1750–6.
122. Talwar S, Cohen S. Her-2 targeting in uterine papillary serous carcinoma. Gynecol Oncol Case Rep. 2012;2(3):94–6.
123. Welcker M, Clurman BE. FBW7 ubiquitin ligase: a tumour suppressor at the crossroads of cell division, growth and differentiation. Nat Rev Cancer. 2008;8(2):83–93.
124. Akhoondi S, Sun D, von der Lehr N, Apostolidou S, Klotz K, Maljukova A, et al. FBXW7/hCDC4 is a general tumor suppressor in human cancer. Can Res. 2007;67 (19):9006–12.
125. Davis RJ, Welcker M, Clurman BE. Tumor suppression by the Fbw7 ubiquitin ligase: mechanisms and opportunities. Cancer Cell. 2014;26(4):455–64.
126. Ono K, Hayashi H, Tateno M, Tanaka R, Suzuki R, Maruyama Y, et al. Uterine superficial serous carcinomas and extensive serous endometrial intraepithelial carcinomas: clinicopathological analysis of 6 patients. Int J Clin Exp Pathol. 2014;7(11):7979–88.
127. Inuzuka H, Shaik S, Onoyama I, Gao DM, Tseng A, Maser RS, et al. SCFFBW7 regulates cellular apoptosis by targeting MCL1 for ubiquitylation and destruction. Nature. 2011;471 (7336):104–9.
128. Teng CL, Hsieh YC, Phan L, Shin J, Gully C, Velazquez-Torres G, et al. FBXW7 is involved in Aurora B degradation. Cell Cycle. 2012;11(21):4059–68.
129. Thompson BJ, Buonamici S, Sulis ML, Palomero T, Vilimas T, Basso G, et al. The SCFFBW7 ubiquitin ligase complex as a tumor suppressor in T cell leukemia. J Exp Med. 2007;204(8):1825–35.
130. Wertz IE, Kusam S, Lam C, Okamoto T, Sandoval W, Anderson DJ, et al. Sensitivity to antitubulin chemotherapeutics is regulated by MCL1 and FBW7. Nature. 2011;471 (7336):110–4.
131. Malyukova A, Dohda T, von der Lehr N, Akhondi S, Corcoran M, Heyman M, et al. The tumor suppressor gene hCDC4 is frequently mutated in human T-cell acute lymphoblastic leukemia with functional consequences for Notch signaling. Cancer Res. 2007;67(12):5611–6.
132. Moberg KH, Bell DW, Wahrer DCR, Haber DA, Hariharan IK. Archipelago regulates cyclin E levels in Drosophila and is mutated in human cancer cell lines. Nature. 2001;413 (6853):311–6.

133. Kuhn E, Bahadirli-Talbott A, Shih IM. Frequent CCNE1 amplification in endometrial intraepithelial carcinoma and uterine serous carcinoma. Mod Pathol. 2014;27(7):1014–9.
134. van Pel DM, Barrett IJ, Shimizu Y, Sajesh BV, Guppy BJ, Pfeifer T, et al. An evolutionarily conserved synthetic lethal interaction network identifies fen1 as a broad-spectrum target for anticancer therapeutic development. PLoS Genet. 2013;9(1).
135. Garnett MJ, Edelman EJ, Heidorn SJ, Greenman CD, Dastur A, Lau KW, et al. Systematic identification of genomic markers of drug sensitivity in cancer cells. Nature. 2012;483 (7391):570–5.
136. He L, Torres-Lockhart K, Forster N, Ramakrishnan S, Greninger P, Garnett MJ, et al. Mcl-1 and FBW7 control a dominant survival pathway underlying HDAC and Bcl-2 inhibitor synergy in squamous cell carcinoma. Cancer Discov. 2013;3(3):324–37.
137. Yokobori T, Yokoyama Y, Mogi A, Endoh H, Altan B, Kosaka T, et al. FBXW7 mediates chemotherapeutic sensitivity and prognosis in NSCLCs. Mol Cancer Res. 2014;12(1):32–7.
138. Eichhorn PJA, Creyghton MP, Bernards R. Protein phosphatase 2A regulatory subunits and cancer. Biochim Biophys Acta. 2009;1795(1):1–15.
139. Westermarck J, Hahn WC. Multiple pathways regulated by the tumor suppressor PP2A in transformation. Trends Mol Med. 2008;14(4):152–60.
140. Ruediger R, Fields K, Walter G. Binding specificity of protein phosphatase 2A core enzyme for regulatory B subunits and T antigens. J Virol. 1999;73(1):839–42.
141. Fitzgerald TW, Gerety SS, Jones WD, van Kogelenberg M, King DA, McRae J, et al. Large-scale discovery of novel genetic causes of developmental disorders. Nature. 2015;519 (7542):223–8.
142. Brinkmann V, Billich A, Baumruker T, Heining P, Schmouder R, Francis G, et al. Fingolimod (FTY720): discovery and development of an oral drug to treat multiple sclerosis. Nat Rev Drug Discov. 2010;9(11):883–97.
143. Walter G, Ruediger R. Mouse model for probing tumor suppressor activity of protein phosphatase 2A in diverse signaling pathways. Cell Cycle. 2012;11(3):451–9.
144. Lai AY, Wade PA. Cancer biology and NuRD: a multifaceted chromatin remodelling complex. Nat Rev Cancer. 2011;11(8):588–96.
145. Torchy MP, Hamiche A, Klaholz BP. Structure and function insights into the NuRD chromatin remodeling complex. Cell Mol Life Sci. 2015;72(13):2491–507.
146. Wang HB, Zhang Y. Mi2, an auto-antigen for dermatomyositis, is an ATP-dependent nucleosome remodeling factor. Nucleic Acids Res. 2001;29(12):2517–21.
147. Gao H, Lukin K, Ramirez J, Fields S, Lopez D, Hagman J. Opposing effects of SWI/SNF and Mi-2/NuRD chromatin remodeling complexes on epigenetic reprogramming by EBF and Pax5. Proc Natl Acad Sci U S A. 2009;106(27):11258–63.
148. Reynolds N, Latos P, Hynes-Allen A, Loos R, Leaford D, O'Shaughnessy A, et al. NuRD suppresses pluripotency gene expression to promote transcriptional heterogeneity and lineage commitment. Cell Stem Cell. 2012;10(5):583–94.
149. Sims JK, Wade PA. Mi-2/NuRD complex function is required for normal S phase progression and assembly of pericentric heterochromatin. Mol Biol Cell. 2011;22(17):3094–102.
150. Larsen DH, Poinsignon C, Gudjonsson T, Dinant C, Payne MR, Hari FJ, et al. The chromatin-remodeling factor CHD4 coordinates signaling and repair after DNA damage. J Cell Biol. 2010;190(5):731–40.
151. Smeenk G, Wiegant WW, Vrolijk H, Solari AP, Pastink A, van Attikum H. The NuRD chromatin-remodeling complex regulates signaling and repair of DNA damage. J Cell Biol. 2010;190(5):741–9.
152. Guillemette S, Serra RW, Peng M, Hayes JA, Konstantinopoulos PA, Green MR, et al. Resistance to therapy in BRCA2 mutant cells due to loss of the nucleosome remodeling factor CHD4. Gene Dev. 2015;29(5):489–94.
153. Pan MR, Hsieh HJ, Dai H, Hung WC, Li K, Peng G, et al. Chromodomain helicase DNA-binding protein 4 (CHD4) regulates homologous recombination DNA repair, and its

deficiency sensitizes cells to poly(ADP-ribose) polymerase (PARP) inhibitor treatment. J Biol Chem. 2012;287(9):6764–72.
154. Polo SE, Kaidi A, Baskcomb L, Galanty Y, Jackson SP. Regulation of DNA-damage responses and cell-cycle progression by the chromatin remodelling factor CHD4. EMBO J. 2010;29(18):3130–9.
155. Pegoraro G, Kubben N, Wickert U, Gohler H, Hoffmann K, Misteli T. Ageing-related chromatin defects through loss of the NURD complex. Nat Cell Biol. 2009;11(10):1261–7.
156. Luijsterburg MS, Acs K, Ackermann L, Wiegant WW, Bekker-Jensen S, Larsen DH, et al. A new non-catalytic role for ubiquitin ligase RNF8 in unfolding higher-order chromatin structure. EMBO J. 2012;31(11):2511–27.
157. Urquhart AJ, Gatei M, Richard DJ, Khanna KK. ATM mediated phosphorylation of CHD4 contributes to genome maintenance. Genome Integr. 2011;2(1):1.
158. Amaya M, Desai M, Gnanapragasam MN, Wang SZ, Zu Zhu S, Williams DC Jr, et al. Mi2beta-mediated silencing of the fetal gamma-globin gene in adult erythroid cells. Blood. 2013;121(17):3493–501.
159. Hosokawa H, Tanaka T, Suzuki Y, Iwamura C, Ohkubo S, Endoh K, et al. Functionally distinct Gata3/Chd4 complexes coordinately establish T helper 2 (Th2) cell identity. Proc Natl Acad Sci U S A. 2013;110(12):4691–6.
160. Williams CJ, Naito T, Arco PG, Seavitt JR, Cashman SM, De Souza B, et al. The chromatin remodeler Mi-2beta is required for CD4 expression and T cell development. Immunity. 2004;20(6):719–33.
161. Morra R, Lee BM, Shaw H, Tuma R, Mancini EJ. Concerted action of the PHD, chromo and motor domains regulates the human chromatin remodelling ATPase CHD4. FEBS Lett. 2012;586(16):2513–21.
162. Ramirez J, Dege C, Kutateladze TG, Hagman J. MBD2 and multiple domains of CHD4 are required for transcriptional repression by Mi-2/NuRD complexes. Mol Cell Biol. 2012;32 (24):5078–88.
163. Watson AA, Mahajan P, Mertens HD, Deery MJ, Zhang W, Pham P, et al. The PHD and chromo domains regulate the ATPase activity of the human chromatin remodeler CHD4. J Mol Biol. 2012;422(1):3–17.
164. Schmidt DR, Schreiber SL. Molecular association between ATR and two components of the nucleosome remodeling and deacetylating complex, HDAC2 and CHD4. Biochemistry. 1999;38(44):14711–7.
165. Shimono Y, Murakami H, Kawai K, Wade PA, Shimokata K, Takahashi M. Mi-2 beta associates with BRG1 and RET finger protein at the distinct regions with transcriptional activating and repressing abilities. J Biol Chem. 2003;278(51):51638–45.
166. Srinivasan R, Mager GM, Ward RM, Mayer J, Svaren J. NAB2 represses transcription by interacting with the CHD4 subunit of the nucleosome remodeling and deacetylase (NuRD) complex. J Biol Chem. 2006;281(22):15129–37.
167. Geyer R, Wee S, Anderson S, Yates J, Wolf DA. BTB/POZ domain proteins are putative substrate adaptors for cullin 3 ubiquitin ligases. Mol Cell. 2003;12(3):783–90.
168. Hernandez-Munoz I, Lund AH, van der Stoop P, Boutsma E, Muijrers I, Verhoeven E, et al. Stable X chromosome inactivation involves the PRC1 Polycomb complex and requires histone MACROH2A1 and the CULLIN3/SPOP ubiquitin E3 ligase. Proc Natl Acad Sci U S A. 2005;102(21):7635–40.
169. An J, Wang CJ, Deng YB, Yu L, Huang HJ. Destruction of full-length androgen receptor by wild-type SPOP, but not prostate-cancer-associated mutants. Cell Rep. 2014;6(4):657–69.
170. Kim B, Nam HJ, Pyo KE, Jang MJ, Kim IS, Kim D, et al. Breast cancer metastasis suppressor 1 (BRMS1) is destabilized by the Cul3-SPOP E3 ubiquitin ligase complex. Biochem Biophys Res Commun. 2011;415(4):720–6.
171. Kwon JE, La M, Oh KH, Oh YM, Kim GR, Seol JH, et al. BTB domain-containing speckle-type POZ protein (SPOP) serves as an adaptor of Daxx for ubiquitination by Cul3-based ubiquitin ligase. J Biol Chem. 2006;281(18):12664–72.

172. La M, Kim K, Park J, Won J, Lee JH, Fu YM, et al. Daxx-mediated transcriptional repression of MMP1 gene is reversed by SPOP. Biochem Biophys Res Commun. 2004;320 (3):760–5.
173. Zhang PZ, Gao K, Tang Y, Jin XF, An J, Yu HX, et al. Destruction of DDIT3/CHOP Protein by Wild-Type SPOP but not prostate cancer-associated mutants. Hum Mutat. 2014;35 (9):1142–51.
174. Wang CB, Pan Y, Wang BL. Suppressor of fused and Spop regulate the stability, processing and function of Gli2 and Gli3 full-length activators but not their repressors. Development. 2010;137(12):2001–9.
175. Zhang Q, Zhang L, Wang B, Ou CY, Chien CT, Jiang J. A hedgehog-induced BTB protein modulates hedgehog signaling by degrading Ci/Gli transcription factor. Dev Cell. 2006;10 (6):719–29.
176. Theurillat JP, Udeshi ND, Errington WJ, Svinkina T, Baca SC, Pop M, et al. Prostate cancer. Ubiquitylome analysis identifies dysregulation of effector substrates in SPOP-mutant prostate cancer. Science. 2014;346(6205):85–9.
177. Byun B, Jung Y. Repression of transcriptional activity of estrogen receptor alpha by a Cullin3/SPOP ubiquitin E3 ligase complex. Mol Cell. 2008;25(2):289–93.
178. Zhang P, Gao K, Jin X, Ma J, Peng J, Wumaier R, et al. Endometrial cancer-associated mutants of SPOP are defective in regulating estrogen receptor-alpha protein turnover. Cell Death Dis. 2015;6:e1687.
179. Takahashi I, Kameoka Y, Hashimoto K. MacroH2A1.2 binds the nuclear protein Spop. Biochem Biophys Acta. 2002;1591(1–3):63–8.
180. Bunce MW, Boronenkov IV, Anderson RA. Coordinated activation of the nuclear ubiquitin ligase Cul3-SPOP by the generation of phosphatidylinositol 5-phosphate. J Biol Chem. 2008;283(13):8678–86.
181. Claiborn KC, Sachdeva MM, Cannon CE, Groff DN, Singer JD, Stoffers DA. Pcif1 modulates Pdx1 protein stability and pancreatic beta cell function and survival in mice. J Clin Investig. 2010;120(10):3713–21.
182. Li C, Ao J, Fu J, Lee DF, Xu J, Lonard D, et al. Tumor-suppressor role for the SPOP ubiquitin ligase in signal-dependent proteolysis of the oncogenic co-activator SRC-3/AIB1. Oncogene. 2011;30(42):4350–64.
183. Li GQ, Ci WM, Karmakar S, Chen K, Dhar R, Fan ZX, et al. SPOP promotes tumorigenesis by acting as a key regulatory hub in kidney cancer. Cancer Cell. 2014;25(4):455–68.
184. Zhuang M, Calabrese MF, Liu J, Waddell MB, Nourse A, Hammel M, et al. Structures of SPOP-substrate complexes: insights into molecular architectures of BTB-Cul3 ubiquitin ligases. Mol Cell. 2009;36(1):39–50.
185. Barbieri CE, Baca SC, Lawrence MS, Demichelis F, Blattner M, Theurillat JP, et al. Exome sequencing identifies recurrent SPOP, FOXA1 and MED12 mutations in prostate cancer. Nat Genet. 2012;44(6):685–9.
186. Blattner M, Lee DJ, O'Reilly C, Park K, MacDonald TY, Khani F, et al. SPOP mutations in prostate cancer across demographically diverse patient cohorts. Neoplasia. 2014;16(1): 14–20.
187. Buckles E, Qian C, Tadros A, Majumdar S, Cvitanovic J, Zabaleta J, et al. Identification of speckle-type POZ protein somatic mutations in African American prostate cancer. Asian J Androl. 2014;16(6):829–32.
188. Garcia-Flores M, Casanova-Salas I, Rubio-Briones J, Calatrava A, Dominguez-Escrig J, Rubio L, et al. Clinico-pathological significance of the molecular alterations of the SPOP gene in prostate cancer. Eur J Cancer. 2014;50(17):2994–3002.
189. Papai G, Weil PA, Schultz P. New insights into the function of transcription factor TFIID from recent structural studies. Curr Opin Genet Dev. 2011;21(2):219–24.
190. Wassarman DA, Sauer F. TAF(II)250: a transcription toolbox. J Cell Sci. 2001; 114(Pt 16):2895–902.

191. Chen JL, Attardi LD, Verrijzer CP, Yokomori K, Tjian R. Assembly of recombinant TFIID reveals differential coactivator requirements for distinct transcriptional activators. Cell. 1994;79(1):93–105.
192. Singh MV, Bland CE, Weil PA. Molecular and genetic characterization of a Taf1p domain essential for yeast TFIID assembly. Mol Cell Biol. 2004;24(11):4929–42.
193. Ohtsuki K, Kasahara K, Shirahige K, Kokubo T. Genome-wide localization analysis of a complete set of Tafs reveals a specific effect of the taf1 mutation on Taf2 occupancy and provides indirect evidence for different TFIID conformations at different promoters. Nucleic Acids Res. 2010;38(6):1805–20.
194. Jacobson RH, Ladurner AG, King DS, Tjian R. Structure and function of a human TAFII250 double bromodomain module. Science. 2000;288(5470):1422–5.
195. Gegonne A, Weissman JD, Singer DS. TAFII55 binding to TAFII250 inhibits its acetyltransferase activity. Proc Natl Acad Sci U S A. 2001;98(22):12432–7.
196. Kloet SL, Whiting JL, Gafken P, Ranish J, Wang EH. Phosphorylation-dependent regulation of cyclin D1 and cyclin A gene transcription by TFIID subunits TAF1 and TAF7. Mol Cell Biol. 2012;32(16):3358–69.
197. Mal TK, Masutomi Y, Zheng L, Nakata Y, Ohta H, Nakatani Y, et al. Structural and functional characterization on the interaction of yeast TFIID subunit TAF1 with TATA-binding protein. J Mol Biol. 2004;339(4):681–93.
198. Maile T, Kwoczynski S, Katzenberger RJ, Wassarman DA, Sauer F. TAF1 activates transcription by phosphorylation of serine 33 in histone H2B. Science. 2004;304(5673):1010–4.
199. Boutet SC, Biressi S, Iori K, Natu V, Rando TA. Taf1 regulates Pax3 protein by monoubiquitination in skeletal muscle progenitors. Mol Cell. 2010;40(5):749–61.
200. Pham AD, Sauer F. Ubiquitin-activating/conjugating activity of TAFII250, a mediator of activation of gene expression in Drosophila. Science. 2000;289(5488):2357–60.
201. Mizzen CA, Yang XJ, Kokubo T, Brownell JE, Bannister AJ, OwenHughes T, et al. The TAF(II)250 subunit of TFIID has histone acetyltransferase activity. Cell. 1996;87(7):1261–70.
202. Morin RD, Mungall K, Pleasance E, Mungall AJ, Goya R, Huff RD, et al. Mutational and structural analysis of diffuse large B-cell lymphoma using whole-genome sequencing. Blood. 2013;122(7):1256–65.
203. Northcott PA, Jones DT, Kool M, Robinson GW, Gilbertson RJ, Cho YJ, et al. Medulloblastomics: the end of the beginning. Nat Rev Cancer. 2012;12(12):818–34.
204. Baudot A, de la Torre V, Valencia A. Mutated genes, pathways and processes in tumours. EMBO Rep. 2010;11(10):805–10.
205. Kandoth C, McLellan MD, Vandin F, Ye K, Niu B, Lu C, et al. Mutational landscape and significance across 12 major cancer types. Nature. 2013;502(7471):333–9.
206. Wang H, Curran EC, Hinds TR, Wang EH, Zheng N. Crystal structure of a TAF1-TAF7 complex in human transcription factor IID reveals a promoter binding module. Cell Res. 2014;24(12):1433–44.
207. McKeown MR, Shaw DL, Fu H, Liu S, Xu X, Marineau JJ, et al. Biased multicomponent reactions to develop novel bromodomain inhibitors. J Med Chem. 2014;57(21):9019–27.
208. Takebe N, McShane L, Conley B. Biomarkers: exceptional responders-discovering predictive biomarkers. Nat Rev Clin Oncol. 2015;12(3):132–4.
209. Mandrekar SJ, Dahlberg SE, Simon R. Improving clinical trial efficiency: thinking outside the box. Available from: http://meetinglibrary.asco.org/content/11500141–156.
210. NCI MPACT. Available from: http://dctd.cancer.gov/MajorInitiatives/NCI-sponsored_trials_in_precision_medicine.htm-h05.
211. Conley BA, Doroshow JH. Molecular analysis for therapy choice: NCI MATCH. Semin Oncol. 2014;41(3):297–9.
212. Rodon J, Soria JC, Berger R, Batist G, Tsimberidou A, Bresson C, et al. Challenges in initiating and conducting personalized cancer therapy trials: perspectives from WINTHER, a worldwide innovative network (WIN) consortium trial. Ann Oncol. 2015.

213. Stelloo E, Bosse T, Nout RA, MacKay HJ, Church DN, Nijman HW, et al. Refining prognosis and identifying targetable pathways for high-risk endometrial cancer; a TransPORTEC initiative. Mod Pathol. 2015;28(6):836–44.
214. McConechy MK, Ding JR, Cheang MCU, Wiegand KC, Senz J, Tone AA, et al. Use of mutation profiles to refine the classification of endometrial carcinomas. J Pathol. 2012;228 (1):20–30.
215. Liang H, Cheung LW, Li J, Ju Z, Yu S, Stemke-Hale K, et al. Whole-exome sequencing combined with functional genomics reveals novel candidate driver cancer genes in endometrial cancer. Genome Res. 2012;22(11):2120–9.
216. Peterson LM, Kipp BR, Halling KC, Kerr SE, Smith DI, Distad TJ, et al. Molecular characterization of endometrial cancer: a correlative study assessing microsatellite instability, MLH1 hypermethylation, DNA mismatch repair protein expression, and PTEN, PIK3CA, KRAS, and BRAF mutation analysis. Int J Gynecol Pathol. 2012;31(3):195–205.
217. Bashir S, Jiang G, Joshi A, Miller C Jr, Matrai C, Yemelyanova A, et al. Molecular alterations of PIK3CA in uterine carcinosarcoma, clear cell, and serous tumors. Inter J Gynecol Cancer. 2014;24(7):1262–7.
218. Han G, Soslow RA, Wethington S, Levine DA, Bogomolniy F, Clement PB, et al. Endometrial carcinomas with clear cells: a study of a heterogeneous group of tumors including interobserver variability, mutation analysis, and immunohistochemistry with HNF-1beta. Int J Gynecol Pathol. 2015;34(4):323–33.
219. McConechy MK, Anglesio MS, Kalloger SE, Yang W, Senz J, Chow C, et al. Subtype-specific mutation of PPP2R1A in endometrial and ovarian carcinomas. J Pathol. 2011;223(5):567–73.
220. Nagendra DC, Burke J 3rd, Maxwell GL, Risinger JI. PPP2R1A mutations are common in the serous type of endometrial cancer. Mol Carcinog. 2012;51(10):826–31.
221. Shih IM, Panuganti PK, Kuo KT, Mao TL, Kuhn E, Jones S, et al. Somatic mutations of PPP2R1A in ovarian and uterine carcinomas. Am J Pathol. 2011;178(4):1442–7.
222. Micci F, Teixeira MR, Haugom L, Kristensen G, Abeler VM, Heim S. Genomic aberrations in carcinomas of the uterine corpus. Gene Chromosomes Cancer. 2004;40(3):229–46.
223. Santin AD, Bellone S, Van Stedum S, Bushen W, Palmieri M, Siegel ER, et al. Amplification of c-erbB2 oncogene: a major prognostic indicator in uterine serous papillary carcinoma. Cancer. 2005;104(7):1391–7.
224. Konecny GE, Santos L, Winterhoff B, Hatmal M, Keeney GL, Mariani A, et al. HER2 gene amplification and EGFR expression in a large cohort of surgically staged patients with nonendometrioid (type II) endometrial cancer. Br J Cancer. 2009;100(1):89–95.

Chapter 6
Uterine Clear Cell Carcinoma

Melissa K. McConechy, Cheng-Han Lee and Blaise A. Clarke

Introduction

Clear cell carcinoma (CCC) is a rare subtype of endometrial cancer [1]. While the frequency of this subtype has been reported to range between 1 and 7%, pure endometrial CCC (excluding cases with mixed subtypes) likely accounts for only 1% of all endometrial cancers [2]. The first reported case of endometrial CCC was described by Dr. De Bonneville in a German report in 1911 [3]. In a comprehensive pathology review by Drs. Clement and Young [2], it is acknowledged that CCCs were not widely recognized until the 1960s and 1970s [3–5]. In 1994, CCC was formally added to the classification of endometrial carcinomas by the World Health Organization (WHO) and the International Society of Gynecologic Pathologists [6]. In 1983, Bokhman proposed the classic dualistic histopathologic model separating endometrial cancer histotypes into two broad types; type 1 as estrogen-dependent endometrioid endometrial carcinoma (EEC), and type 2 non-endometrioid endometrial carcinoma (NEEC) [7]. This was based on pathogenetic features including clinical, metabolic, and endocrine characteristics. However, Bokhman did not acknowledge all endometrial subtypes in his dualistic model; for example CCC,

M.K. McConechy
Department of Human Genetics, Research Institute of the McGill University Health Centre, McGill University, 1001 Décarie Boulevard, Montreal, QC H4A 3J1, Canada

C.-H. Lee
Department of Laboratory Medicine and Pathology, University of Alberta, 4B1.21 Walter Mackenzie Centre 8440-112 Street, Edmonton AB T6G 2B7, Canada

B.A. Clarke (✉)
Department of Laboratory Medicine and Pathobiology, University of Toronto, University Health Network, Toronto, ON M5G 2C4, Canada
e-mail: blaise.clarke@uhn.ca

M.T. Deavers and D.M. Coffey (eds.), *Precision Molecular Pathology of Uterine Cancer*, Molecular Pathology Library,
DOI 10.1007/978-3-319-57985-6_6

carcinosarcoma, and undifferentiated carcinoma were not included [8, 9]. While endometrial CCC was never included in this model, most studies have grouped endometrial CCC together with serous carcinoma in this dualistic historical classification [10].

Clinically, CCC of the endometrium has a poor prognosis with a tendency to metastasize to lymph nodes and the peritoneal cavity, and has a poor response to standard chemotherapy [11–14]. The overall five-year survival rate for stages I–IV is 79, 77, 47, and 21%, respectively [14]. Driven by the clinical need for more effective systemic therapies, there are ongoing and emerging clinical trials evaluating the efficacy of targeted therapies (i.e., Temsirolimus or Sunitinib) on both ovarian and endometrial CCCs (clinical trial NCT01396408) [15]. Accurate classification and diagnosis of endometrial CCC is therefore important. However, it is increasingly recognized that a subset of other more common subtypes of endometrial carcinoma, such as endometrioid adenocarcinoma and serous carcinoma, can display significant morphologic overlap with CCC. Therefore, it can be difficult to differentiate CCC from its mimics in some instances, and this contributes to significant interobserver variability in the diagnosis of CCC [16–18]. In addition, there are also tumors that exhibit a mixture of different histologic subtypes, thus prompting the diagnosis of mixed-type carcinoma that includes a CCC component [2]. However, there is emerging evidence that most such mixed-type endometrial carcinomas with a CCC component may not be clinically and biologically the same as pure endometrial CCC.

The relative rarity of endometrial CCC and the diagnostic difficulties present significant challenges to a better understanding of endometrial CCC. As such, most of our current understanding about endometrial CCC was advanced through study of its ovarian counterpart. In this chapter, we will review the molecular features of endometrial CCC, with an emphasis on recent and emerging findings that will likely impact the management of this disease.

Histopathologic Features

Like its ovarian counterpart, endometrial CCC can exhibit a range of architectural patterns (papillary, glandular, solid, and cystic) and cytoplasmic features (clear and oxyphilic) [19]. In the largest series of rigorously reviewed pure endometrial CCCs to date [19], about 90% of endometrial CCCs display a mixture of architectural patterns, with the glandular pattern being the most common and predominant, followed by papillary, solid, and cystic patterns in decreasing order of frequency (Fig. 6.1). The tumor cells are cuboidal in shape and may display a hobnail appearance in the glandular, papillary, and cystic areas. The cytoplasm can be clear or eosinophilic in tincture and the great majority of cases have a mix of clear and eosinophilic cytoplasm. About 10% of the cases have purely eosinophilic cytoplasm (eosinophilic variant of clear cell carcinoma). There is typically moderate nuclear atypia with most tumors containing focally prominent nucleoli. Nuclear stratification is uncommon and focal if present. Mitotic activity is typically low (<5 mitotic figures per 10 high power fields). Stromal hyalinization and hyaline bodies are seen in a subset of cases. It is important to note that the above descriptions are for histologically conventional and unambiguous cases of pure endometrial CCCs. It is also well recognized that the two most common subtypes of endometrial carcinoma—endometrioid adenocarcinoma and serous carcinoma can exhibit varying amounts and varying degrees of clear cell features in some cases [20]. Thus, there are morphologically ambiguous cases that can display hybrid histology (features intermediate between different histologic subtypes) or spatially mixed cases with different areas exhibiting different histotypes (potential collision tumor).

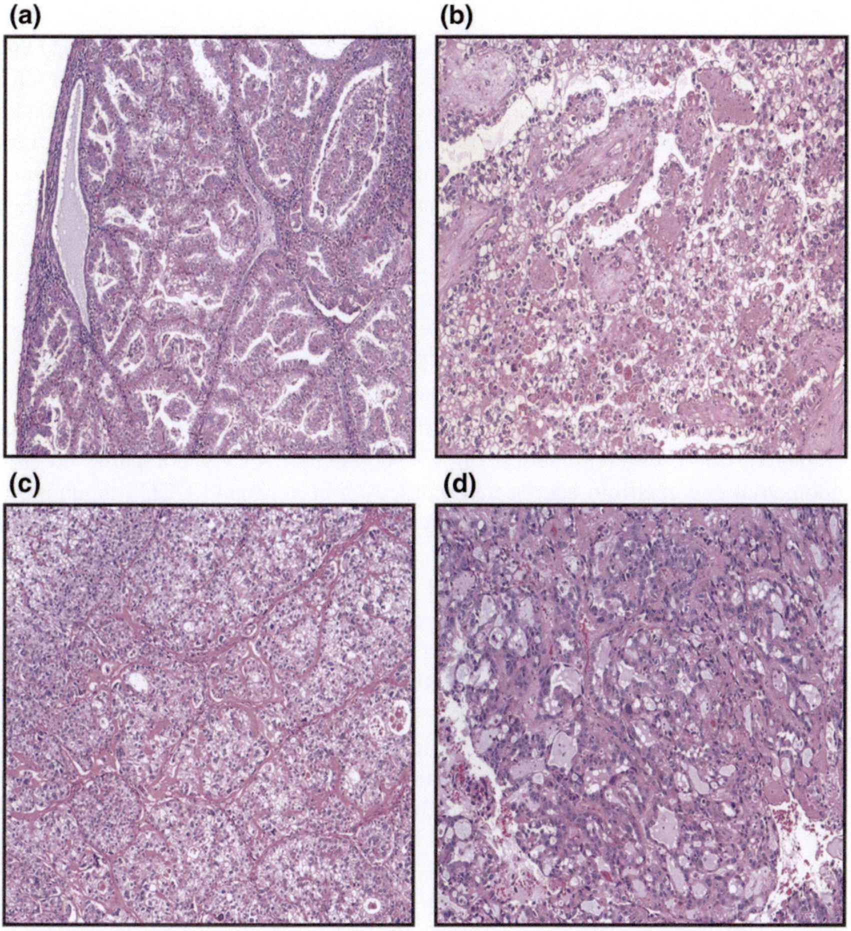

Fig. 6.1 Histologic features of pure endometrial clear cell carcinoma. **a** Clear cell carcinoma with glandular architecture, **b** clear cell carcinoma with papillary architecture and prominent stromal hyalinization, **c** clear cell carcinoma with solid growth pattern, **d** clear cell carcinoma with tubulocystic growth pattern

Immunophenotypic Features

Given the routine use of immunohistochemistry in diagnostic pathology, significant effort has been made to determine the immunophenotype of endometrial CCC in an attempt to identify a panel of immunomarkers that may aid in its diagnosis. This section provides a description of immunohistochemical markers that have been used to define endometrial CCC, although not all markers are considered clinically useful. The studies discussed herein summarized in Table 6.1.

One of the first immunoprofiles of CCC by Lax et al. characterized tumors by ER and PR immunonegativity, low p53 immunoreactivity, and a high Ki67 proliferation index [21] (Fig. 6.2a). The first comprehensive study to determine the immunohistochemical profiles of CCCs came from Vang et al. in 2001, in which they studied 13 different markers in a small number of ovarian CCC (n = 11) and uterine CCC (n = 5) [22]. Uterine clear cell tumors were immunopositive for CK7 (100%), CAM5.2 (100%), 34βE12 (80%), CEA (100%), Leu-MI (100%), Vimentin (100%), bcl-2 (80%), p53 (100%), CA-125 (100%), and Her-2/neu (20%). Markers that were negative included CK20, ER, and PR. These immunoprofiles were found to be similar in the ovary, endometrium, and genitourinary tract, and therefore, they are generally not useful in distinguishing the primary site of origin [22]. A second immunohistochemical study by Vang et al., tested a panel of immunomarkers with the of goal distinguishing Arias-Stella reaction from high-grade endometrial carcinomas, in particular CCCs [23]. In this series, the majority of uterine clear cell carcinomas were Ki67 positive (82%), p53 positive (73%), and ER and PR negative. These markers, although helpful in the differential diagnosis of CCC and Arias-Stella reaction, did not aid in distinguishing endometrial CCC from serous carcinoma. In a different series of 13 endometrial CCCs compared to 144 endometrial endometrioid adenocarcinomas, Arai et al., found CCC immunopositivity for p53, cyclin A, Ki67, and P-glycoprotein, but low or no expressivity of cyclin E, E-cadherin, and PR [24].

The gene *HNF1β* was first described to be associated with ovarian CCC and ovarian endometriosis using DNA microarray gene expression analysis [25, 26]. Using this association, Yamamoto et al., first described strong immunoreactivity of HNF-1β in a small number of endometrial CCC (n = 5), with all other endometrial histologies negative [27]. All ovarian CCCs were also strongly positive for HNF-1β, with other ovarian histologies mostly negative. Hoang et al., described the use of a panel of HNF-1β, ER, and p53 immunomarkers to distinguish prototypical endometrial CCC (n = 15) from endometrial serous and endometrioid carcinomas [28]. All prototypical CCC were HNF-1β positive (diffuse moderate to strong nuclear staining), all except one was ER negative, and 33% displayed aberrant p53 staining (Fig. 6.2). In contrast, endometrioid adenocarcinomas were all HNF-1β negative, the majority ER positive, and 20% had an abnormal p53. Serous carcinomas exhibited HNF-1β positive or negative staining, all except one was ER positive, and all had aberrant p53 staining. In this study, a prototypical CCC was

Table 6.1 A subset of immunohistochemical markers used in endometrial clear cell carcinomas diagnosis

Study	*N*	HNF-1β positive (%)	ER positive (%)	p53 positive (%)	Napsin A positive (%)	PR positive (%)	Loss of BAF250a (%)	Ki67 (%)
Vang et al. [22]	5	NA	0	5 (100)	NA	0	NA	NA
Arai et al. [24][a]	13	NA	NA	46.4 ± 24.3	NA	0	NA	52.1 ± 20.5
Vang et al. [23]	11	NA	0	8 (73)	NA	1 (9)	NA	9 (82)
Yamamoto et al. [27]	5	5 (100)	NA	NA	NA	NA	NA	NA
Wiegand et al. [31]	23	NA	NA	NA	NA	NA	6 (26)	NA
Fadare et al. [32]	22	NA	NA	NA	NA	NA	5 (23)	NA
Fadare et al. [35]	50	NA	NA	17 (34)	NA	NA	10 (20)	NA
Fadare et al. [94]	15	11 (73%)	NA	NA	NA	NA	NA	NA
Hoang et al. [28][b]	15	15 (100)	1 (7)	5 (33)[c]	NA	NA	NA	NA
Lim et al. [34]	24	20 (83)	5 (21)	NA	18 (75)	3 (13)	3 (13)	NA
Fadare et al. [38]	49	NA	NA	NA	43 (88)	NA	NA	NA
Hoang et al. [33][b]	15	15 (100)	1 (7)	5 (33)[c]	14 (93)	NA	2 (13)	NA
Iwamoto et al. [39]	15	NA	NA	NA	10 (67)	NA	NA	NA
Overall Summary	247	51 (86)	6 (15)	35 (43)	85 (83)	4 (11)	26 (19)	9 (82)

NA indicates marker was not used in the study. The overall summary percentages are a reflection of the column, and only accounts for the studies in which the marker was evaluated

[a]This study expressed results as LI (labeling index) based on the percentages of positive nuclei of at least 1200 cells and is not included in the overall summary

[b]These two studies use the same cohort of prototypical endometrial clear cell carcinomas and are not duplicated in the overall summary numbers and percentages

[c]Four of these tumors had diffuse strong staining indicating presence of a *TP53* missense mutation, and one tumor had complete absence of p53 nuclear staining indicating a truncating or nonsense *TP53* mutation

characterized by a profile with HNF-1β positive, ER negative, and either p53 diffuse or absent immunostaining [28].

Mutations in the gene *ARID1A* results in loss of the BAF250a protein, which was originally identified in 46–57% of ovarian CCCs and endometriosis precursors [29, 30]. The histologic similarities of ovarian and endometrial CCC, also led to the exploration of loss of BAF250a in endometrial CCC. In a study of BAF250a loss in a number of different tumor types, 26% (6 of 23 cases) of endometrial CCC were found to be immunonegative for BAF250a [31]. In a subsequent study, 23% of pure endometrial CCC were BAF250a negative and these tumors were significantly more likely to present with advanced stage disease [32]. Additional studies have displayed loss of BAF250a in 13% of endometrial CCC [33, 34]. In a follow-up study by Fadre et al., the authors set out to determine if loss of BAF250a expression and p53 immunopositive staining was associated with prognostic significance. They discovered that 20% of endometrial CCC were BAF250a negative, but that this was not prognostically significant despite earlier studies reporting the association of protein loss in advanced stage tumors [35].

Immunohistochemical expression of the protein napsin A has been reported in 8–10% of endometrial carcinomas [36, 37]. In endometrial CCC, the expression of napsin A is frequent (88%), with napsin A being negative or low in endometrial endometrioid and serous carcinomas [38]. Expression is not associated with outcome or other clinicopathologic factors. In a separate study, 75% of endometrial CCC were napsin A immunopositive, with no expression in endometrioid adenocarcinoma or endometrioid adenocarcinoma with clear cell changes [34]. Napsin A alone as a diagnostic marker for CCC had high specificity (93%) and sensitivity (87.5%). Iwamoto et al., reported a series of endometrial CCC (n = 15) with 67% napsin A positive expression, 100% PAX8 positive, 80% CA125 positive, and 93% TTF-1 (thyroid transcription factor 1) negative. These markers were used to distinguish CCC from other ovarian and endometrial histotypes [39]. Lastly, in a consensus-reviewed cohort of 15 prototypical CCC, an immunoanalysis of napsin A and ARID1A/BAF250a, and a mutational analysis were performed [33]. Napsin A positivity was observed in 93% of clear cell tumors and 13% had loss of BAF250a. Thus, napsin A immunoexpression has the potential for being a diagnostic adjunct in distinguishing typical CCC from endometrial histological mimics. Furthermore, it has been suggested that the expression of napsin A may provide insight into why clear cell carcinoma patients may be at increased risk for venous thromboembolic events [38, 40].

Early immunohistochemical analyses of p53 were difficult to interpret [41, 42], as they predate subsequent studies that better defined the relationship between *TP53* mutation status and protein expression patterns by immunohistochemistry [43, 44]. Missense mutations in *TP53* cause accumulation of nuclear p53 and they typically result in strong diffuse nuclear p53 immunopositivity [45]. In contrast, null mutations (nonsense, deletions, and insertions) typically result in a complete loss of p53 immunostaining, though this can be difficult to interpret if there is no internal positive control present [46]. In studies that applied the more up-to-date interpretation of p53 immunohistochemistry, abnormal p53 immunostaining that suggests

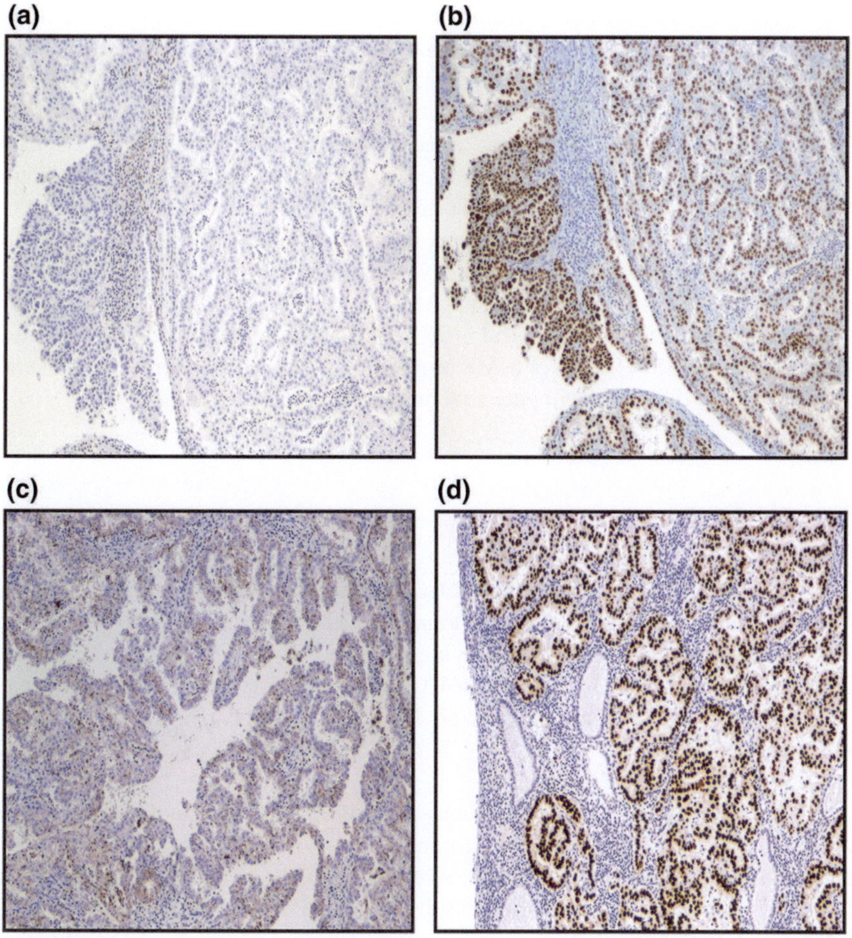

Fig. 6.2 Immunohistochemical features of pure endometrial clear cell carcinoma. **a** Negative estrogen receptor (*ER*) with internal stroma positive control, **b** diffuse HNF-1β nuclear staining, **c** cytoplasmic Napsin A staining, **d** diffuse strong nuclear p53 staining in a clear cell carcinoma harboring a R141C missense TP53 mutation (in contrast to the wild-type p53 staining pattern in the adjacent normal endometrial glands)

the presence of *TP53* mutation was observed in about a third of endometrial CCC [33, 35].

Overall, it is clear that at present, no single immunomarker marker alone is sufficient to support an unequivocal diagnosis of endometrial clear cell carcinoma. One therefore has to make use of a combination of markers. The majority of pure endometrial clear cell carcinomas have an HNF-1β-positive, napsin A-positive, and ER-negative immunoprofile, while exhibiting a wild-type p53 staining pattern. As such, tumors that exhibit the histologic features and the prototypical immunoprofile of clear cell carcinoma can be classified as endometrial clear cell carcinoma.

The diagnostic challenge lies with tumors that exhibit an atypical immunophenotype. For instance, about a third of pure endometrial clear cell carcinomas have a mutated p53 immunostaining pattern, and within this TP53-mutated subset some exhibit a mutational profile that is identical to endometrial serous carcinoma (with concurrent TP53 and PPP2R1A mutations, and a lack of ARID1A mutation). It is therefore plausible that some of these TP53-mutated endometrial clear cell carcinomas may actually be serous carcinomas. On that note, there is also evidence to suggest that TP53-mutated endometrial clear cell carcinomas behave more aggressive clinically than tumors with wild-type TP53 [35]. As for mixed histotype endometrial carcinomas with a clear cell carcinoma component, MSI or MMR protein immunohistochemical studies may provide useful insight into the nature of these tumors, as those having identical MSI-H status or MMR protein deficiency in the different components are molecularly different from pure endometrial clear cell carcinoma.

Genetic Features

Given the rarity of pure endometrial CCC, there are only a few studies in the literature that have examined pure endometrial CCC. The mutation frequencies for each of the studies described herein are found in Table 6.2. The first study to identify DNA mutations in endometrial CCC (n = 14) described *PTEN* mutations in 21% of tumors, 9% of pure tumors with *TP53* mutations [47], and 4 (29%) mixed tumors with clear cell components with *TP53* mutations. Microsatellite instability (MI) was identified in 2 cases (14%).

Mutations in *PIK3CA* and other genes in the PI3K pathway have been identified in all subtypes of endometrial carcinoma [48, 49], with a high frequency in endometrioid adenocarcinomas [50]. Few studies have identified *PIK3CA* mutations in CCC, with frequencies ranging from 9 to 30% [33, 50–52]. In a study by Bashir et al. [51] 17% (3 of 18 cases) harbored *PIK3CA* mutations, all identified in exon 4, which is outside of the hotspot helical (exon 9) and kinase (exon 20) domains. Moreover in all other studies, *PIK3CA* mutations were found in multiple exons as well as the classic hotspot regions.

A study by Rudd et al. sequenced serous and clear cell carcinomas to determine the mutational landscape of tyrosine kinases in an effort to provide targets for therapeutics [53]. Mutations in these genes were rare, as only 1 of 21 (5%) CCC harbored a mutation in the gene *TNK2* (Tyrosine kinase non-receptor protein 2). This particular tumor was also MSI positive; therefore, the *TNK2* mutation could have been a passenger mutation as a consequence of mismatch repair deficiency. The MSI status of theses tumors was previously reported as 3 of 23 tumors (13%) being MSI positive [54]. Additionally, 1 of 21 (5%) tumors harbored a *POLE* mutation in the exonuclease domain; this event was mutually exclusive from the *TNK2* mutation and MSI positivity [53].

Gallo et al. was the first to perform whole exome sequencing in endometrial serous carcinomas to identify recurrent mutations in chromatin remodeling and ubiquitin ligase complex genes [54]. From this group of genes, endometrial CCC were resequenced to identify 22% (5 of 23) harboring mutations in ubiquitin ligase complex genes (*FBXW7, SPOP*) and 22% (5 of 23) with mutations in chromatin-remodeling genes (*CHD4, EP300, ARID1A, BAZ1B*).

To study the molecular genetic features of pure endometrial CCC, Hoang et al. [33] sequenced a panel of genes previously identified to be recurrently mutated in ovarian and endometrial carcinomas [49, 54, 55]. In this series, 29% (4 of 14) harbored *TP53* mutations, 29% (4 of 14) *SPOP* mutations, 21% (3 of 14) *PPP2R1A* mutations, and 7% (1 of 14) with *FBXW7* mutations. This mutational profile is similar to serous-type carcinoma. While previous studies have found mutations in the PI3K pathway, only 14% (2 of 14) of tumors contained *PIK3CA* mutations and no mutations were identified in *PTEN.* ARID1A mutations were identified in 14% of tumors (2 of 14), 1 had a *KRAS* mutation (non-hotspot), and no *CTNNB1* mutations were found. In addition, all 14 pure CCC had intact mismatch repair protein expression by immunohistochemistry. Therefore, the authors concluded that most endometrial CCC lack mutations that are more commonly seen in endometrioid adenocarcinomas. Interestingly, *TP53*-mutated endometrial CCC demonstrate overlap with serous carcinomas, with half of the *TP53*-mutated CCC having a serous-type mutation profile (concurrent *TP53* and *PPP2R1A* mutations).

Recently, gain-of-function mutations at the telomerase reverse transcriptase TERT promoter has been identified in a subset (21%) of endometrial CCC [56]. Upregulated expression of TERT is believed to aid in the maintenance of telomere length and tumor development.

To date, there have been no published reports of whole genome or exome sequencing performed on pure endometrial CCC. This rare tumor was not included in the TCGA endometrial sequencing project [55], therefore more genetic analysis is needed to fully determine its genetic landscape. However, based on targeted sequencing efforts and the limited mutation profile obtained thus far, pure endometrial CCC as a group do not appear to fit well into a single TCGA endometrial molecular type category [33]. An extensive genetic profile using whole genome or exome sequencing may also aid in characterizing the distinction between serous and clear cell carcinomas.

Biological Function of Immunohistochemical and Genetic Markers

HNF-1β

Hepatocyte nuclear factor-1β or transcription factor 2 (*HNF-1β, TCF2*) is a homeodomain transcription factor that is related to hepatocyte nuclear factor-1α [57]. This gene is important in the embryonic development of kidney, pancreas, liver, and bile duct differentiation and organogenesis [58–60]. HNF-1β is a major

Table 6.2 Molecular genetic features of endometrial clear cell carcinomas

Study	*N*	*PTEN* (%)	*PIK3CA* (%)	*TP53* (%)	*POLE* (%)	MSI (%)	*SPOP* (%)	*FBXW7* (%)	*PPP2R1A* (%)	*ARID1A* (%)	*CHD4* (%)	*EP300* (%)
An et al. [47]	14	3 (21)	NA	1 (9), 4 (29)[a]	NA	2 (14)	NA	NA	NA	NA	NA	NA
Rudd et al. [50]	20	NA	6 (30)	NA	NA	NA	NA	NA	NA	NA	NA	NA
Gallo et al. [54]	23	NA	NA	NA	NA	3 (13)	2 (9)	3 (13)	NA	3 (13)	1 (4)	1 (4)
Bashir et al. [51]	18	NA	3 (17)	NA	NA	NA	NA	NA	NA	NA	NA	NA
McIntrye et al. [52]	11	NA	1 (9)	NA	NA	NA	NA	NA	NA	NA	NA	NA
Rudd et al. [53]	21	NA	NA	NA	1 (5)	NA	NA	NA	NA	NA	NA	NA
Hoang et al. [33]	14	0	2 (14)	4 (29)[c]	1 (7)[b]	0	4 (29)	1 (7)	3 (21)	2 (14)	0	0
Overall Summary	121	3 (11)	12 (19)	9 (32)	2 (6)	5 (14)	6 (16)	4 (11)	3 (21)	5 (14)	1 (4)	1 (4)

NA indicates marker was not used in the study. The overall summary percentages are a reflection of the column, and only accounts for the studies in which the marker was evaluated

[a]These tumors were mixed tumors with clear cell components

[b]*POLE* missense mutation falls outside of the exonuclease domain (K777T)

[c]All 4 tumors with missense mutations showed p53 diffuse strong nuclear expression, and a fifth tumor did not harbor a detectable mutation but showed complete loss of p53 IHC expression

regulator of glucose homeostasis [61] and mutations are associated with multi-system disorders such as kidney and pancreatic disease, genital tract malformations, and abnormal liver function [62]. Upregulation of HNF-1β by expression analysis was first documented in ovarian CCC [25, 26] and has since been used as an immunohistochemical marker to distinguish ovarian clear cell from endometrioid and serous carcinomas [63, 64]. Epigenetic genome-wide studies have identified DNA SNPs (single nucleotide polymorphisms) within HNF-1β that are associated with differing risks of developing ovarian clear cell or serous cancers [65, 66].

Napsin A

Napsin A, aspartic peptidase (*NAPSA*), is a peptide segment of aspartic proteinase that is important for the control and activation of these enzymes. This gene was first discovered to be expressed in lung and kidney tissue [67] and is identical to the TAO1/TAO2 peptides previously discovered in lung adenocarcinomas [68]. This stimulated interest in its use as a diagnostic marker, and it is now used in the classification of lung and renal carcinomas [69, 70]. Ovarian CCC were also identified as expressing napsin A [36], with potential utility as a diagnostic marker [71, 72]. As described previously, napsin A immunohistochemical expression may be used as a diagnostic aid for endometrial CCC when combined with additional markers in a panel [33, 38, 39] (Table 6.1). Napsin A expression also may be an important link to increased risk for venous thromboembolic events in CCC patients [38, 40].

Bax and Bcl-2

Bax is an apoptosis promoting gene from the *bcl-2* family, whereas bcl-2 acts to prolong survival and counteract apoptosis [73]. Studies have shown the expression of bcl-2 and Bax in normal endometrium [74] and the expression of bcl-2 in endometrial carcinomas (14, 15). However, Kakawa et al, found that bcl-2 expression is low to negative in endometrial CCC and that there is an increased number of Bax positive cells [75]. Therefore, the process of apoptosis may be increased in CCC, although this is still uncertain. In epithelial ovarian cancer, Bax expression has been reported as a prognostic indicator in *TP53* mutation positive tumors [76].

TP53/p53

Tumor protein 53 (*TP53*, p53) is a tumor suppressor protein that plays a role in transcriptional activation in response to cellular stresses. The *TP53* gene is the most highly studied gene in cancer biology, as it is the most commonly mutated gene in human cancer [77]. As previously described, it took many years to understand how different patterns of p53 protein staining were associated with mutation status. *TP53* mutations and p53 abnormal staining have been associated with clinical prognosis in endometrial tumor types [55, 78], primarily serous carcinoma, but this has not been adequately verified in endometrial CCC. The abnormal expression of p53 and *TP53* mutations has been reported in about a third of endometrial CCC (Tables 6.1 and 6.2); this is considerably greater than that observed in ovarian CCC. It is possible that some *TP53*-mutated endometrial CCC may represent typical *TP53* wild-type CCC that subsequently acquired *TP53* mutations. However, it is also possible that some of the TP53-mutated endometrial tumors thought to be CCC may actually be serous carcinomas that exhibit diffuse clear cell changes closely mimicking CCC [33].

ARID1A/BAF250a

The gene *ARID1A* (AT-Rich Interacting Domain containing protein 1A—SWI-like) encodes a protein subunit of the SWI/SNF complex BAF250a that acts as a tumor suppressor. The SWI/SNF chromatin remodeling complex is a multi-subunit ATP-dependent protein complex that acts in transcriptional regulation, DNA replication and repair, and cellular differentiation [79]. *ARID1A* mutations were first described in 46–57% of ovarian clear cell carcinomas [29, 30] and have since been identified in endometrial, gastric, breast, pancreatic, hepatocellular, bladder, and other cancer types [80]. Loss of BAF250a or mutations of *ARID1A* are present at a lower frequency of 13–26% in endometrial clear cell carcinomas (Table 6.1 and 6.2). In ovarian clear cell carcinoma, the majority of the mutations are truncating inactivating mutations that lead to loss of the BAF250a protein that can be identified by immunohistochemistry [31]. *ARID1A* mutations also have been identified in adjacent endometriosis, the putative precursor to ovarian clear cell carcinoma, raising the possibility that mutations in the gene are an early-cancer causing event [29].

PPP2R1A

Protein phosphatase 2A, regulatory subunit Aα (*PPP2R1A*), is the scaffolding protein subunit of the heterotrimeric protein phosphatase 2A complex (PP2A). PP2A is a serine/threonine phosphatase complex that makes up about 1% of all cellular proteins and is involved in numerous cellular processes such as differentiation, development, and growth [81, 82]. The PP2A holoenzyme is composed of a scaffolding A subunit, a catalytic C subunit, and a regulatory B subunit, in which the B subunit family is composed of many protein members and is the key component for substrate-specificity, cellular functions, and localization [83]. Mutations in *PPP2R1A* were first identified in ovarian clear cell carcinoma at a low frequency (7%) [30]. In subsequent studies, subtype-specific *PPP2R1A* mutations were identified in 19–40% of endometrial serous carcinoma and in 5–7% of endometrial endometrioid adenocarcinomas [84, 85]. In ovarian endometrioid adenocarcinomas, *PPP2R1A* mutations were identified in 10–12% of cases, with no mutations identified in ovarian serous carcinomas, suggesting that ovarian and endometrial serous carcinomas are different entities with similar histologic features. *PPP2R1A* mutations have also been identified in endometrial clear cell carcinoma (21%), which show mutational profiles that overlap with serous carcinoma [33].

PIK3CA

PIK3CA (phosphoinositide-3-kinase, catalytic alpha) is a kinase that acts at the cell membrane to phosphorylate PIP2 (phosphatidylinositol 4,5-bisphosphate) to PIP3 (phosphatidylinositol 3,4,5-trisphosphate) that in turn activates the PI3K-AKT-mTOR pathway. This signal transduction pathway is highly deregulated in many cancer types and acts to promote cell survival and proliferation [86]. *PIK3CA* is the second most frequently mutated oncoprotein, and mutations have been identified in all subtypes of endometrial and ovarian cancers; however, the frequency of mutations in endometrial clear cell is variable (9–30%). PI3K inhibitors have been proposed to target cancers with alterations in the PI3K pathway, although clinical trials have been limited and faced challenges [87].

PTEN

The tumor suppressor phosphatase with tensin homology (*PTEN*) is involved in suppressing the PI3K pathway and is one of the most frequently altered (by mutation or promoter methylation) genes in cancer [87]. *PTEN* opposes *PIK3CA* by dephosphorylating PIP3 to PIP2 to inhibit progression of the PI3K pathway [88]. Although mutations in *PTEN* are identified at high frequency in endometrial endometrioid adenocarcinomas, *PTEN* mutations in pure endometrial clear cell carcinoma are infrequent.

Precursor Lesion and Oncogenesis

Clear cell endometrial intraepithelial carcinoma has been proposed as a putative precursor lesion of clear cell carcinoma of the endometrium [89, 90]. This is described an atypical cellular proliferation on the endometrial surface and/or within superficial glands that exhibits cytologic features of clear cell carcinoma. This putative precursor lesion has been identified in about 50–90% of endometrial clear cell carcinomas [19, 90] and shares immunophenotypic similarity with clear cell carcinoma (i.e., reduced hormone receptor expression and wild-type p53 staining pattern). There has not been genetic characterization of this putative precursor lesion to date. In the absence of more definitive characterization, it remains unclear whether this intraepithelial proliferation is truly a precursor lesion.

Similarity and Differences of Molecular Features of Endometrial and Ovarian Clear Cell Carcinoma

Endometrial clear cell carcinoma is uncommon compared to its ovarian counterpart. Due to its rarity, many of the molecular characteristics of endometrial clear cell carcinoma have been extrapolated from ovarian clear cell carcinoma. There is considerable similarity in the immunophenotype and mutation profiles of ovarian and endometrial clear cell carcinoma, although the frequencies can vary. For example, the expression of HNF-1β [26] and napsin A [71] is frequent in both ovarian and endometrial clear cell carcinomas. Mutations in *ARID1A* and the loss of protein BAF250a were first discovered in ovarian clear cell carcinoma [29, 30] and subsequently also identified in endometrial clear cell carcinoma albeit at lower frequency [31, 32].

One of the major differences between endometrial and ovarian clear cell carcinoma is the presence of *TP53* mutations leading to loss or overexpression of the p53 protein. *TP53* mutations have been identified in about one-third of endometrial clear cell carcinomas (Tables 6.1 and 6.2). In ovarian clear cell carcinomas, *TP53* mutations are infrequent events [91, 92]. While this may reflect true biologic differences between ovarian and endometrial clear cell carcinomas, it is possible as discussed earlier that some of these *TP53*-mutated endometrial clear cell carcinomas may in fact represent serous carcinomas with diffuse clear cell changes [33, 93].

Conclusion and Future Directions

Significant progress has been made in our understanding of endometrial clear cell carcinoma over the past decade, and this has prompted some changes in our approach to its diagnosis. There remains, however, a significant gap in our understanding of the underlying oncobiology of endometrial clear cell carcinoma. For pure endometrial clear cell carcinoma, it is unclear what the underlying genetic/epigenetic abnormalities are aside from *ARID1A* that contribute to their oncogenesis. It is also unclear whether *TP53*-mutated endometrial clear cell carcinomas are truly clear cell carcinomas or whether they should be considered as serous carcinoma or perhaps copy number high serous-like molecular type based on the TCGA endometrial cancer molecular subtype classification [55]. Furthermore, is MSI-H/MMR protein-deficient clear cell carcinoma (either in its pure form or as a component of a mixed histotype carcinoma) biologically and clinically the same as pure endometrial clear cell carcinoma that is MSI/MMR-intact? These are all scientifically important questions that have far reaching clinical implications. With the application of increasingly robust high throughput genetic, epigenetic, and proteomic analytical tools, it is hopeful that we will soon gain more clarity on the oncobiology of endometrial clear cell carcinoma.

References

1. Gadducci A, Cosio S, Spirito N, Cionini L. Clear cell carcinoma of the endometrium: a biological and clinical enigma. Anticancer Res. 2010;30(4):1327–34.
2. Clement PB, Young RH. Non-endometrioid carcinomas of the uterine corpus: a review of their pathology with emphasis on recent advances and problematic aspects. Adv Anat Pathol. 2004;11(3):117–42.
3. Silverberg SG, De Giorgi LS. Clear cell carcinoma of the endometrium. Clinical, pathologic, and ultrastructural findings. Cancer. 1973;31(5):1127–40.
4. Kay S. Clear-cell carcinoma of the endometrium. Cancer. 1957;10(1):124–30.
5. Kurman RJ, Scully RE. Clear cell carcinoma of the endometrium: an analysis of 21 cases. Cancer. 1976;37(2):872–82.
6. Scully RE, Poulsen HE. Histological typing of female genital tract tumours. International histological classification of tumours. 2nd ed. New York: Springer; 1994.
7. Bokhman JV. Two pathogenetic types of endometrial carcinoma. Gynecol Oncol. 1983;15 (1):10–7.
8. Voss MA, Ganesan R, Ludeman L, McCarthy K, Gornall R, Schaller G et al. Should grade 3 endometrioid endometrial carcinoma be considered a type 2 cancer—a clinical and pathological evaluation. Gynecol oncol. 2012;124(1):15–20. doi:10.1016/J.Ygyno.2011.07.030.
9. Zannoni GF, Scambia G, Gallo D. The dualistic model of endometrial cancer: the challenge of classifying grade 3 endometrioid carcinoma. Gynecol Oncol. 2012;127(1):262–3. doi:10.1016/j.ygyno.2011.09.036.
10. Murali R, Soslow RA, Weigelt B. Classification of endometrial carcinoma: more than two types. Lancet Oncol. 2014;15(7):e268–78. doi:10.1016/S1470-2045(13)70591-6.
11. Olawaiye AB, Boruta DM 2nd. Management of women with clear cell endometrial cancer: a Society of Gynecologic Oncology (SGO) review. Gynecol Oncol. 2009;113(2):277–83. doi:10.1016/j.ygyno.2009.02.003.
12. Amant F, Moerman P, Neven P, Timmerman D, Van Limbergen E, Vergote I. Treatment modalities in endometrial cancer. Curr Opin Oncol. 2007;19(5):479–85. doi:10.1097/CCO.0b013e32827853c0.
13. Soslow RA, Bissonnette JP, Wilton A, Ferguson SE, Alektiar KM, Duska LR et al. Clinicopathologic analysis of 187 high-grade endometrial carcinomas of different histologic subtypes: similar outcomes belie distinctive biologic differences. Am J Surg Pathol. 2007;31 (7):979-87. doi:10.1097/PAS.0b013e31802ee494; [pii] 00000478-200707000-00001.
14. Thomas M, Mariani A, Wright JD, Madarek EO, Powell MA, Mutch DG, et al. Surgical management and adjuvant therapy for patients with uterine clear cell carcinoma:

a multi-institutional review. Gynecol Oncol. 2008;108(2):293–7. doi:10.1016/j.ygyno.2007.11.008.

15. McMeekin DS, Filiaci VL, Thigpen JT, Gallion HH, Fleming GF, Rodgers WH, et al. The relationship between histology and outcome in advanced and recurrent endometrial cancer patients participating in first-line chemotherapy trials: a gynecologic oncology group study. Gynecol Oncol. 2007;106(1):16–22. doi:10.1016/j.ygyno.2007.04.032.
16. Tan DS, Miller RE, Kaye SB. New perspectives on molecular targeted therapy in ovarian clear cell carcinoma. Br J Cancer. 2013;108(8):1553–9. doi:10.1038/bjc.2013.126.
17. Fadare O, Parkash V, Dupont WD, Acs G, Atkins KA, Irving JA, et al. The diagnosis of endometrial carcinomas with clear cells by gynecologic pathologists: an assessment of interobserver variability and associated morphologic features. Am J Surg Pathol. 2012;36(8):1107–18. doi:10.1097/PAS.0b013e31825dd4b3.
18. Gilks CB, Oliva E, Soslow R. Poor interobserver reproducibility in the diagnosis of high-grade endometrial carcinoma. Mod Pathol. 2011;24:248A-A.
19. Han G, Sidhu D, Duggan MA, Arseneau J, Cesari M, Clement PB, et al. Reproducibility of histological cell type in high-grade endometrial carcinoma. Mod Pathol. 2013;26(12):1594–604. doi:10.1038/modpathol.2013.102.
20. Fadare O, Zheng W, Crispens MA, Jones HW, Khabele D, Gwin K, et al. Morphologic and other clinicopathologic features of endometrial clear cell carcinoma: a comprehensive analysis of 50 rigorously classified cases. Am J Cancer Res. 2013;3(1):70–95.
21. Bartosch C, Manuel Lopes J, Oliva E. Endometrial carcinomas: a review emphasizing overlapping and distinctive morphological and immunohistochemical features. Adv anat pathol. 2011;18(6):415–37. doi:10.1097/PAP.0b013e318234ab18.
22. Lax SF, Pizer ES, Ronnett BM, Kurman RJ. Clear cell carcinoma of the endometrium is characterized by a distinctive profile of p53, Ki-67, estrogen, and progesterone receptor expression. Hum Pathol. 1998;29(6):551–8.
23. Vang R, Whitaker BP, Farhood AI, Silva EG, Ro JY, Deavers MT. Immunohistochemical analysis of clear cell carcinoma of the gynecologic tract. Int J Gynecol Pathol. 2001;20(3):252–9.
24. Vang R, Barner R, Wheeler DT, Strauss BL. Immunohistochemical staining for Ki-67 and p53 helps distinguish endometrial Arias-Stella reaction from high-grade carcinoma, including clear cell carcinoma. Int J Gynecol Pathol. 2004;23(3):223–33.
25. Arai T, Watanabe J, Kawaguchi M, Kamata Y, Nishimura Y, Jobo T, et al. Clear cell adenocarcinoma of the endometrium is a biologically distinct entity from endometrioid adenocarcinoma. Int J Gynecol Cancer. 2006;16(1):391–5. doi:10.1111/j.1525-1438.2006.00494.x.
26. Schwartz DR, Kardia SL, Shedden KA, Kuick R, Michailidis G, Taylor JM, et al. Gene expression in ovarian cancer reflects both morphology and biological behavior, distinguishing clear cell from other poor-prognosis ovarian carcinomas. Can Res. 2002;62(16):4722–9.
27. Tsuchiya A, Sakamoto M, Yasuda J, Chuma M, Ohta T, Ohki M, et al. Expression profiling in ovarian clear cell carcinoma: identification of hepatocyte nuclear factor-1 beta as a molecular marker and a possible molecular target for therapy of ovarian clear cell carcinoma. Am J Pathol. 2003;163(6):2503–12.
28. Yamamoto S, Tsuda H, Aida S, Shimazaki H, Tamai S, Matsubara O. Immunohistochemical detection of hepatocyte nuclear factor 1beta in ovarian and endometrial clear-cell adenocarcinomas and nonneoplastic endometrium. Hum Pathol. 2007;38(7):1074–80. doi:10.1016/j.humpath.2006.12.018.
29. Hoang LN, Han G, McConechy M, Lau S, Chow C, Gilks CB, et al. Immunohistochemical characterization of prototypical endometrial clear cell carcinoma–diagnostic utility of HNF-1beta and oestrogen receptor. Histopathology. 2014;64(4):585–96. doi:10.1111/his.12286.
30. Wiegand KC, Shah SP, Al-Agha OM, Zhao Y, Tse K, Zeng T, et al. ARID1A mutations in endometriosis-associated ovarian carcinomas. New Engl J Med. 2010;363(16):1532–43. doi:10.1056/NEJMoa1008433.

31. Jones S, Wang TL, Shih Ie M, Mao TL, Nakayama K, Roden R, et al. Frequent mutations of chromatin remodeling gene ARID1A in ovarian clear cell carcinoma. Science. 2010;330 (6001):228–31. doi:10.1126/science.1196333.
32. Wiegand KC, Lee AF, Al-Agha OM, Chow C, Kalloger SE, Scott DW, et al. Loss of BAF250a (ARID1A) is frequent in high-grade endometrial carcinomas. J Pathol. 2011;224 (3):328–33. doi:10.1002/path.2911.
33. Fadare O, Renshaw IL, Liang SX. Does the loss of ARID1A (BAF-250a) expression in endometrial clear cell carcinomas have any clinicopathologic significance? Pilot Assess J Cancer. 2012;3:129–36. doi:10.7150/jca.4140.
34. Hoang LN, McConechy MK, Meng B, McIntyre JB, Ewanowich C, Gilks CB, et al. Targeted mutation analysis of endometrial clear cell carcinoma. Histopathology. 2015;66 (5):664–74. doi:10.1111/his.12581.
35. Lim D, Ip PP, Cheung AN, Kiyokawa T, Oliva E. Immunohistochemical comparison of ovarian and uterine endometrioid carcinoma, endometrioid carcinoma with clear cell change, and clear cell carcinoma. Am J Surg Pathol. 2015;39(8):1061–9. doi:10.1097/PAS.0000000000000436.
36. Fadare O, Gwin K, Desouki MM, Crispens MA, Jones HW 3rd, Khabele D, et al. The clinicopathologic significance of p53 and BAF-250a (ARID1A) expression in clear cell carcinoma of the endometrium. Mod Pathol. 2013;26(8):1101–10. doi:10.1038/modpathol.2013.35.
37. Kadivar M, Boozari B. Applications and limitations of immunohistochemical expression of "Napsin-A" in distinguishing lung adenocarcinoma from adenocarcinomas of other organs. Appl Immunohistochem Mol Morphol Aimm/Off Publ Soc Appl Immunohistochem. 2013;21(3):191–5. doi:10.1097/PAI.0b013e3182612643.
38. Turner BM, Cagle PT, Sainz IM, Fukuoka J, Shen SS, Jagirdar J. Napsin A, a new marker for lung adenocarcinoma, is complementary and more sensitive and specific than thyroid transcription factor 1 in the differential diagnosis of primary pulmonary carcinoma: evaluation of 1674 cases by tissue microarray. Arch Pathol Lab Med. 2012;136(2):163–71. doi:10.5858/arpa.2011-0320-OA.
39. Fadare O, Desouki MM, Gwin K, Hanley KZ, Jarboe EA, Liang SX, et al. Frequent expression of napsin A in clear cell carcinoma of the endometrium: potential diagnostic utility. Am J Surg Pathol. 2014;38(2):189–96. doi:10.1097/PAS.0000000000000085.
40. Iwamoto M, Nakatani Y, Fugo K, Kishimoto T, Kiyokawa T. Napsin A is frequently expressed in clear cell carcinoma of the ovary and endometrium. Hum Pathol. 2015;46 (7):957–62. doi:10.1016/j.humpath.2015.03.008.
41. Lee L, Garrett L, Lee H, Oliva E, Horowitz N, Duska LR. Association of clear cell carcinoma of the endometrium with a high rate of venous thromboembolism. J Reprod Med. 2009;54(3):133–8.
42. Wynford-Thomas D. P53 in tumour pathology: can we trust immunocytochemistry? J Pathol. 1992;166(4):329–30. doi:10.1002/path.1711660402.
43. Hall PA, Lane DP. p53 in tumour pathology: can we trust immunohistochemistry?Revisited! J Pathol. 1994;172(1):1–4. doi:10.1002/path.1711720103.
44. Marks JR, Davidoff AM, Kerns BJ, Humphrey PA, Pence JC, Dodge RK, et al. Overexpression and mutation of p53 in epithelial ovarian cancer. Can Res. 1991;51 (11):2979–84.
45. Lepelley P, Preudhomme C, Vanrumbeke M, Quesnel B, Cosson A, Fenaux P. Detection of p53 mutations in hematological malignancies: comparison between immunocytochemistry and DNA analysis. Leukemia. 1994;8(8):1342–9.
46. Bartek J, Iggo R, Gannon J, Lane DP. Genetic and immunochemical analysis of mutant p53 in human breast cancer cell lines. Oncogene. 1990;5(6):893–9.
47. Fadare O, Liang SX. Diagnostic utility of hepatocyte nuclear factor 1-beta immunoreactivity in endometrial carcinomas: lack of specificity for endometrial clear cell carcinoma. Appl Immunohistochem Mol Morphol Aimm/Off Publ Soc Appl Immunohistochem. 2012;20 (6):580–7. doi:10.1097/PAI.0b013e31824973d1.

48. An HJ, Logani S, Isacson C, Ellenson LH. Molecular characterization of uterine clear cell carcinoma. Mod Pathol. 2004;17(5):530–7. doi:10.1038/modpathol.3800057.
49. Cheung LW, Hennessy BT, Li J, Yu S, Myers AP, Djordjevic B, et al. High frequency of PIK3R1 and PIK3R2 mutations in endometrial cancer elucidates a novel mechanism for regulation of PTEN protein stability. Cancer Discov. 2011;1(2):170–85. doi:10.1158/2159-8290.CD-11-0039.
50. McConechy MK, Ding J, Cheang MC, Wiegand KC, Senz J, Tone AA, et al. Use of mutation profiles to refine the classification of endometrial carcinomas. J Pathol. 2012;228 (1):20–30. doi:10.1002/path.4056.
51. Rudd ML, Price JC, Fogoros S, Godwin AK, Sgroi DC, Merino MJ, et al. A unique spectrum of somatic PIK3CA (p110alpha) mutations within primary endometrial carcinomas. Clin Cancer Res Off J Am Assoc Cancer Res. 2011;17(6):1331–40. doi:10.1158/1078-0432.CCR-10-0540.
52. Bashir S, Jiang G, Joshi A, Miller C Jr, Matrai C, Yemelyanova A, et al. Molecular alterations of PIK3CA in uterine carcinosarcoma, clear cell, and serous tumors. Int J Gynecol Cancer. 2014;24(7):1262–7. doi:10.1097/IGC.0000000000000183.
53. McIntyre JB, Nelson GS, Ghatage P, Morris D, Duggan MA, Lee CH, et al. PIK3CA missense mutation is associated with unfavorable outcome in grade 3 endometrioid carcinoma but not in serous endometrial carcinoma. Gynecol Oncol. 2014;132(1):188–93. doi:10.1016/j.ygyno.2013.11.015.
54. Rudd ML, Mohamed H, Price JC, O'Hara AJ, Le Gallo M, Urick ME, et al. Mutational analysis of the tyrosine kinome in serous and clear cell endometrial cancer uncovers rare somatic mutations in TNK2 and DDR1. BMC Cancer. 2014;14:884. doi:10.1186/1471-2407-14-884.
55. Gallo ML, O'Hara AJ, Rudd ML, Urick ME, Hansen NF, O'Neil NJ, et al. Exome sequencing of serous endometrial tumors identifies recurrent somatic mutations in chromatin-remodeling and ubiquitin ligase complex genes. Nat Genet. 2012;. doi:10.1038/ng.2455.
56. Kandoth C, Schultz N, Cherniack AD, Akbani R, Liu Y, Shen H, et al. Integrated genomic characterization of endometrial carcinoma. Nature. 2013;497(7447):67–73. doi:10.1038/nature12113.
57. Huang HN, Chiang YC, Cheng WF, Chen CA, Lin MC, Kuo KT. Molecular alterations in endometrial and ovarian clear cell carcinomas: clinical impacts of telomerase reverse transcriptase promoter mutation. Mod Pathol. 2015;28(2):303–11. doi:10.1038/modpathol.2014.93.
58. Mendel DB, Hansen LP, Graves MK, Conley PB, Crabtree GR. HNF-1 alpha and HNF-1 beta (vHNF-1) share dimerization and homeo domains, but not activation domains, and form heterodimers in vitro. Genes Dev. 1991;5(6):1042–56.
59. Coffinier C, Gresh L, Fiette L, Tronche F, Schutz G, Babinet C, et al. Bile system morphogenesis defects and liver dysfunction upon targeted deletion of HNF1beta. Development. 2002;129(8):1829–38.
60. Bohn S, Thomas H, Turan G, Ellard S, Bingham C, Hattersley AT, et al. Distinct molecular and morphogenetic properties of mutations in the human HNF1beta gene that lead to defective kidney development. J Am Soc Nephrol. 2003;14(8):2033–41.
61. Coffinier C, Barra J, Babinet C, Yaniv M. Expression of the vHNF1/HNF1beta homeoprotein gene during mouse organogenesis. Mech Dev. 1999;89(1–2):211–3.
62. Pontoglio M. Hepatocyte nuclear factor 1, a transcription factor at the crossroads of glucose homeostasis. J Am Soc Nephrol. 2000;11(Suppl 16):S140–3.
63. Clissold RL, Hamilton AJ, Hattersley AT, Ellard S, Bingham C. HNF1B-associated renal and extra-renal disease-an expanding clinical spectrum. Nat Rev Nephrol. 2015;11(2):102–12. doi:10.1038/nrneph.2014.232.
64. Kao YC, Lin MC, Lin WC, Jeng YM, Mao TL. Utility of hepatocyte nuclear factor-1beta as a diagnostic marker in ovarian carcinomas with clear cells. Histopathology. 2012;61(5):760–8. doi:10.1111/j.1365-2559.2012.04267.x.

65. Kalloger SE, Kobel M, Leung S, Mehl E, Gao D, Marcon KM, et al. Calculator for ovarian carcinoma subtype prediction. Mod Pathol. 2011;24(4):512–21. doi:10.1038/modpathol.2010.215.
66. Shen H, Fridley BL, Song H, Lawrenson K, Cunningham JM, Ramus SJ, et al. Epigenetic analysis leads to identification of HNF1B as a subtype-specific susceptibility gene for ovarian cancer. Nat Commun. 2013;4:1628. doi:10.1038/ncomms2629.
67. Painter JN, O'Mara TA, Batra J, Cheng T, Lose FA, Dennis J, et al. Fine-mapping of the HNF1B multicancer locus identifies candidate variants that mediate endometrial cancer risk. Hum Mol Genet. 2015;24(5):1478–92. doi:10.1093/hmg/ddu552.
68. Tatnell PJ, Powell DJ, Hill J, Smith TS, Tew DG, Kay J. Napsins: new human aspartic proteinases. Distinction between two closely related genes. FEBS Lett. 1998;441(1):43–8.
69. Hirano T, Franzen B, Uryu K, Okuzawa K, Alaiya AA, Vanky F, et al. Detection of polypeptides associated with the histopathological differentiation of primary lung carcinoma. Br J Cancer. 1995;72(4):840–8.
70. Chuman Y, Bergman A, Ueno T, Saito S, Sakaguchi K, Alaiya AA, et al. Napsin A, a member of the aspartic protease family, is abundantly expressed in normal lung and kidney tissue and is expressed in lung adenocarcinomas. FEBS Lett. 1999;462(1–2):129–34.
71. Ueno T, Linder S, Elmberger G. Aspartic proteinase napsin is a useful marker for diagnosis of primary lung adenocarcinoma. Br J Cancer. 2003;88(8):1229–33. doi:10.1038/sj.bjc.6600879.
72. Skirnisdottir I, Bjersand K, Akerud H, Seidal T. Napsin A as a marker of clear cell ovarian carcinoma. BMC Cancer. 2013;13:524. doi:10.1186/1471-2407-13-524.
73. Yamashita Y, Nagasaka T, Naiki-Ito A, Sato S, Suzuki S, Toyokuni S, et al. Napsin A is a specific marker for ovarian clear cell adenocarcinoma. Mod Pathol. 2015;28(1):111–7. doi:10.1038/modpathol.2014.61.
74. Oltvai ZN, Milliman CL, Korsmeyer SJ. Bcl-2 heterodimerizes in vivo with a conserved homolog, Bax, that accelerates programmed cell death. Cell. 1993;74(4):609–19.
75. Tao XJ, Tilly KI, Maravei DV, Shifren JL, Krajewski S, Reed JC, et al. Differential expression of members of the bcl-2 gene family in proliferative and secretory human endometrium: glandular epithelial cell apoptosis is associated with increased expression of bax. J Clin Endocrinol Metab. 1997;82(8):2738–46. doi:10.1210/jcem.82.8.4146.
76. Kokawa K, Shikone T, Otani T, Nishiyama R, Ishii Y, Yagi S, et al. Apoptosis and the expression of Bcl-2 and Bax in patients with endometrioid, clear cell, and serous carcinomas of the uterine endometrium. Gynecol Oncol. 2001;81(2):178–83. doi:10.1006/gyno.2001.6138.
77. Kupryjanczyk J, Szymanska T, Madry R, Timorek A, Stelmachow J, Karpinska G, et al. Evaluation of clinical significance of TP53, BCL-2, BAX and MEK1 expression in 229 ovarian carcinomas treated with platinum-based regimen. Br J Cancer. 2003;88(6):848–54. doi:10.1038/sj.bjc.6600789.
78. Greenblatt MS, Bennett WP, Hollstein M, Harris CC. Mutations in the p53 tumor suppressor gene: clues to cancer etiology and molecular pathogenesis. Can Res. 1994;54(18):4855–78.
79. Talhouk A, McConechy MK, Leung S, Li-Chang HH, Kwon JS, Melnyk N, et al. A clinically applicable molecular-based classification for endometrial cancers. Br J Cancer. 2015;113(2):299–310. doi:10.1038/bjc.2015.190.
80. Wilson BG, Roberts CW. SWI/SNF nucleosome remodellers and cancer. Nat Rev Cancer. 2011;11(7):481–92. doi:10.1038/nrc3068.
81. Wu JN, Roberts CW. ARID1A mutations in cancer: another epigenetic tumor suppressor? Cancer Discov. 2013;3(1):35–43. doi:10.1158/2159-8290.CD-12-0361.
82. Eichhorn PJ, Creyghton MP, Bernards R. Protein phosphatase 2A regulatory subunits and cancer. Biochem Biophys Acta. 2009;1795(1):1–15. doi:10.1016/j.bbcan.2008.05.005.
83. Virshup DM. Protein phosphatase 2A: a panoply of enzymes. Curr Opin Cell Biol. 2000;12(2):180–5.
84. Xu Y, Xing Y, Chen Y, Chao Y, Lin Z, Fan E, et al. Structure of the protein phosphatase 2A holoenzyme. Cell. 2006;127(6):1239–51. doi:10.1016/j.cell.2006.11.033.

85. McConechy MK, Anglesio MS, Kalloger SE, Yang W, Senz J, Chow C, et al. Subtype-specific mutation of PPP2R1A in endometrial and ovarian carcinomas. J Pathol. 2011;223(5):567–73. doi:10.1002/path.2848.
86. Shih Ie M, Panuganti PK, Kuo KT, Mao TL, Kuhn E, Jones S, et al. Somatic mutations of PPP2R1A in ovarian and uterine carcinomas. Am J Pathol. 2011;178(4):1442–7. doi:10.1016/j.ajpath.2011.01.009.
87. Samuels Y, Wang Z, Bardelli A, Silliman N, Ptak J, Szabo S, et al. High frequency of mutations of the PIK3CA gene in human cancers. Science. 2004;304(5670):554. doi:10.1126/science.1096502.
88. Fruman DA, Rommel C. PI3K and cancer: lessons, challenges and opportunities. Nat Rev Drug Discov. 2014;13(2):140–56. doi:10.1038/nrd4204.
89. Hoang LN, McConechy MK, Kobel M, Anglesio M, Senz J, Maassen M, et al. polymerase epsilon exonuclease domain mutations in ovarian endometrioid carcinoma. Int J Gynecol Cancer. 2015;25(7):1187–93. doi:10.1097/IGC.0000000000000492.
90. Moid F, Berezowski K. Pathologic quiz case: a 70-year-old woman with postmenopausal bleeding. Endometrial intraepithelial carcinoma, clear cell type. Arch Pathol Lab Med. 2004;128(11):e157–8. doi:10.1043/1543-2165(2004)128<e157:PQCAYW>2.0.CO;2.
91. Kobel M, Meng B, Hoang LN, Almadani N, Li X, Soslow RA, et al. Molecular analysis of mixed endometrial carcinomas shows clonality in most cases. Am J Surg Pathol. 2016;40(2):166–80. doi:10.1097/PAS.0000000000000536.
92. Kobel M, Kalloger SE, Carrick J, Huntsman D, Asad H, Oliva E, et al. A limited panel of immunomarkers can reliably distinguish between clear cell and high-grade serous carcinoma of the ovary. Am J Surg Pathol. 2009;33(1):14–21. doi:10.1097/PAS.0b013e3181788546.
93. Varughese J, Hui P, Lu L, Yu H, Schwartz PE. Clear cell cancer of the uterine corpus: the association of clinicopathologic parameters and treatment on disease progression. J Oncol. 2011;2011:628084. doi:10.1155/2011/628084.
94. Shahin MS, Hughes JH, Sood AK, Buller RE. The prognostic significance of p53 tumor suppressor gene alterations in ovarian carcinoma. Cancer. 2000;89(9):2006–17.

Chapter 7
Mucinous Adenocarcinoma of the Endometrium

Kyu-Rae Kim and Stanley J. Robboy

Clinical Features

The clinical features of mucinous adenocarcinoma including age, body mass index, menopausal status, nulliparity, and clinical symptoms are similar to those of endometrioid adenocarcinoma [1–10]. Hormone use has been implicated as a possible cause of this histologic feature, as approximately half of patients had a history of exogenous hormones (estrogen, progesterone, or combined) in one study [1]. HPV DNA has not been detected by PCR amplification of tumor DNA; thus, this tumor does not seem to be caused by HPV infection [11].

No significant differences are observed in baseline characteristics of the tumor, including tumor diameter, lymphvascular invasion, deep myometrial invasion, cervical involvement, disease-free survival, and overall survival compared to endometrioid adenocarcinoma. However, in a few studies, including one using the SEER database, patients with mucinous histology were more likely to have pelvic lymph nodes metastases at the time of surgery compared to endometrioid adenocarcinoma [9, 10, 12]. The overall prognosis of patients with mucinous adenocarcinoma appears similar to those with low-grade endometrioid adenocarcinoma of the same stage.

K.-R. Kim (✉)
Department of Pathology, Asan Medical Center, 88, Olympic-ro 43-gil,
Songpa-gu, Seoul 05505, Republic of Korea
e-mail: krkim@amc.seoul.kr

S.J. Robboy
Department of Pathology, Duke University Medical Center,
40 Medical Center Dr, Durham, NC 27517, USA
e-mail: Stanley.robboy@duke.edu

M.T. Deavers and D.M. Coffey (eds.), *Precision Molecular Pathology of Uterine Cancer*, Molecular Pathology Library,
DOI 10.1007/978-3-319-57985-6_7

Histopathologic Features

Mucinous adenocarcinoma of the endometrium includes a typical type and several rare variants, including microglandular adenocarcinoma and low-grade mucinous adenocarcinoma, which simulate non-neoplastic endocervical tissue and adenoma malignum of the uterine cervix, respectively. Histologically, the tumor forms cribriform or confluent glands, similar to typical endometrioid adenocarcinoma, but with abundant mucinous cytoplasm (Fig. 7.1a, b). Often, they have papillary or villoglandular architecture. Nuclear atypia is only mild to moderate, and mitotic activity is not prominent. Endometrial hyperplasia/endometrial intraepithelial neoplasia (EIN) or papillary/complex mucinous metaplasia is sometimes present in the adjacent endometrium.

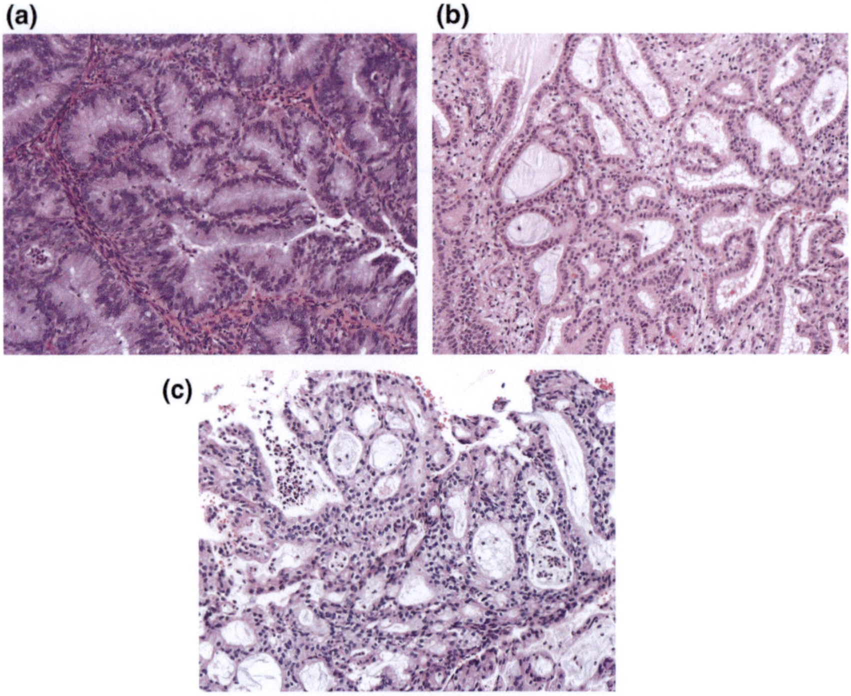

Fig. 7.1 Mucinous adenocarcinoma of the endometrium. **a** Typical pattern of mucinous adenocarcinoma with cribriform or confluent glands lined by cells with mucinous cytoplasm. **b** Low-grade carcinoma showing a moderately complex architecture with absent-to-mild cytologic atypia. **c** Microglandular adenocarcinoma of the endometrium composed of a tightly packed proliferation of small mucinous glands simulating endocervical glandular hyperplasia. These glands are architecturally irregular and display tall columnar cells with stratification and atypia, prominent nucleoli and pale to eosinophilic cytoplasm. Numerous neutrophils lie within glandular lumens and in the stroma

Microglandular adenocarcinoma of the endometrium simulates microglandular hyperplasia of the endocervix because of its closely packed small glands typically lined by one to several layers of bland, flattened, or cuboidal to columnar cells, with low mitotic activity [7, 11, 13–15]. Cystically dilated glands are often interspersed. In some cases, solid sheets of epithelial cells are formed around the microglandular spaces, which mimic immature squamous metaplasia. The cells contain pale to eosinophilic or amphophilic cytoplasm and the glandular lumina contain eosinophilic or basophilic secretory material. There are acute inflammatory cells in the glandular lumina and intervening stroma, which enhance the resemblance to microglandular hyperplasia of the endocervix. The remaining endometrial mucosa frequently contains complex hyperplasia with atypia/EIN [11].

Features that may help distinguish microglandular adenocarcinoma from microglandular hyperplasia in a curettage specimen are postmenopausal age of the patient, transition to typical endometrioid adenocarcinoma, and nuclear atypia and mitotic activity exceeding that usually found in microglandular hyperplasia. Microglandular hyperplasia of the endocervix is rare in postmenopausal women if they are not receiving hormonal treatment and the glands are typically lined by bland, flattened, or cuboidal cells, usually with very little mitotic activity. However, atypical variants of microglandular hyperplasia may have reticular, solid (sheet-like), or pseudo-infiltrative growth pattern, nuclear pleomorphism, hobnail and signet ring cells, and increased mitotic activity [16, 17]. Thus, KRAS mutation status and a PAX2 negative immunophenotype can be helpful in the differential diagnosis [17, 18].

Another rare histologic variant of mucinous endometrial adenocarcinoma has been described under the name "low-grade mucinous adenocarcinoma" [1]. It has deceptively bland cytology resembling adenoma malignum of the cervix [1]. The clinical features, however, are not significantly different from other types of endometrial mucinous adenocarcinoma [1].

Histologically, these tumors have simple or branched papillary epithelium with eosinophilic-to-basophilic mucin containing cytoplasm (Fig. 7.1c). The nuclei are basally located and are either cytologically bland or exhibit only mild-to-moderate atypia with prominent nucleoli. Neutrophils may infiltrate the mucinous glands, but a microglandular pattern is not present, which distinguishes it from microglandular adenocarcinoma.

The chief differential diagnoses for "low-grade mucinous endometrial adenocarcinoma" include endocervical glandular hyperplasia, minimal deviation adenocarcinoma (adenoma malignum) of the cervix, endometrial mucinous metaplasia, and mucinous hyperplasia.

Immunohistochemical Profile

The typical immunohistochemical profile of mucinous endometrial adenocarcinoma, including the variants microglandular adenocarcinoma and low-grade adenocarcinoma, includes strong, diffuse immunoreactivity for cytokeratin CAM5.2 and strong positivity for estrogen, but no p53 reactivity. Expression of progesterone receptor is variable [7, 11, 19]. P16 is negative or patchy, which is a distinguishing feature from cervical adenocarcinoma, in which the reactivity is diffuse and strong [1]. Vimentin and CEA are also useful immunohistochemical markers for distinguishing endometrial and endocervical adenocarcinomas. Vimentin is strong in the great majority of endometrial mucinous adenocarcinomas, whereas only a small percentage of cervical adenocarcinomas are vimentin positive (commonly as focal membranous reactivity). CEA is either not expressed [15], may be reactive in rare cells, or can have luminal positivity in glands [11, 14]. The Ki-67 proliferation index ranges from 5 to 27% [19].

Differential Diagnosis

Mucinous endometrial adenocarcinoma should be differentiated from endocervical adenocarcinoma, atypical endometrial hyperplasia with mucinous metaplasia, papillary or complex mucinous metaplasia, and non-neoplastic endocervical tissue including microglandular hyperplasia.

Infrequently, endocervical adenocarcinoma can spread intramucosally and colonize the endometrium, which may lead to a misdiagnosis of endometrial mucinous or endometrioid adenocarcinoma [20]. Histologically, endocervical adenocarcinoma usually has greater cytologic atypia and more prominent mitotic activity compared to endometrial mucinous adenocarcinoma. Frequently, benign or uninvolved endometrial glands are noted beneath or among the neoplastic glands in cases of endocervical adenocarcinoma involving the endometrium [20]. Diffuse immunoreactivity for $p16^{INK4}$, at least focal reactivity for monoclonal CEA, non-reactivity for vimentin, and no more than focal expression of estrogen receptor (ER) or progesterone receptor (PR) helps with the diagnosis of endocervical adenocarcinoma [8, 21, 22].

Rarely, mucinous material from a low-grade appendiceal mucinous neoplasm spreads transtubally, which may lead to a misdiagnosis of a primary mucinous tumor of the endometrium secondary to mucinous substance in cytology or in biopsy specimens [23, 24]. The recognition of this phenomenon can be extremely difficult in the absence of a clinical history, but the presence of epithelium containing goblet cells that are cytokeratin (CK) 20 positive and CK 7 negative, plus absence of coexisting typical endometrioid adenocarcinoma or endometrial hyperplasia are important clues in the differentiation from primary mucinous endometrial adenocarcinoma.

Microglandular adenocarcinoma of the endometrium can closely mimic microglandular hyperplasia of the endocervix in a curettage specimen when there is a complex proliferation of glands lined by columnar or cuboidal epithelial cells. KRAS reportedly can separate the two lesions, as KRAS mutation was absent in all cases of microglandular hyperplasia, but found in 60% (9 of 15) of cases of microglandular adenocarcinoma [18].

Papillary Mucinous Metaplasia, a Possible Precursor of Mucinous Endometrial Adenocarcinoma

Mucinous differentiation of the endometrium occurs in a spectrum that ranges from simple tubular glands to complex glands, some of which are architecturally indistinguishable from low-grade mucinous adenocarcinomas (Fig. 7.2a–d).

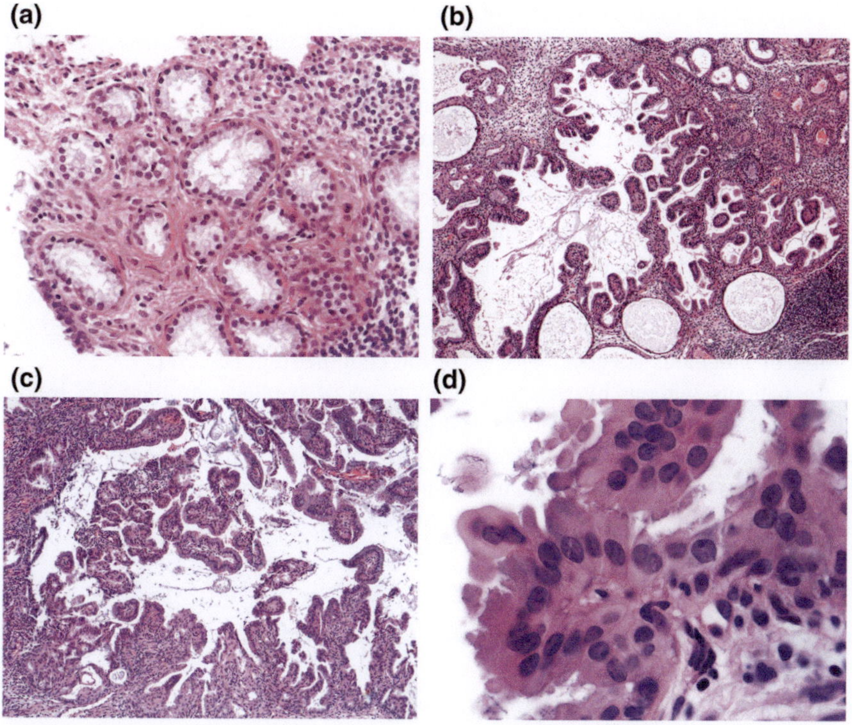

Fig. 7.2 Variable morphologic features of mucinous metaplasia from simple mucinous metaplasia (**a**) to complex/papillary mucinous metaplasia (**b**, **c**). Although some glands are architecturally indistinguishable from mucinous adenocarcinomas (**d**), the nuclear features of simple and papillary mucinous metaplasia are similar, with round uniform nuclei, finely dispersed chromatin, and one or two small conspicuous nucleoli

Various diagnostic terms describe architecturally complex lesions, such as complex hyperplastic papillary proliferation [25], complex mucinous metaplasia [26], papillary mucinous metaplasia [27], and atypical mucinous proliferation. Regardless of the term chosen, architecturally complex mucinous lesions are associated with an increased rate of subsequent endometrial adenocarcinoma [28, 29].

Histologically, simple mucinous metaplasia of endometrium is composed of simple tubular endometrial glands of varying size, lined by a single layer of columnar or cuboidal epithelium containing intracytoplasmic mucin (Fig. 7.2a). In some areas, the glandular epithelium is slightly raised above the surrounding flat mucinous epithelium. More complex forms have a spectrum of architectural alterations including tufts, micropapillary or papillary infoldings with or without fibrovascular cores (Fig. 7.2b), cystically dilated glands with intraluminal projecting papillary structures (Fig. 7.2c) and complex cribriform-like glandular arrangements at the periphery of the glands. The nuclei are uniformly round with finely dispersed chromatin and one or two small conspicuous nucleoli, but no nuclear pleomorphism or mitoses are identified (Fig. 7.2d). In endometrial biopsy or curettage specimens, distinguishing complex endometrial mucinous lesions from mucinous adenocarcinoma often poses a significant diagnostic challenge. In our experience, the Ki-67 proliferation index is usually low, close to zero, even in the most complex papillary mucinous structures [27].

Mucinous metaplasia may represent a monoclonal alteration of the endometrium, as suggested by the presence of non-random X-chromosome inactivation [30]. In our previous study [27] and in others [31], KRAS mutation was found to be frequent (67–89%) in papillary mucinous metaplasia (Fig. 7.3), but low (0–14%) in simple mucinous metaplasia. It was associated with overexpression of $P16^{INK4A}$ and loss of PAX2 and PR expression in intraglandular papillary tufts, suggesting that papillary mucinous metaplasia may represent a precancerous state for a certain subset of mucinous adenocarcinomas of the endometrium [27, 32].

In patients without hysterectomy, follow-up of papillary proliferative lesions lacking obvious malignant nuclear features showed an uneventful long-term outcome [25]. Therefore, a lesion with complex papillary architecture should not be diagnosed as well-differentiated mucinous adenocarcinoma solely because of the architecture in the absence of cytologic atypia [25].

Pyloric/Gastric Metaplasia of the Endometrium

Patients with Peutz–Jeghers syndrome (PJS) may have both lobular endocervical glandular hyperplasia and adenoma malignum in the uterine cervix, but they may also have multiple mucinous lesions in other genital organs, including the endometrium, vagina, fallopian tube, and ovary [33, 34] as well as extragenital organs such as the urinary bladder, pelvic serosa, and small intestine [35]. The same multifocal mucinous lesions found in the female genital organs have been described

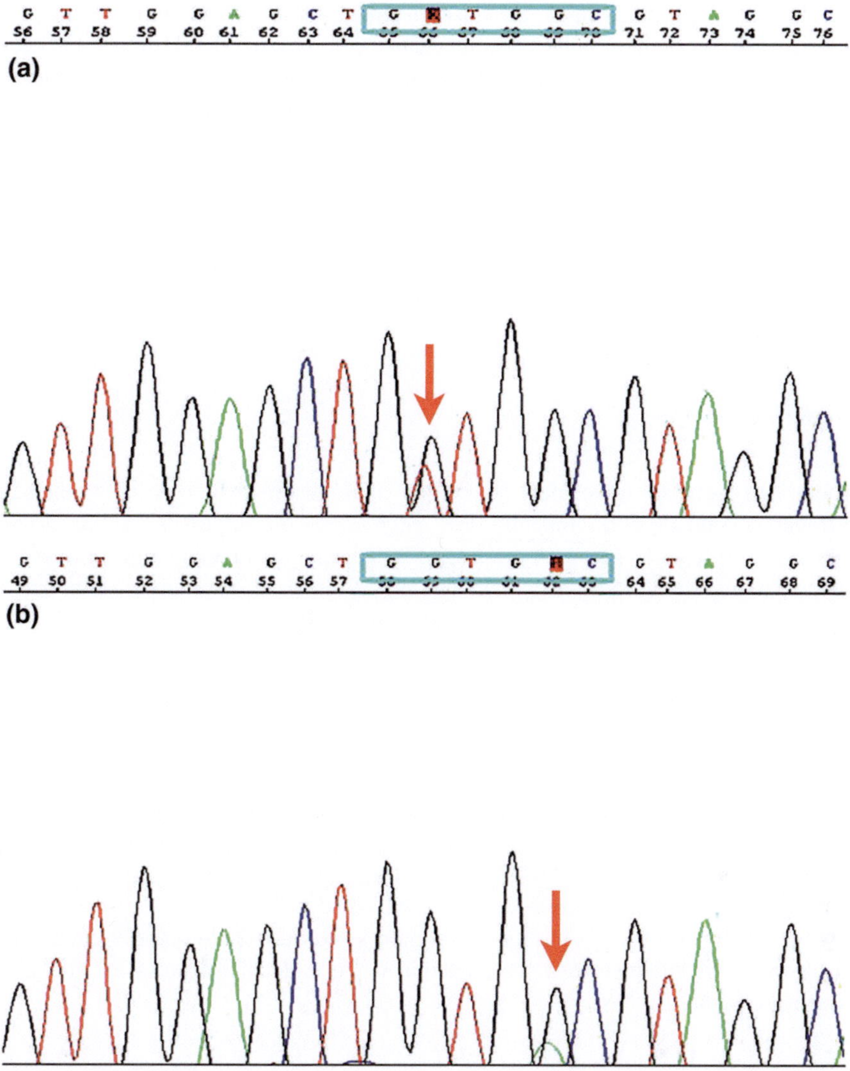

Fig. 7.3 Point mutations in the KRAS gene from GGT to GTT in codon 12 (**a** *arrow*) and from GGC to GAC in codon 13 (**b** *arrow*), causing single amino-acid substitutions from glycine to valine, and glycine to aspartic acid, respectively

in non-PJS patients [36, 37]. Interestingly, the multiple mucinous lesions found in the genital organs almost exclusively show pyloric gland/gastric metaplasia, containing intracytoplasmic gastric-type mucin (of neutral type), and express gastric markers including MUC5AC, MUC6, carbonic anhydrase IX, and HIK1083 [35, 37, 38]. The mucinous epithelium in PJS shows marked morphologic diversity, including benign, malignant, and non-neoplastic (metaplastic) features in the same patient [39]. The tumorigenic mechanism in patients with PJS is not understood, but there may be a common underlying mechanism for pyloric gland metaplasia, such as sporadic or germ line mutation of a STK11/LKB1 gene. The protein product of STK11 involves chromatin remodeling, cellular energy metabolism, cellular arrest and cell proliferation, cell polarity, p53-dependent apoptosis, the regulation of VEGF and Wnt signal transduction [40, 41]. P53 mutations [42] or KRAS mutations have been associated with PJS-associated endocervical [39] and lung cancers [43]. Further study of the cellular function of *STK11/LKB1* may explain why pyloric gland/gastric metaplasia of the endometrium has malignant potential and the pathogenetic link between pyloric gland/gastric metaplasia and neoplasia.

Genetics

There are several molecular alterations that distinguish type I (generally estrogen-dependent and clinically less aggressive, encompassing endometrioid tumors) and type II (generally estrogen-independent and clinically aggressive, encompassing serous and clear cell tumors) endometrial carcinomas, although a substantial overlap exists between the two types [44].

The most common alterations in type I endometrial carcinomas are microsatellite instability and mutations in PTEN, K-RAS, PIK3CA, FGFR2, and beta-catenin genes (CTNNBs), whereas type II carcinomas are more often associated with altered *CDKN2A, TP53*, and *ERBB2* gene functions.

The Cancer Genome Atlas (TCGA) data identified four groups of endometrial carcinoma based on an integrated genomic characterization, including POLE ultramutated, microsatellite instability-high, copy number-low, and copy number-high (serous-like) [45–47]. While these results promise to provide independent prognostic information beyond established risk factors, molecular studies have generally focused on the more common serous and endometrioid carcinoma histotypes, and relatively few have examined the molecular aspects of mucinous adenocarcinoma.

KRAS

Mutations in *KRAS*, which cause aberrant activation, are found in 10–30% of endometrioid adenocarcinomas [48–50], but more than 80% of mucinous adenocarcinomas [31, 32]. More than 95% of pathogenic mutations localize to hotspots in exon 2 (codons 12 and 13). A similar high prevalence of *KRAS* mutations occur in endometrioid adenocarcinomas with prominent mucinous differentiation and complex mucinous proliferation/complex mucinous metaplasia. It is significantly higher in these than in endometrial adenocarcinomas without mucinous components or atypical endometrial hyperplasia [27, 32, 50, 51]. This suggests that KRAS mutational activation is important in the pathogenesis of mucinous endometrial adenocarcinoma. No significant differences in *KRAS* mutation between complex mucinous proliferation/complex mucinous metaplasia and mucinous adenocarcinoma suggests that somatic *KRAS* mutation might occur at an early stage in mucinous carcinogenesis. However, KRAS mutation is not specific for mucinous endometrial adenocarcinoma, as it is common in various human cancers, including those in the pancreas (90%), colon (50%), thyroid (50%), and lung (30%) [52].

Recently, KRAS status has been used to compare pre-treatment and post-treatment changes in a randomized phase II study of the antitumor efficacy of a MEK inhibitor alone vs. a MEK inhibitor in combination with an AKT inhibitor, in patients with recurrent or persistent endometrial cancer [53].

KRAS mutational status may also help refine the risk stratification of patients with endometrial mucinous lesions. KRAS mutation in a biopsy has a positive predictive value of 88% for complex atypical hyperplasia or adenocarcinoma in the follow-up hysterectomy [32]. Simple mucinous metaplasia is not associated with KRAS mutation [27, 31, 32], and the chance of finding endometrial adenocarcinoma in a hysterectomy following a diagnosis of simple mucinous metaplasia on biopsy is negligible [28, 29, 32]. KRAS mutation status also helps differentiate endometrial mucinous adenocarcinoma from endocervical microglandular hyperplasia. Because endometrial and endocervical biopsy/curettage specimens often contain only small amounts of tissue, a highly sensitive and specific test for KRAS mutation is essential.

PTEN

PTEN is the most common genetic alteration in Type I endometrial cancer, being inactivated in 83% of sporadic cases associated with a coexisting or prior premalignant lesion [54]. *PTEN* mutation is one of the earliest known events in the tumorigenesis of endometrioid endometrial adenocarcinoma, occurring in 20–27% of endometrial hyperplasias and 55% of EIN [54]. No PTEN mutations have been seen in either simple or complex mucinous metaplasia of the endometrium [27].

Genetic alterations found in other endometrial carcinomas, including *PIK3CA, PIK3R1*, and *PTEN, ARID1A*, KRAS, FGFR2, ARID1A (BAF250a), CTNNB1 (beta-catenin), and microsatellite instability, have not been properly studied in mucinous adenocarcinoma.

References

1. Fujiwara M, Longacre TA. Low-grade mucinous adenocarcinoma of the uterine corpus: a rare and deceptively bland form of endometrial carcinoma. Am J Surg Pathol. 2011;35:537–44.
2. Ross JC, Eifel PJ, Cox RS, et al. Primary mucinous adenocarcinoma of the endometrium. a clinicopathologic and histochemical study. Am J Surg Pathol. 1983;7:715–29.
3. Melhem MF, Tobon H. Mucinous adenocarcinoma of the endometrium: a clinico-pathological review of 18 cases. Int J Gynecol Pathol. 1987;6:347–55.

4. Zaino R, Carinelli SG, Ellenson LH, et al. Tumours of the uterine corpus. In: Kurman RJ, Carcangiu ML, Herrington CS, et al., editors. WHO classification of tumours of female reproductive organs. 4th ed. Geneva: WHO Press; 2014. p. 128–30.
5. Vang R, Tavassoli FA. Proliferative mucinous lesions of the endometrium: analysis of existing criteria for diagnosing carcinoma in biopsies and curettings. Int J Surg Pathol. 2003;11:261–70.
6. Young RH, Scully RE. Uterine carcinomas simulating microglandular hyperplasia. A report of six cases. Am J Surg Pathol. 1992;16:1092–7.
7. Zaloudek C, Hayashi GM, Ryan IP, et al. Microglandular adenocarcinoma of the endometrium: a form of mucinous adenocarcinoma that may be confused with microglandular hyperplasia of the cervix. Int J Gynecol Pathol. 1997;16:52–9.
8. Qiu W, Mittal K. Comparison of morphologic and immunohistochemical features of cervical microglandular hyperplasia with low-grade mucinous adenocarcinoma of the endometrium. Int J Gynecol Pathol. 2003;22:261–5.
9. Rauh-Hain JA, Vargas RJ, Clemmer J, et al. Mucinous adenocarcinoma of the endometrium compared with endometrioid endometrial cancer: a SEER analysis. Am J Clin Oncol. 2014.
10. Gungorduk K, Ozdemir A, Ertas IE, et al. Is mucinous adenocarcinoma of the endometrium a risk factor for lymph node involvement? A multicenter case–control study. Int J Clin Oncol. 2015;20:782–9.
11. Giordano G, D'Adda T, Gnetti L, et al. Endometrial mucinous microglandular adenocarcinoma: morphologic, immunohistochemical features, and emphasis in the human papillomavirus status. Int J Gynecol Pathol. 2006;25:77–82.
12. Musa F, Huang M, Adams B, et al. Mucinous histology is a risk factor for nodal metastases in endometrial cancer. Gynecol Oncol. 2012;125:541–5.
13. Fukunaga M. Mucinous endometrial adenocarcinoma simulating microglandular hyperplasia of the cervix. Pathol Int. 2000;50:541–5.
14. Zamecnik M, Skalova A, Opatrny V. Microglandular adenocarcinoma of the uterus mimicking microglandular cervical hyperplasia. Ann Diagn Pathol. 2003;7:180–6.
15. Karateke A, Haliloglu B, Atay V, et al. A case of microglandular adenocarcinoma of the endometrium. Gynecol Oncol. 2005;99:778–81.
16. Young RH, Scully RE. Atypical forms of microglandular hyperplasia of the cervix simulating carcinoma. A report of five cases and review of the literature. Am J Surg Pathol. 1989;13:50–6.
17. Stewart CJ, Crook ML. PAX2 and cyclin D1 expression in the distinction between cervical microglandular hyperplasia and endometrial microglandular-like carcinoma: a comparison with p16, vimentin, and Ki67. Int J Gynecol Pathol. 2015;34:90–100.
18. Hong W, Abi-Raad R, Alomari AK, et al. Diagnostic application of KRAS mutation testing in uterine microglandular proliferations. Hum Pathol. 2015;46:1000–5.
19. Lax SF, Pizer ES, Ronnett BM, et al. Comparison of estrogen and progesterone receptor, Ki-67, and p53 immunoreactivity in uterine endometrioid carcinoma and endometrioid carcinoma with squamous, mucinous, secretory, and ciliated cell differentiation. Hum Pathol. 1998;29:924–31.
20. Reyes C, Murali R, Park KJ. Secondary involvement of the adnexa and uterine corpus by carcinomas of the uterine cervix: a detailed morphologic description. Int J Gynecol Pathol. 2015.
21. Yemelyanova A, Vang R, Seidman JD, et al. Endocervical adenocarcinomas with prominent endometrial or endomyometrial involvement simulating primary endometrial carcinomas: utility of HPV DNA detection and immunohistochemical expression of p16 and hormone receptors to confirm the cervical origin of the corpus tumor. Am J Surg Pathol. 2009;33:914–24.
22. Staebler A, Sherman ME, Zaino RJ, et al. Hormone receptor immunohistochemistry and human papillomavirus in situ hybridization are useful for distinguishing endocervical and endometrial adenocarcinomas. Am J Surg Pathol. 2002;26:998–1006.

23. Tanaka H, Kobayashi T, Yoshida K, et al. Low-grade appendiceal mucinous neoplasm with disseminated peritoneal adenomucinosis involving the uterus, mimicking primary mucinous endometrial adenocarcinoma: a case report. J Obstet Gynaecol Res. 2011;37:1726–30.
24. Shaw KC, Kokh D, Ioffe OB, et al. "Pseudomyxoma Endometrii": endometrial deposition of acellular mucin from a low-grade appendiceal mucinous neoplasm as a rare mimic of myxoid uterine tumors. Int J Gynecol Pathol. 2015;34:351–6.
25. Lehman MB, Hart WR. Simple and complex hyperplastic papillary proliferations of the endometrium: a clinicopathologic study of nine cases of apparently localized papillary lesions with fibrovascular stromal cores and epithelial metaplasia. Am J Surg Pathol. 2001;25: 1347–54.
26. Nicolae A, Goyenaga P, McCluggage WG, et al. Endometrial intestinal metaplasia: a report of two cases, including one associated with cervical intestinal and pyloric metaplasia. Int J Gynecol Pathol. 2011;30:492–6.
27. Yoo SH, Park BH, Choi J, et al. Papillary mucinous metaplasia of the endometrium as a possible precursor of endometrial mucinous adenocarcinoma. Mod Pathol. 2012;25: 1496–507.
28. Nucci MR, Prasad CJ, Crum CP, et al. Mucinous endometrial epithelial proliferations: a morphologic spectrum of changes with diverse clinical significance. Mod Pathol. 1999;12:1137–42.
29. Ip PP, Irving JA, McCluggage WG, et al. Papillary proliferation of the endometrium: a clinicopathologic study of 59 cases of simple and complex papillae without cytologic atypia. Am J Surg Pathol. 2013;37:167–77.
30. Jovanovic AS, Boynton KA, Mutter GL. Uteri of women with endometrial carcinoma contain a histopathological spectrum of monoclonal putative precancers, some with microsatellite instability. Cancer Res. 1996;56:1917–21.
31. He M, Jackson CL, Gubrod RB, et al. KRAS mutations in mucinous lesions of the uterus. Am J Clin Pathol. 2015;143:778–84.
32. Alomari A, Abi-Raad R, Buza N, et al. Frequent KRAS mutation in complex mucinous epithelial lesions of the endometrium. Mod Pathol. 2014;27:675–80.
33. Seidman JD. Mucinous lesions of the fallopian tube. a report of seven cases. Am J Surg Pathol. 1994;18:1205–12.
34. Young RH, Scully RE. Mucinous ovarian tumors associated with mucinous adenocarcinomas of the cervix. A clinicopathological analysis of 16 cases. Int J Gynecol Pathol. 1988;7: 99–111.
35. Kato N, Sugawara M, Maeda K, et al. Pyloric gland metaplasia/differentiation in multiple organ systems in a patient with Peutz-Jegher's syndrome. Pathol Int. 2011;61:369–72.
36. Anjarwalla S, Rollason TP, Rooney N, et al. Atypical mucinous metaplasia and intraepithelial neoplasia of the female genital tract–a case report and review of the literature. Int J Gynecol Cancer. 2007;17:1147–50.
37. Mikami Y, Kiyokawa T, Sasajima Y, et al. Reappraisal of synchronous and multifocal mucinous lesions of the female genital tract: a close association with gastric metaplasia. Histopathology. 2009;54:184–91.
38. Liao SY, Rodgers WH, Kauderer J, et al. Endocervical glandular neoplasia associated with lobular endocervical glandular hyperplasia is HPV-independent and correlates with carbonic anhydrase-IX expression: a gynaecological oncology group study. Br J Cancer. 2013;108:613–20.
39. Ito S, Tase T, Satoh K, et al. Gastric-type endocervical glandular neoplasms associated with aberrant p16 expression and K-RAS gene mutation in Peutz-Jeghers syndrome. Pathol Int. 2014;64:283–8.
40. Marignani PA. LKB1, the multitasking tumour suppressor kinase. J Clin Pathol. 2005;58: 15–9.
41. Banno K, Kisu I, Yanokura M, et al. Hereditary gynecological tumors associated with Peutz-Jeghers syndrome (Review). Oncol Lett. 2013;6:1184–8.

42. Korsse SE, Biermann K, Offerhaus GJ, et al. Identification of molecular alterations in gastrointestinal carcinomas and dysplastic hamartomas in Peutz–Jeghers syndrome. Carcinogenesis. 2013;34:1611–9.
43. Zaba O, Holbe D, Aretz S, et al. LKB1 mutant in a KRAS activated adenocarcinoma of the lung associated with Peutz-Jeghers syndrome: a case report. Lung Cancer. 2013;82:368–9.
44. Setiawan VW, Yang HP, Pike MC, et al. Type I and II endometrial cancers: have they different risk factors? J Clin Oncol. 2013;31:2607–18.
45. Cancer Genome Atlas Research N, Kandoth C, Schultz N, et al. Integrated genomic characterization of endometrial carcinoma. Nature. 2013;497:67–73.
46. Le Gallo M, Bell DW. The emerging genomic landscape of endometrial cancer. Clin Chem. 2014;60:98–110.
47. Talhouk A, McConechy MK, Leung S, et al. A clinically applicable molecular-based classification for endometrial cancers. Br J Cancer. 2015;113:299–310.
48. Sasaki H, Nishii H, Takahashi H, et al. Mutation of the Ki-ras protooncogene in human endometrial hyperplasia and carcinoma. Cancer Res. 1993;53:1906–10.
49. Lax SF, Kendall B, Tashiro H, et al. The frequency of p53, K-ras mutations, and microsatellite instability differs in uterine endometrioid and serous carcinoma: evidence of distinct molecular genetic pathways. Cancer. 2000;88:814–24.
50. Feng YZ, Shiozawa T, Miyamoto T, et al. BRAF mutation in endometrial carcinoma and hyperplasia: correlation with KRAS and p53 mutations and mismatch repair protein expression. Clin Cancer Res. 2005;11:6133–8.
51. Dobrzycka B, Terlikowski SJ, Mazurek A, et al. Mutations of the KRAS oncogene in endometrial hyperplasia and carcinoma. Folia Histochem Cytobiol. 2009;47:65–8.
52. Mirkovic J, Sholl LM, Garcia E, et al. Targeted genomic profiling reveals recurrent KRAS mutations and gain of chromosome 1q in mesonephric carcinomas of the female genital tract. Mod Pathol. 2015.
53. Frantz VK. Tumors of the pancreas. In: Atlas of tumor pathology, vol. 7. Washington: Armed Forces Institute of Pathology, 1959. p. 32–3.
54. Mutter GL, Lin MC, Fitzgerald JT, et al. Altered PTEN expression as a diagnostic marker for the earliest endometrial precancers. J Natl Cancer Inst. 2000;92:924–30.

Chapter 8
Molecular Pathology of Uterine Carcinosarcoma

Susanna Leskelä, Belen Pérez-Mies, Juan Manuel Rosa-Rosa, Eva Cristóbal, Michele Biscuola and José Palacios

Clinicopathologic Features of Uterine Carcinosarcoma

Uterine carcinosarcoma (UCS, also known as malignant mixed Müllerian tumor, MMMT) is a rare aggressive neoplasm accounting for approximately 2% of all malignancies of the uterine corpus [1]. It is by definition a high-grade tumor, characterized by a biphasic growth of malignant epithelial and mesenchymal components that are distinct at the histologic or ultrastructural level (Fig. 8.1) [1].

S. Leskelä · B. Pérez-Mies · J.M. Rosa-Rosa · E. Cristóbal · J. Palacios (✉)
Servicio de Anatomía Patológica, Hospital Universitario Ramón y Cajal (IRYCIS), Departamento de Medicina y Especialidades Médicas, Universidad de Alcalá, Madrid, Spain
e-mail: jose.palacios@salud.madrid.org

S. Leskelä
e-mail: susanna.leskela@salud.madrid.org

B. Pérez-Mies
e-mail: bperezm@salud.madrid.org

J.M. Rosa-Rosa
e-mail: juanm.rosa@gmail.com

E. Cristóbal
e-mail: evamaria.cristobal@salud.madrid.org

S. Leskelä · B. Pérez-Mies · J.M. Rosa-Rosa · E. Cristóbal · J. Palacios
Red Temática de Investigación Cooperativa en Cáncer (RTICC), CIBERONC, Carr. Colmenar km.9.100, 28034 Madrid, Spain

M. Biscuola
Department of Pathology, Instituto de Biomedicina de Sevilla (IBiS), Hospital Universitario Virgen del Rocío/CSIC/Universidad de Sevilla, Calle Antonio Maura Montaner, 41013 Seville, Spain
e-mail: michele.biscuola@gmail.com

M.T. Deavers and D.M. Coffey (eds.), *Precision Molecular Pathology of Uterine Cancer*, Molecular Pathology Library,
DOI 10.1007/978-3-319-57985-6_8

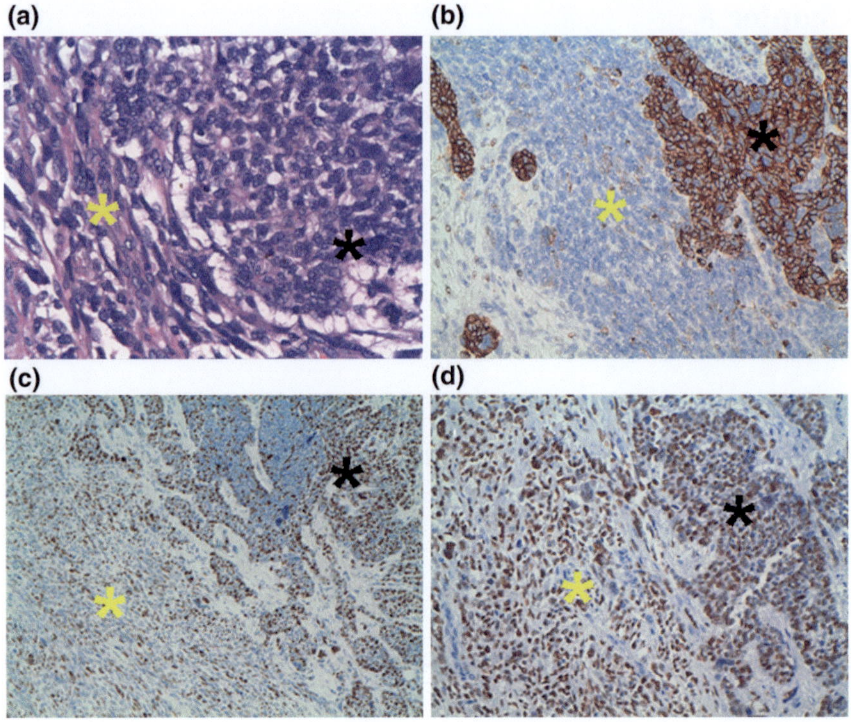

Fig. 8.1 Carcinosarcoma. **a** Hematoxylin & eosin staining showing the epithelial component (*black asterisk*) surrounded by mesenchymal component (*yellow asterisk*). **b** Cytokeratin AE1/AE3 immunohistochemical staining positive in the epithelial component, negative in the mesenchymal component. **c** Ki67 and **d** P53 staining positive in both components

The epithelial component of uterine carcinosarcoma can be endometrioid (most common in most series) or non-endometrioid (serous, clear cell or mixed) [2–7]. The mesenchymal component can be minimal or extensive and can be subdivided into homologous or heterologous, the latter including skeletal muscle, cartilage, fat, or osteoid (in up to 60% of tumors) [2–8].

Uterine carcinosarcoma shares similar risk factors with endometrial carcinoma, such as obesity, nulliparity, smoking, and exogenous estrogen use, but overall it is detected at more advanced stages and has a significantly worse survival rate than high-grade endometrial carcinomas [2, 6, 9–12].

Clonality is crucial in establishing the histogenesis of carcinosarcoma [10]. The hypotheses proposed concerning the pathogenesis of this tumor include combination, conversion, and collision theories. The first proposes that a single stem cell undergoes divergent differentiation early in tumor development, while the conversion theory places divergence at a later stage during the evolution of the tumor [13]. As stated by Abeln and colleagues, early divergence would result in high somatic-genetic discordance of the carcinoma and sarcoma due to the stochastic nature of the evolutionary process, thus divergent transformation at a later stage of tumor development is favored in the majority of the tumors (conversion theory) [14]. In a minority of tumors, the two components are seen in juxtaposition and in these cases, the collision theory may be favored [13].

Molecular studies support that the epithelial and mesenchymal components of carcinosarcoma are related as they show similar genetic alterations. These include identical patterns of chromosome X inactivation [10, 15], loss of heterozygosity in identical alleles [14, 16], uniform pattern of chromosomal gains, losses or aberrations [17], similar loss of expression of mismatch repair (MMR) proteins and microsatellite instability (MSI-high) [6, 18–21], similar angiogenic activity by VEGF and angiopoietins [22, 23], comparable cyclo-oxygenase-2 (COX-2), EGFR and Her2neu overexpression [22, 24, 25], identical *KRAS* gene mutations [15, 26, 27], identical *TP53* gene mutations and p53 pattern of expression [3, 6, 14, 16, 28–30], and similar alterations in the p16-retinoblastoma pathway [3, 31–33].

Thus, it is now generally accepted that most carcinosarcomas are carcinomas with divergent differentiation, as their malignant behavior is most often driven by the carcinomatous component, with lymphvascular invasion and distant metastases mostly represented by the epithelial component [4, 5, 34, 35]. Although most carcinosarcomas are carcinomas with divergent differentiation, with an admixture of malignant epithelial and mesenchymal elements, a small percentage of these tumors probably represent real collision tumors. This particular subset of MMMTs is shown to be biclonal and most likely develops from two independent cell populations [10, 15].

The sarcomatous component in monoclonal UCS is thought to be derived from the carcinomatous component as a result of transdifferentiation (epithelial-to-mesenchymal transition, EMT) during the evolution of the tumor [36, 37]. EMT involves the acquisition of a mesenchymal/stem cell-like phenotype by the malignant epithelial cells, endowing these cells with migratory and invasive properties, promoting cancer progression, preventing cell death and senescence, and inducing resistance to chemotherapy [38].

UCS follows an aggressive clinical course and accounts for 16% of deaths caused by uterine malignancy [6, 39]. Patients with International Federation of Gynecology and Obstetrics (FIGO) stage I–II disease have a 5-year disease-free survival of 59%, while those with stages 3 and 4 disease have a 5-year disease-free survival of 22 and 9%, respectively [39]. The most important prognostic factors in these tumors include FIGO stage and depth of myometrial invasion [4, 7, 9, 11, 12, 28]. Other known clinicopathologic features associated with worse outcome are grade and histology of the epithelial component and lymphvascular invasion [4, 6, 9, 12], while grade and amount of the sarcomatous component and presence of heterologous elements are not related to overall outcome in most studies [4, 8, 10, 28]. A recent study, however, reported an increased rate of recurrence and decreased rate of survival in stage I carcinosarcoma with heterologous differentiation [2].

Table 8.1 Comparison of gene mutation frequency among different histologic types of endometrial cancer

GENE	Endometrioid adenocarcinoma (%)	Serous carcinoma (%)	Carcinosarcoma (%)
PTEN	79	2	19
PIK3CA	55	43	35
PIK3R1	39	4	10
CTNNB1	37	0	0
ARID1A	39	9	14
KRAS	26	2	12
CTCF	22	0	5
TP53	14	89	91
FBXW7	12	32	39
PPP2R1A	7	27	28
CHD4	14	13	17

Genetic Alterations

p53 Pathway

The most common mutational event in UCS is *TP53* mutation (Table 8.1). Several studies have focused on *TP53* in uterine carcinosarcoma, using p53 protein overexpression, as well as *TP53* mutation analysis, to detect alterations in this pathway [3, 6, 14, 15, 28–30, 33]. In these studies, around 60 and 50% of uterine carcinosarcoma showed p53 protein overexpression and/or *TP53* gene mutation. Moreover, the degree of concordance between the carcinomatous and sarcomatous components was 85% for protein overexpression and 96% for gene mutation, providing strong evidence for monoclonal origin of both components (Fig. 8.1).

Most recent studies using next-generation sequencing (NGS) techniques have demonstrated that the frequency of *TP53* mutation in UCS is in fact higher, between 64 and 90% [40–42]. According to data generated by the TCGA Research Network (http://cancergenome.nih.gov/), the most frequent mutations are R248Q and R273C/H (12 and 7%, respectively), while 32% of mutations are located on known hotspot residues in the DNA binding domain (Fig. 8.2) [43].

Most of the tumors harboring missense *TP53* mutations showed diffuse nuclear p53 immunostaining (although there are exceptions). Complete loss of nuclear p53 expression is usually detected in cases with indel or nonsense mutations.

In most human tumors with *TP53* mutation, p16 overexpression is a common event. In accordance with this observation, it has been reported that about 60% of UCS overexpress p16. Concordance of p16 overexpression between the carcinomatous and sarcomatous components was 85% [3, 31–33, 44].

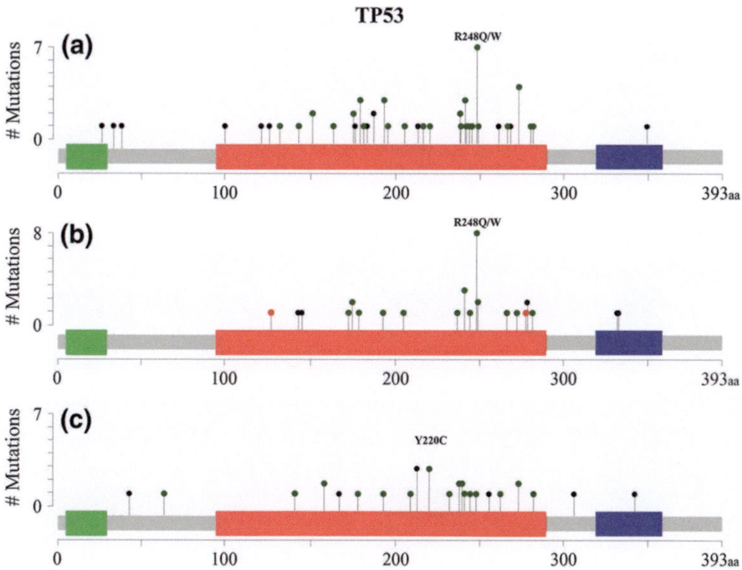

Fig. 8.2 Schematic representation of *TP53* mutations in endometrial carcinoma. **a** UCS (n = 57), **b** ESC (n = 115), and **c** EEC (n = 409). Mutations are indicated as *lollipop plots* along the domains of *TP53*. *Green dots* indicate missense mutations, *red dots* indicate frameshift mutations and *black dots* truncating mutations. *Green boxes* represent the transactivation motif, *red boxes* the DNA binding domain, and *blue boxes* the tetramerization motif. Most mutations have been detected in the DNA binding domain. The mutation plot was constructed based on data from TCGA using the cBioPortal visualization tool MutationMapper v1.0 [65, 66]

PI3K/AKT Pathway

In UCS, mutations involving genes that encode the kinase or regulatory proteins of the PI3K/AKT pathway have been detected in up to 67% of cases [42], including multiple PI3K/AKT pathway proteins mutated in the same tumor. *PIK3CA* mutations have been found in 11 to 40% [27, 40, 41, 45, 46] of the tumors, which were scattered throughout the different functional domains of *PIK3CA* (Fig. 8.3). In addition to both traditional *PIK3CA* hotspot (exons 9 and 20) mutations, a lower proportion of UCS carry mutations in exon 1, in the adaptor binding domain, helical domain, and C2 domain that can also enhance kinase enzymatic activity [42, 46]. *PI3KCA* mutations have been found in the carcinoma and sarcoma components of the primary tumor, as well as in the metastatic tumor. This indicates that these mutations occur relatively early in the tumorigenesis of carcinosarcoma and likely represent important oncogenic driver events that could be targeted with PIK3CA/mTOR inhibitors [41].

PTEN mutations occur in a subset of UCS. Although Jones et al. [40] reported that 47% of 17 UCS cases in their series carried a *PTEN* mutation, this figure is significantly higher than that observed in the McConechy et al. (17%)

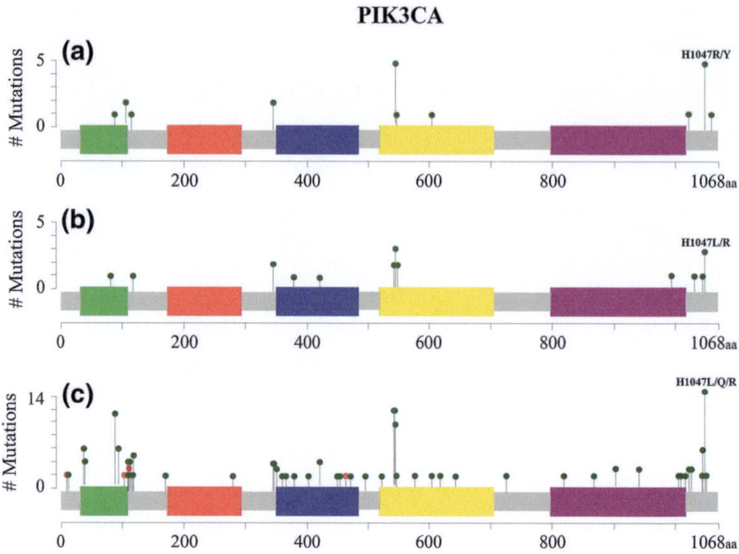

Fig. 8.3 Schematic representation of *PIK3CA* mutations in endometrial carcinoma. **a** UCS (n = 57), **b** ESC (n = 115) and **c** EEC (n = 409). Mutations are indicated as *lollipop plots* along the domains of *PIK3CA*. *Green dots* indicate missense mutations and *red dots* indicate frameshift mutations. *Green boxes* represent the p68-binding domain, *red boxes* the ras-binding domain, *blue boxes* the Phosphoinositide 3-kinase C2 motif, *yellow boxes* the accessory domain, and *purple boxes* the Phosphatidylinositol 3- and 4-kinase domain. Mutations are found throughout the different functional domains of *PIK3CA*. The mutation plot was constructed based on data from TCGA using the cBioPortal visualization tool MutationMapper v1.0 [65, 66]

and TCGA (19%) series. *PTEN* mutations in UCS frequently coexist with *PIK3CA* mutations [41].

Other genes of the PI3K/AKT pathway that are mutated at lower frequencies in UCS include *PIK3R1* (10–17%), *PIK3R2*, *AKT1*, *AKT2,* and *AKT3* (less than 5% for each gene) [40, 42, 46].

Other Mutated Genes in UCS

UCS can carry mutations that are typically detected in endometrial serous carcinoma (ESC). For example, mutations of *FBXW7* and *PPP2R1A* have been reported in 20 to 39% and 1 to 38% of cases, respectively [40, 42].

As to genes recurrently mutated in endometrioid endometrial cancer (EEC), mutation in *ARID1A* occurs in 10 to 15% of UCS. This mutation is frequently associated with loss of protein expression. CTNNB1 mutations are infrequent in UCS [40, 45]. Regarding *POLE* mutations, Hembree et al. [47] identified a *POLE* proofreading-domain mutation, V411L, in a UCS. After reviewing uterine carcinosarcoma data from TCGA, a single sample with a *POLE* mutation in the same region, P286R, was reported. Thus, although mutations in *POLE* are uncommon, these findings suggest that they are present in a small proportion of UCS.

Mismatch Repair (MMR) Deficiency

The expression or the presence of mutations in *MLH1*, *PMS2*, *MSH2,* and *MSH6* has been evaluated in a number of studies. The frequency of MMR deficiency ranged between 3 and 23%. Lower frequencies were observed in series analyzing a larger number of samples [41, 48], compared to studies with a smaller sample size [21, 40]. In most tumors, MMR deficiency is probably due to *MLH1* methylation [48], although in some cases, it might be associated with Lynch syndrome [49].

Copy Number Variations

The amplification frequencies for relevant oncogenes are shown in Table 8.2. The most frequently amplified oncogene in UCS is *CCNE1.* This amplification is associated with poor prognosis and resistance to chemotherapy in various tumors, such as ovarian high-grade serous carcinoma, according to data in TCGA Research Network. Regarding C-MYC amplification, Schipf et al. analyzed a series of 30 paraffin-embedded carcinosarcomas of the ovary and of the uterus by FISH and reported gene amplification in 78% of the cases. The amplification had a lower frequency in the sarcomatous component compared to the carcinomatous component [17].

In the few studies that analyzed HER2 amplification in UCS, the frequencies ranged from 3 to 20% [50–52]. Given the significant fraction of UCS with *ERBB2* amplification, it has been suggested that anti-HER2 therapies, such as trastuzumab may represent a treatment option for a subset of patients. Results from recent studies indicate that UCS cell lines and derived xenografts with HER2 amplification are very responsive to T-DM1; hence, it has been suggested that T-DM1 may represent a novel treatment option for the subset of carcinosarcoma patients who harbor disease refractory to traditional salvage chemotherapy and/or are unresponsive to trastuzumab [53].

Table 8.2 Comparison of gene amplification frequency among different histologic types of endometrial cancer

Gene	Endometrioid adenocarcinoma (%)	Serous carcinoma (%)	Carcinosarcoma (%)
CCNE1	2	31	42
MYC	5	26	23
MECOM	6	38	21
PIK3CA	3	27	14
ERBB2	2	23	10

Other oncogenes frequently amplified in UCS, but not reported in TCGA data set, are *ZNF217*, *EGFR*, and *URI*. Schipf et al. reported amplification of *ZNF217* in 87% of gynecologic CS, which was seen in both tumor components [17]. EGFR protein overexpression has been reported in 45 to 82% of UCS, always at a higher rate in the sarcomatous component, supporting biological differences with respect to the carcinomatous component [22, 50, 54]. However, the only study analyzing a large number of UCSs for *EGFR* amplification by FISH reported that only 19% of tumors carried this molecular alteration [46].

Wang et al. reported *URI1* (unconventional prefolding RPB5 interactor 1) amplification in 40% of UCS [55]. UCS patients with *URI1* amplification had 13% tumor-free survival compared to 41% in the absence of *URI* amplification. Importantly, the patients with *URI1* amplification had poor response to adjuvant treatment compared to a control group. Tumors with *URI1* amplification displayed decreased transcription of genes encoding tumor suppressor and apoptotic regulators and increased expression of genes regulating oncogenesis, survival and metastasis. Overexpression of *URI1* in a cultured cell model induced *ATM* expression and resistance to cisplatin [55].

mRNA and miRNA Expression Profiles

Few studies have analyzed mRNA and miRNA expression profiles in UCS. Gene expression studies have shown changes in the expression of genes modulating processes such as EMT (see below), muscle differentiation, cancer testis antigens (CTAs), and immune response. In the study by Romero-Pérez et al., a large proportion of the differentially expressed genes were involved in muscle differentiation, probably due to the rhabdomyoblastic differentiation seen in most tumors studied [56]. UCS is also characterized by the overexpression of many members of the CTA family, including *CTCF*, also known as *brother of the regulator of imprinted sites* (*BORIS*), an oncogene that deregulates the cancer epigenome. *CTCFL* expression is thought to mediate the demethylation of other CTA genes, resulting in activation via repression [57]. Given the immunogenicity and tissue-restricted expression of CTA, it is reasonable to suggest that UCS patients might benefit from immunotherapy based on CTA vaccines [56].

Carcinosarcomas have a unique microRNA (miRNA) signature that differs from both endometrioid and serous carcinomas [58]. Certain miRNAs appear to be consistently altered in carcinosarcoma compared to both EEC and ESC. For instance, miR-518b is down-regulated in carcinosarcoma compared to both endometrioid and serous tumors, while miR-20b, miR-301, and miR-487 are up-regulated. It has been suggested that low expression of miR-20b inhibits tumor cell growth but gives the tumor cell more resistance to apoptosis in hypoxia [59]. Additionally, Hovey et al. reported miR-888 overexpression in UCS and found that the progesterone receptor is one of its direct targets [60].

We have analyzed the microRNA signatures associated with EMT in human UCS and determined their relationships with EMT markers and repressors of

E-cadherin transcription [36, 61]. The expression of E-, P- and N-cadherin, cadherin-11, p120, vimentin, SPARC, fascin, and caveolin-1 was studied in a group of 76 UCS by immunohistochemistry. In addition, real-time PCR was used to measure differences in the expression of 384 miRNAs, *E-cadherin*, *cadherin-11*, *SPARC, SNAIL*, *ZEB1*, *ZEB2*, *TWIST-1*, *TCF4*, *TGFβ1,* and *TGFβ2* between the epithelial and mesenchymal components of 23 ECSs. Loss of epithelial characteristics, including cadherin switching (loss of E-cadherin and expression of N-cadherin and/or cadherin 11) and the acquisition of a mesenchymal phenotype, was accompanied by changes in the profile of miRNA expression and the up-regulation of all the E-cadherin repressors analyzed. A greater than five-fold difference in expression of 14 miRNAs between both neoplastic components was seen. Members of the miR-200 family were down-regulated in the mesenchymal part of the ECS. In addition, miR-23b and miR-29c, which are involved in the inhibition of mesenchymal markers, and miR-203, which is involved in the inhibition of cell stemness, were also down-regulated. Up-regulated miRNAs included miR-155, miR-369-5p, miR-370, miR-450a, and miR-542-5p. These data suggest that in human UCS the interplay between transcriptional repressors of E-cadherin and miRNAs provides a link between EMT-activation and the maintenance of stemness [56, 61].

Regulation of miRNA expression via methylation has been observed for miR-200 and miR-205 loci in both cancer and normal tissue [62, 63]. We have detected down-regulation of the miR-200 cluster and miR-205 during EMT both in vitro (MDCK transfectants) and in vivo (ECS) models of EMT [61].

Molecular Types of UCS

Given the mutational profile previously described (Table 8.1), it is obvious that most UCS show a serous-like, copy number high molecular type. In the study by McConechy et al., part of the tumors showed endometrial serous carcinoma-like mutation profiles (characterized by the presence of *TP53* mutation with *PPP2R1A* and/or *FBXW7* mutations, and the absence of *PTEN*, *CTNNB1*, *KRAS,* or *ARID1A* mutations), while other tumors displayed endometrioid adenocarcinoma-like mutation profiles (characterized by the presence of *PTEN*, *CTNNB1*, *KRAS,* and/or *ARID1A* mutations). Based on the combined genetic and immunohistochemical profiles in that cohort, 18 tumors had serous-like and 11 tumors had endometrioid-like molecular profiles. Good correlation was found between histologic subtyping (based on the morphology of the epithelial component) and molecular subtyping in 27 of 29 UCS (93%) [41].

Most of the UCS that had an endometrioid adenocarcinoma-like mutation profile also had *TP53* mutations, suggesting that *TP53* can be involved in the progression of some copy number low endometrioid adenocarcinomas to UCS, as has been previously reported in undifferentiated endometrial carcinoma [64]. Finally, only a few UCS belong to the microsatellite-unstable hypermutated molecular type and the *POLE*-mutated ultramutated molecular type. This molecular heterogeneity among UCS may have treatment implications with emerging therapies.

Acknowledgements The group has funding from Instituto Carlos III (ISCIII) (CIBERONC, PI13/02477, RD12/0036/0064 and CB16/12/00316), co-financed by the European Development Regional Fund. 'A way to achieve Europe' FEDER, and by Fundació La Marató de TV3 (2/C2013). SL is a PhD investigator funded by Asociación Española Contra el Cáncer (AECC). JMRR and EC are PhD investigators, JMRR is funded by ISCII (CIBERONC) and EC is funded by ISCIII (RD12/0036/0064) and MB by ISCII (RD12/0036/0017).

References

1. Kurman R. WHO classification of tumours of female reproductive organs. In: Kurman Robert, editor. Lyon: IARC Press; 2014.
2. Ferguson SE, Tornos C, Hummer A, Barakat RR, Soslow RA. Prognostic features of surgical stage I uterine carcinosarcoma. Am J Surg Pathol. 2007;31(11):1653–61.
3. Buza N, Tavassoli FA. Comparative analysis of P16 and P53 expression in uterine malignant mixed mullerian tumors. Int J Gynecol Pathol. 2009;28(6):514–21.
4. Silverberg SG, Major FJ, Blessing JA, Fetter B, Askin FB, Liao SY, et al. Carcinosarcoma (malignant mixed mesodermal tumor) of the uterus. A gynecologic oncology group pathologic study of 203 cases. Int J Gynecol Pathol. 1990;9(1):1–19.
5. Sreenan JJ, Hart WR. Carcinosarcomas of the female genital tract. A pathologic study of 29 metastatic tumors: further evidence for the dominant role of the epithelial component and the conversion theory of histogenesis. Am J Surg Pathol. 1995;19(6):666–74.
6. de Jong RA, Nijman HW, Wijbrandi TF, Reyners AK, Boezen HM, Hollema H. Molecular markers and clinical behavior of uterine carcinosarcomas: focus on the epithelial tumor component. Mod Pathol. 2011;24(10):1368–79.
7. Costa MJ, Vogelsan J, Young LJ. p53 gene mutation in female genital tract carcinosarcomas (malignant mixed mullerian tumors): a clinicopathologic study of 74 cases. Mod Pathol. 1994;7(6):619–27.
8. Costa MJ, Khan R, Judd R. Carcinoma (malignant mixed mullerian [mesodermal] tumor) of the uterus and ovary. Correlation of clinical, pathologic, and immunohistochemical features in 29 cases. Arch Pathol Lab Med. 1991;115(6):583–90.
9. Amant F, Cadron I, Fuso L, Berteloot P, de Jonge E, Jacomen G, et al. Endometrial carcinosarcomas have a different prognosis and pattern of spread compared to high-risk epithelial endometrial cancer. Gynecol Oncol. 2005;98(2):274–80.
10. George E, Lillemoe TJ, Twiggs LB, Perrone T. Malignant mixed mullerian tumor versus high-grade endometrial carcinoma and aggressive variants of endometrial carcinoma: a comparative analysis of survival. Int J Gynecol Pathol. 1995;14(1):39–44.
11. Callister M, Ramondetta LM, Jhingran A, Burke TW, Eifel PJ. Malignant mixed mullerian tumors of the uterus: analysis of patterns of failure, prognostic factors, and treatment outcome. Int J Radiat Oncol Biol Phys. 2004;58(3):786–96.
12. Bansal N, Herzog TJ, Seshan VE, Schiff PB, Burke WM, Cohen CJ, et al. Uterine carcinosarcomas and grade 3 endometrioid cancers: evidence for distinct tumor behavior. Obstet Gynecol. 2008;112(1):64–70.
13. McCluggage WG. Malignant biphasic uterine tumours: carcinosarcomas or metaplastic carcinomas? J Clin Pathol. 2002;55(5):321–5.

14. Abeln EC, Smit VT, Wessels JW, de Leeuw WJ, Cornelisse CJ, Fleuren GJ. Molecular genetic evidence for the conversion hypothesis of the origin of malignant mixed mullerian tumours. J Pathol. 1997;183(4):424–31.
15. Wada H, Enomoto T, Fujita M, Yoshino K, Nakashima R, Kurachi H, et al. Molecular evidence that most but not all carcinosarcomas of the uterus are combination tumors. Cancer Res. 1997;57(23):5379–85.
16. Fujii H, Yoshida M, Gong ZX, Matsumoto T, Hamano Y, Fukunaga M, et al. Frequent genetic heterogeneity in the clonal evolution of gynecological carcinosarcoma and its influence on phenotypic diversity. Cancer Res. 2000;60(1):114–20.
17. Schipf A, Mayr D, Kirchner T, Diebold J. Molecular genetic aberrations of ovarian and uterine carcinosarcomas–a CGH and FISH study. Virchows Arch. 2008;452(3):259–68.
18. Jin Z, Ogata S, Tamura G, Katayama Y, Fukase M, Yajima M, et al. Carcinosarcomas (malignant mullerian mixed tumors) of the uterus and ovary: a genetic study with special reference to histogenesis. Int J Gynecol Pathol. 2003;22(4):368–73.
19. Lax SF. Molecular genetic pathways in various types of endometrial carcinoma: from a phenotypical to a molecular-based classification. Virchows Arch. 2004;444(3):213–23.
20. South SA, Hutton M, Farrell C, Mhawech-Fauceglia P, Rodabaugh KJ. Uterine carcinosarcoma associated with hereditary nonpolyposis colorectal cancer. Obstet Gynecol. 2007;110(2 Pt 2):543–5.
21. Taylor NP, Zighelboim I, Huettner PC, Powell MA, Gibb RK, Rader JS, et al. DNA mismatch repair and TP53 defects are early events in uterine carcinosarcoma tumorigenesis. Mod Pathol. 2006;19(10):1333–8.
22. Cimbaluk D, Rotmensch J, Scudiere J, Gown A, Bitterman P. Uterine carcinosarcoma: immunohistochemical studies on tissue microarrays with focus on potential therapeutic targets. Gynecol Oncol. 2007;105(1):138–44.
23. Emoto M, Iwasaki H, Ishiguro M, Kikuchi M, Horiuchi S, Saito T, et al. Angiogenesis in carcinosarcomas of the uterus: differences in the microvessel density and expression of vascular endothelial growth factor between the epithelial and mesenchymal elements. Hum Pathol. 1999;30(10):1232–41.
24. Amant F, Vloeberghs V, Woestenborghs H, Debiec-Rychter M, Verbist L, Moerman P, et al. ERBB-2 gene overexpression and amplification in uterine sarcomas. Gynecol Oncol. 2004;95 (3):583–7.
25. Bland AE, Stone R, Heuser C, Shu J, Jazaeri A, Shutter J, et al. A clinical and biological comparison between malignant mixed mullerian tumors and grade 3 endometrioid endometrial carcinomas. Int J Gynecol Cancer. 2009;19(2):261–5.
26. Caduff RF, Johnston CM, Frank TS. Mutations of the Ki-ras oncogene in carcinoma of the endometrium. Am J Pathol. 1995;146(1):182–8.
27. Murray S, Linardou H, Mountzios G, Manoloukos M, Markaki S, Eleutherakis-Papaiakovou E, et al. Low frequency of somatic mutations in uterine sarcomas: a molecular analysis and review of the literature. Mutat Res. 2010;686(1–2):68–73.
28. Iwasa Y, Haga H, Konishi I, Kobashi Y, Higuchi K, Katsuyama E, et al. Prognostic factors in uterine carcinosarcoma: a clinicopathologic study of 25 patients. Cancer. 1998;82(3):512–9.
29. Kounelis S, Jones MW, Papadaki H, Bakker A, Swalsky P, Finkelstein SD. Carcinosarcomas (malignant mixed mullerian tumors) of the female genital tract: comparative molecular analysis of epithelial and mesenchymal components. Hum Pathol. 1998;29(1):82–7.
30. Liu FS, Kohler MF, Marks JR, Bast RC Jr, Boyd J, Berchuck A. Mutation and overexpression of the p53 tumor suppressor gene frequently occurs in uterine and ovarian sarcomas. Obstet Gynecol. 1994;83(1):118–24.
31. Reid-Nicholson M, Iyengar P, Hummer AJ, Linkov I, Asher M, Soslow RA. Immunophenotypic diversity of endometrial adenocarcinomas: implications for differential diagnosis. Mod Pathol. 2006;19(8):1091–100.
32. Robinson-Bennett B, Belch RZ, Han AC. Loss of p16 in recurrent malignant mixed mullerian tumors of the uterus. Int J Gynecol Cancer. 2006;16(3):1354–7.

33. Kanthan R, Senger JL, Diudea D. Malignant mixed Mullerian tumors of the uterus: histopathological evaluation of cell cycle and apoptotic regulatory proteins. World J Surg Oncol. 2010;8:60.
34. Nordal RR, Kristensen GB, Stenwig AE, Nesland JM, Pettersen EO, Trope CG. An evaluation of prognostic factors in uterine carcinosarcoma. Gynecol Oncol. 1997;67(3): 316–21.
35. Nicotina PA, Ferlazzo G, Vincelli AM. Proliferation indices and p53-immunocytochemistry in uterine mixed mullerian tumors. Histol Histopathol. 1997;12(4):967–72.
36. Castilla MA, Moreno-Bueno G, Romero-Perez L, Van De Vijver K, Biscuola M, Lopez-Garcia MA, et al. Micro-RNA signature of the epithelial-mesenchymal transition in endometrial carcinosarcoma. J Pathol. 2011;223(1):72–80.
37. Chiyoda T, Tsuda H, Tanaka H, Kataoka F, Nomura H, Nishimura S, et al. Expression profiles of carcinosarcoma of the uterine corpus-are these similar to carcinoma or sarcoma? Genes Chromosomes Cancer. 2012;51(3):229–39.
38. Thiery JP, Acloque H, Huang RY, Nieto MA. Epithelial–mesenchymal transitions in development and disease. Cell. 2009;139(5):871–90.
39. Gonzalez Bosquet J, Terstriep SA, Cliby WA, Brown-Jones M, Kaur JS, Podratz KC, et al. The impact of multi-modal therapy on survival for uterine carcinosarcomas. Gynecol Oncol. 2010;116(3):419–23.
40. Jones S, Stransky N, McCord CL, Cerami E, Lagowski J, Kelly D, et al. Genomic analyses of gynaecologic carcinosarcomas reveal frequent mutations in chromatin remodelling genes. Nat Commun. 2014;5:5006.
41. McConechy MK, Hoang LN, Chui MH, Senz J, Yang W, Rozenberg N, et al. In-depth molecular profiling of the biphasic components of Uterine Carcinosarcomas. J Pathol Clin Res. 2015;1(3):173–85.
42. Cherniack, Shen, Walter, Stewart, Murray, Bowlby, et al. Integrated molecular characterization of Uterine Carcinosarcoma. Cancer Cell. 2017;31(3):411–23.
43. D'Brot A, Kurtz P, Regan E, Jakubowski B, Abrams JM. A platform for interrogating cancer-associated p53 alleles. Oncogene. 2016;36(2):286–91.
44. Semczuk A, Skomra D, Chyzynska M, Szewczuk W, Olcha P, Korobowicz E. Immunohistochemical analysis of carcinomatous and sarcomatous components in the uterine carcinosarcoma: a case report. Pathol Res Pract. 2008;204(3):203–7.
45. Growdon WB, Roussel BN, Scialabba VL, Foster R, Dias-Santagata D, Iafrate AJ, et al. Tissue-specific signatures of activating PIK3CA and RAS mutations in carcinosarcomas of gynecologic origin. Gynecol Oncol. 2011;121(1):212–7.
46. Biscuola M, Van de Vijver K, Castilla MA, Romero-Perez L, Lopez-Garcia MA, Diaz-Martin J, et al. Oncogene alterations in endometrial carcinosarcomas. Hum Pathol. 2013;44(5): 852–9.
47. Hembree TN, Teer JK, Hakam A, Chiappori AA. Genetic investigation of uterine carcinosarcoma: case report and cohort analysis. Cancer Control. 2016;23(1):61–6.
48. Hoang LN, Ali RH, Lau S, Gilks CB, Lee CH. Immunohistochemical survey of mismatch repair protein expression in uterine sarcomas and carcinosarcomas. Int J Gynecol Pathol. 2014;33(5):483–91.
49. Mills AM, Liou S, Ford JM, Berek JS, Pai RK, Longacre TA. Lynch syndrome screening should be considered for all patients with newly diagnosed endometrial cancer. Am J Surg Pathol. 2014;38(11):1501–9.
50. Livasy CA, Reading FC, Moore DT, Boggess JF, Lininger RA. EGFR expression and HER2/neu overexpression/amplification in endometrial carcinosarcoma. Gynecol Oncol. 2006;100(1):101–6.
51. Raspollini MR, Susini T, Amunni G, Paglierani M, Taddei A, Marchionni M, et al. COX-2, c-KIT and HER-2/neu expression in uterine carcinosarcomas: prognostic factors or potential markers for targeted therapies? Gynecol Oncol. 2005;96(1):159–67.

52. Sawada M, Tsuda H, Kimura M, Okamoto S, Kita T, Kasamatsu T, et al. Different expression patterns of KIT, EGFR, and HER-2 (c-erbB-2) oncoproteins between epithelial and mesenchymal components in uterine carcinosarcoma. Cancer Sci. 2003;94(11):986–91.
53. Nicoletti R, Lopez S, Bellone S, Cocco E, Schwab CL, Black JD, et al. T-DM1, a novel antibody-drug conjugate, is highly effective against uterine and ovarian carcinosarcomas overexpressing HER2. Clin Exp Metastasis. 2015;32(1):29–38.
54. Hayes MP, Douglas W, Ellenson LH. Molecular alterations of EGFR and PIK3CA in uterine serous carcinoma. Gynecol Oncol. 2009;113(3):370–3.
55. Wang Y, Garabedian MJ, Logan SK. URI1 amplification in uterine carcinosarcoma associates with chemo-resistance and poor prognosis. Am J Cancer Res. 2015;5(7):2320–9.
56. Romero-Perez L, Castilla MA, Lopez-Garcia MA, Diaz-Martin J, Biscuola M, Ramiro-Fuentes S, et al. Molecular events in endometrial carcinosarcomas and the role of high mobility group AT-hook 2 in endometrial carcinogenesis. Hum Pathol. 2013;44(2):244–54.
57. Risinger JI, Chandramouli GV, Maxwell GL, Custer M, Pack S, Loukinov D, et al. Global expression analysis of cancer/testis genes in uterine cancers reveals a high incidence of BORIS expression. Clin Cancer Res. 2007;13(6):1713–9.
58. Ratner ES, Tuck D, Richter C, Nallur S, Patel RM, Schultz V, et al. MicroRNA signatures differentiate uterine cancer tumor subtypes. Gynecol Oncol. 2010;118(3):251–7.
59. Lei Z, Li B, Yang Z, Fang H, Zhang GM, Feng ZH, et al. Regulation of HIF-1alpha and VEGF by miR-20b tunes tumor cells to adapt to the alteration of oxygen concentration. PLoS ONE. 2009;4(10):e7629.
60. Hovey AM, Devor EJ, Breheny PJ, Mott SL, Dai D, Thiel KW, et al. miR-888: a novel cancer-testis antigen that targets the progesterone receptor in endometrial cancer. Transl Oncol. 2015;8(2):85–96.
61. Diaz-Martin J, Diaz-Lopez A, Moreno-Bueno G, Castilla MA, Rosa-Rosa JM, Cano A, et al. A core microRNA signature associated with inducers of the epithelial-to-mesenchymal transition. J Pathol. 2014;232(3):319–29.
62. Vrba L, Garbe JC, Stampfer MR, Futscher BW. Epigenetic regulation of normal human mammary cell type-specific miRNAs. Genome Res. 2011;21(12):2026–37.
63. Wiklund ED, Gao S, Hulf T, Sibbritt T, Nair S, Costea DE, et al. MicroRNA alterations and associated aberrant DNA methylation patterns across multiple sample types in oral squamous cell carcinoma. PLoS ONE. 2011;6(11):e27840.
64. Rosa-Rosa JM, Leskela S, Cristobal-Lana E, Santon A, Lopez-Garcia MA, Munoz G, et al. Molecular genetic heterogeneity in undifferentiated endometrial carcinomas. Mod Pathol. 2016;29(11):1390–98.
65. Cerami E, Gao J, Dogrusoz U, Gross BE, Sumer SO, Aksoy BA, et al. The cBio cancer genomics portal: an open platform for exploring multidimensional cancer genomics data. Cancer Discov. 2012;2(5):401–4.
66. Gao J, Aksoy BA, Dogrusoz U, Dresdner G, Gross B, Sumer SO, et al. Integrative analysis of complex cancer genomics and clinical profiles using the cBioPortal. Sci Signal. 2013;6(269):pl1.

Chapter 9
Hereditary Endometrial Carcinoma

Anne M. Mills and Teri A. Longacre

Introduction

Advances in molecular testing have both increased recognition of heritable cancer syndromes and provided tools for their clinical diagnosis. Familial cancer syndromes that manifest in endometrial cancer include Lynch syndrome and Cowden syndrome, with very rare contributions by Cowden-like syndromes. Germline *BRCA* mutations have not yet been directly associated with increased endometrial cancer risk, but do appear to predispose patients to endometrial carcinogenesis indirectly through high rates of tamoxifen exposure.

An underlying cancer syndrome should always be considered in very young endometrial cancer patients, particularly in the setting of aberrant tumor morphologies or endometrioid adenocarcinoma without concomitant obesity or other evidence of estrogen excess. A personal or family history of relevant malignancies should also provoke concern. That said, some syndromic cancers manifest outside of a clinicopathologically concerning context and may warrant universal tumor screening. As the interpreter and caretaker of the tumor tissue, the pathologist is positioned to synthesize clinical, morphologic, and molecular data and suggest a work-up for an underlying germline mutation, and should therefore be well-acquainted with the features of heritable cancer in the endometrium.

A.M. Mills
Department of Pathology, University of Virginia, Charlottesville, VA, USA
e-mail: amm7r@virginia.edu

T.A. Longacre (✉)
Department of Pathology, Stanford Medicine, Stanford, CA, USA
e-mail: longacre@stanford.edu

M.T. Deavers and D.M. Coffey (eds.), *Precision Molecular Pathology of Uterine Cancer*, Molecular Pathology Library,
DOI 10.1007/978-3-319-57985-6_9

Lynch Syndrome

Lynch syndrome is among the most common heritable cancer syndromes and predisposes patients to malignancies at a variety of sites, most notably the endometrium and lower gastrointestinal tract, and less commonly the ovaries, skin, renal pelvis, stomach, and brain. Endometrial carcinomas occur in 60–80% of women with Lynch syndrome and represent the sentinel malignancy in many of these patients. Between 2 and 5% of all endometrial cancers are associated with Lynch syndrome, and recognizing them as such allows for the identification and prevention of subsequent malignancies through increased surveillance and intervention programs [1–5].

Molecular Basis

Lynch syndrome is most often attributable to germline mutations in one of four mismatch repair genes: *MLH1*, *PMS2*, *MSH2*, and *MSH6*. These four genes encode proteins which dimerize into a MLH1–PMS2 complex and an MSH2–MSH6 complex. The two dimerized pairs form a four-protein complex that recognizes DNA mismatches and recruits repair machinery for excision and replacement of aberrant nucleotides. The prevalence and disease penetrance of endometrial cancer varies according to the implicated gene. *MSH2* and *MSH6* mutations are more commonly associated with endometrial carcinomas than are *MLH1* and *PMS2* mutations, a distribution that contrasts with Lynch syndrome-associated colorectal carcinoma. *MSH6* mutations impart a particularly high risk of endometrial cancer development, with up to 71% of patients developing disease by age 70. Lifetime risk is considerably lower for *PMS2* mutations at 12% by age 70, and ranges from 21 to 54% for *MLH1* and *MSH2* mutations [6].

In rare instances, the heritable defect lies not in one of these four mismatch repair genes, but in the related gene *EPCAM*. Mutations in the 3′ end of the *EPCAM* gene lead to hypermethylation of the *MSH2* promotor region, disabling *MSH2* and leading to dual loss of MSH2 and MSH6 [7–9]. Still more uncommon are recently described heritable mutations in *MLH1* promoter mechanisms. In such patients the *MLH1* gene is intact however MLH1 protein production is inhibited by hypermethlyation [10].

It is critical to emphasize that the vast majority of hypermethylated endometrial cancers are sporadic and are not associated with the exceedingly rare inheritance pattern described above. In fact, epigenetic methylation of the *MLH1* promoter region is by far the most common cause of deficient mismatch repair in the uterus, underlying approximately 25% of endometrial carcinomas [11, 12].

Clinical Features

Lynch syndrome-related endometrial carcinomas, on average, develop a decade earlier in life when compared to sporadic endometrial malignancies [13–17]. However, these tumors are not exclusive to younger women, and a significant proportion occur in women over 50 years of age [18, 19]. Although prior and simultaneous malignancies may flag a subset of endometrial carcinomas that arise in women with Lynch syndrome, the endometrium is often the initial site of disease in these patients, and only a minority of Lynch patients identified on universal screening will have a history of colorectal or other cancers [18–22].

Pathologic Features

The anatomic localization of Lynch syndrome-related endometrial cancers varies. Although some studies have shown a predilection for the lower uterine segment when compared to their mismatch repair-competent counterparts, these tumors are by no means restricted to a lower uterine locale, and many arise in the fundus and surrounding uterine walls [19, 20, 23–25].

Reproducible histomorphologic features have been noted in a subset of Lynch syndrome-associated endometrial cancers. Perhaps most striking are the dedifferentiated and undifferentiated carcinomas; the former is characterized by areas of well-formed glands immediately juxtaposed with confluent sheets of markedly atypical tumor, while the latter contains no glandular structures (Figs. 9.1 and 9.2) [23, 26–30]. Such abrupt deviations in morphology make ontological sense given that tumors with incompetent DNA repair mechanisms are expected to acquire mutations rapidly. It is important to emphasize these morphologies that have been described in Lynch syndrome-related endometrial malignancies have also been recorded in both sporadically methylated and in "Lynch-like" endometrial carcinomas (e.g., cancers with mismatch repair protein patterns suggestive of Lynch syndrome, but without demonstrable mutations on germline sequencing) [31]. This suggests that these features are not an intrinsic feature of germline mutations themselves, but rather a marker of mismatch repair dysfunction at the protein level, irrespective of whether it is acquired through somatic or heritable mechanisms.

Not all Lynch syndrome-associated endometrial tumors exhibit remarkable morphologies. In fact the majority display a conventional, well to moderately differentiated endometrioid phenotype without notable demarcations in differentiation or distinct intratumoral morphologies [18–20, 22]. Pure serous, clear cell, and carcinosarcoma phenotypes are not typical of endometrial cancers arising in the setting of Lynch syndrome, but may occasionally occur.

As in the colorectum, Lynch syndrome-related endometrial cancers have been associated with increased tumor-infiltrating and peritumoral lymphocytes in some

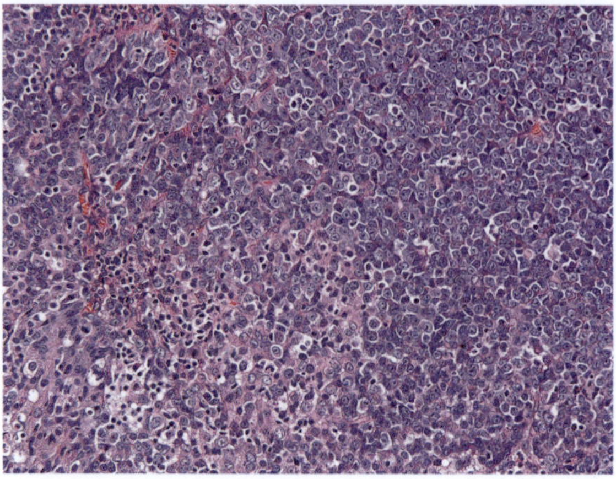

Fig. 9.1 Undifferentiated endometrial adenocarcinoma is uncommon, but often associated with microsatellite instability due to epigenetic methylation and less commonly, to germline mutation in *MLH1*

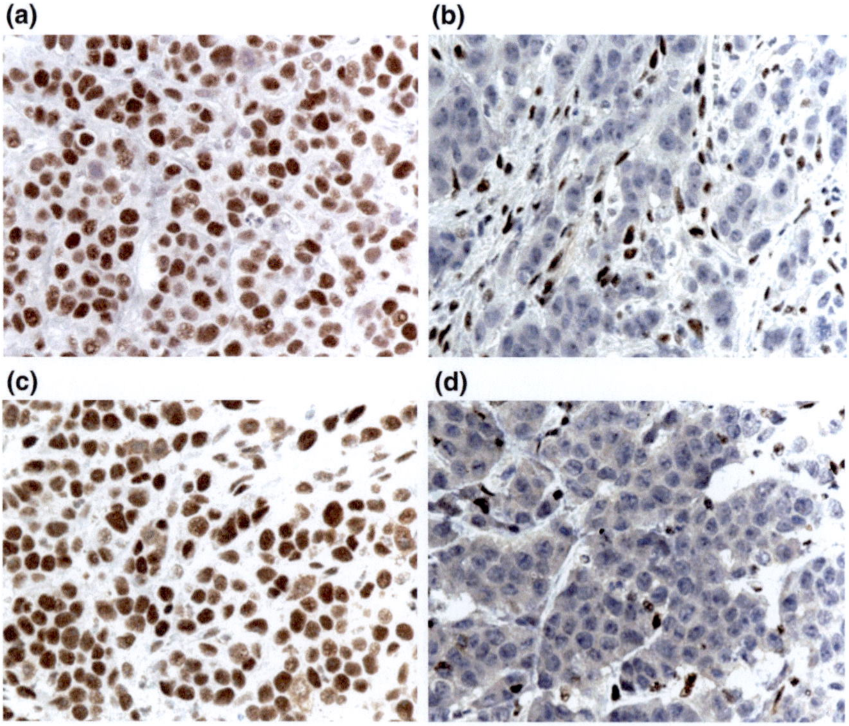

Fig. 9.2 Undifferentiated endometrial adenocarcinoma (depicted in Fig. 9.1) exhibits intact expression of mismatch repair proteins **a** MHS2 and **c** MSH6, with loss of expression of mismatch repair proteins **b** MLH1 and **d** PMS2. In this tumor, loss of mismatch repair proteins is secondary to epigenetic methylation of the *MLH1* promotor

cases [19, 23, 26, 29, 32]. Although thresholds vary across the literature, most data suggest >40–42 intratumoral lymphocytes per 10 high-power fields [19, 23].

Screening and Confirmatory Testing

Because Lynch syndrome-associated endometrial carcinomas can serve as a harbinger of carcinogenesis at other sites, screening and confirmatory testing programs are of utmost clinical importance. Screening algorithms rely on mismatch repair immunohistochemistry, *MLH1* promoter hypermethylation analysis, and microsatellite instability (MSI) testing in a variety of combinations. Diagnostic confirmation can be achieved through germline sequencing, with selective enlistment of somatic tumor sequencing in cases without identified germline mutations.

Mismatch Repair Protein Immunohistochemistry

Immunohistochemistry for the mismatch repair proteins MLH1, PMS2, MSH2, and MSH6 is the preferred initial screen for Lynch syndrome. This methodology has multiple benefits: firstly, immunohistochemistry is relatively inexpensive, technically simple, and readily accessible for most practicing pathologists [33, 34]. Sensitivity for the presence of MSI exceeds 90% [35]. Furthermore, the immunohistochemical loss pattern provides information as to the underlying mismatch repair defect: because MSH6 has an obligate reliance on MSH2 for expression (but the reverse does not hold), dual nuclear loss of MSH2 and MSH6 suggests an *MSH2* mutation. Notably, this pattern can also be seen with 3′ *EPCAM* mutations due to the hypermethylation of the *MSH2* promoter region (Fig. 9.3). On the other hand, isolated MSH6 loss indicates a possible *MSH6* mutation.

A similar pattern is observed with the MLH1/PMS2 pairing: because PMS2 is not expressed in the absence of MLH1 (MLH1 can be expressed in absence of PMS2), simultaneous loss of tumor nuclear expression of MLH1 and PMS2 signals a deficiency in the MLH1 protein. Importantly, this can be due to either epigenetic *MLH1* methylation (Fig. 9.2) or, much less commonly, *MLH1* germline mutations (Fig. 9.4). Isolated loss of PMS2 suggests a germline *PMS2* mutation.

A variety of algorithms have been proposed for the screening of endometrial carcinomas for Lynch syndrome. It is well-established that limiting screening to patients with age and history-based clinical risk as defined by the Amsterdam and Bethesda criteria misses affected patients [19, 22, 25, 31, 36]. Although screening methodologies for endometrial cancers remain a subject of debate, most experts in the field advocate some form of universal testing as is currently recommended for colorectal cancer (Fig. 9.5) [18, 19, 22, 25, 37].

Screening approaches also differ with respect to the antibodies enlisted. Although many centers screen using a 4-antibody panel including MLH1, PMS2, MSH2, and MSH6, mismatch repair protein dimerization patterns allow for an

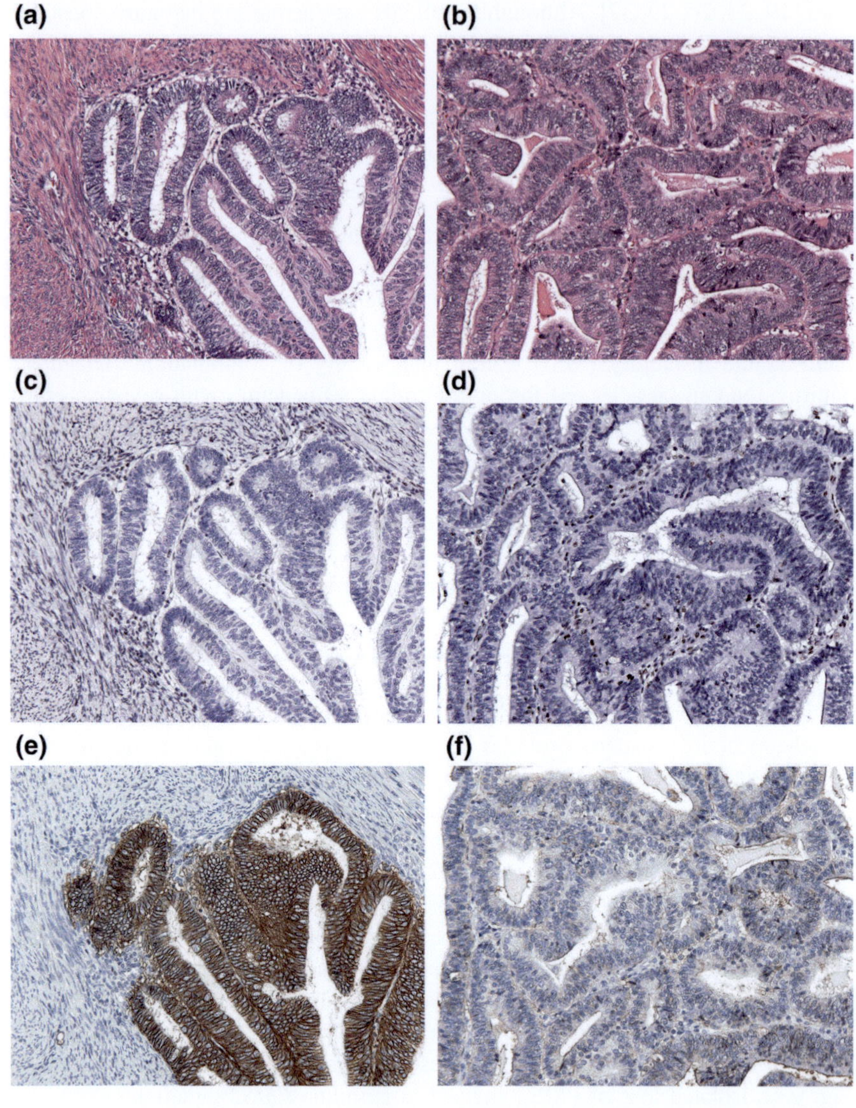

Fig. 9.3 Endometrial carcinomas may exhibit loss of MSH2 and MSH6 mismatch repair proteins due to germline mutation in **a**, **c**, **e** *MSH2* or in **b**, **d**, **f** *EPCAM.* In both cases **c**, **d** MSH2 protein is not expressed, but in cases with mutations in *EPCAM,* expression for **f** EPCAM is also lost, while it is retained in tumors with **e** MSH2 mutations

alternative 2-antibody approach that enlists PMS2 and MSH6 as an initial screen. Current data suggests that the 2 and 4-antibody approaches show comparable efficacy in the detection of mismatch repair deficits [38, 39]. Given the relative rarity of *MLH1* and *PMS2* mutations in Lynch syndrome-related endometrial carcinomas, MSH6-only screening has also been proposed, although some evidence

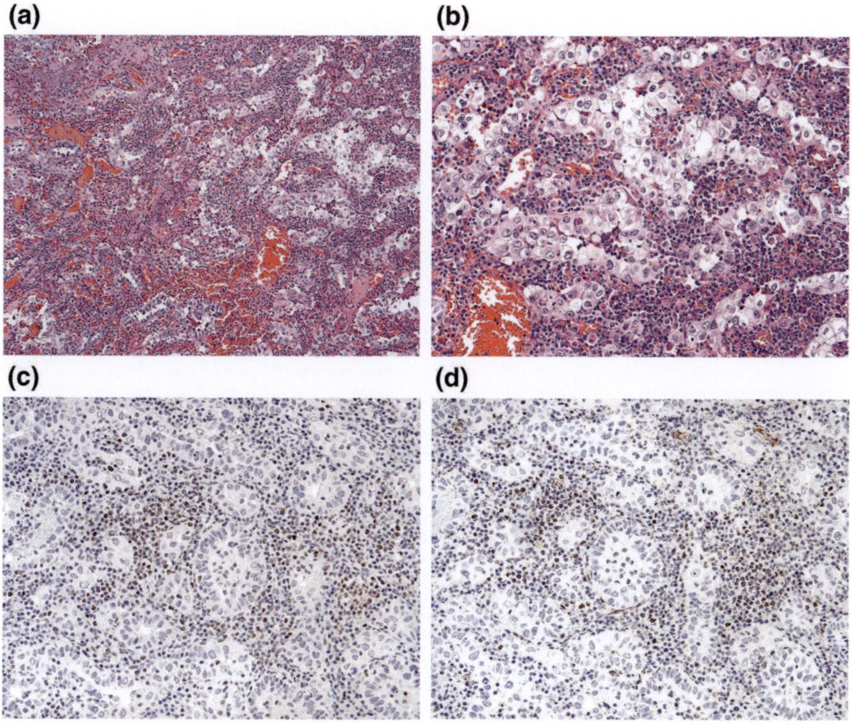

Fig. 9.4 **a**, **b** Clear cell carcinoma of the endometrium with loss of **c** MLH1 and **d** PMS2 proteins secondary to germline mutation in *MLH1*

suggests that such focused panels will miss occasional Lynch syndrome patients [19, 25].

Mismatch repair immunohistochemistry interpretation is relatively straightforward, but is not without caveats. Intact expression is defined as the presence of any nuclear staining within the tumor, but sometimes staining is patchy and may be faint, particularly for the MSH6 antibody. MSH6 staining is prone to patchy, irregular staining and may pose problems on small biopsy samples. External positive and negative controls are desirable, but absence (or deficiency) of mismatch repair protein in a tumor can only be diagnosed in the presence of internal positive control staining with the antibody under evaluation. Care must be taken to specifically evaluate tumor cell nuclei as some mismatch repair deficient tumors may contain numerous intraepithelial lymphocytes that may lead to an erroneous diagnosis of intact expression. Cases that continue to present diagnostic difficulty on careful review should be classified as equivocal and subjected to second-line testing (such as MSI testing or, if clinical suspicion for heritable cancer is high, directed germline testing).

Occasionally, aberrant mismatch repair protein expression patterns may be observed. Loss of all 4 mismatch repair proteins may occur in tumors with

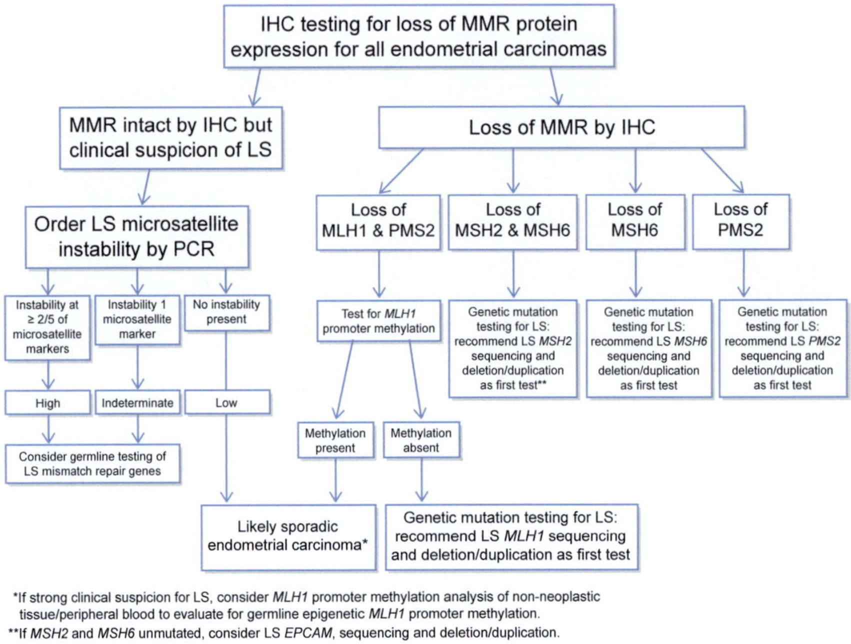

Fig. 9.5 Algorithm for evaluating endometrial cancer for possible Lynch syndrome. A more cost effective approach utilizing only 2 mismatch repair antibodies (MSH6 and PMS2) will capture most cases

underlying germline *MSH2* mutations and concomitant *MLH1* epigenetic methylation (Fig. 9.6) [40]. Also, some tumors with underlying *MLH1* germline mutations may contain a nonfunctional protein that continues to be expressed on immunohistochemistry [41]. This latter aberrant expression pattern appears to be more common in colorectal cancer, in which *MLH1* germline mutations are more common. Zonal loss of MLH1 and PMS2 may also be encountered [42]. This is easily recognized in the hysterectomy specimen, but may not be apparent in an endometrial sampling. It has been suggested this may reflect increased tumor aggressiveness, but that has not been our experience. Apparent isolated loss of PMS2 protein expression may be associated with *MLH1* hypermethylation with heterogeneous MLH1 protein expression [43].

Microsatellite Instability Analysis

Mismatch repair defects lead to frequent replicative errors in short repetitive genomic regions known as microsatellites. The finding of MSI therefore serves as an indirect proxy for the presence of dysfunctional mismatch repair. PCR-based MSI testing measures repeat lengths of dinucleotide and mononucleotide markers

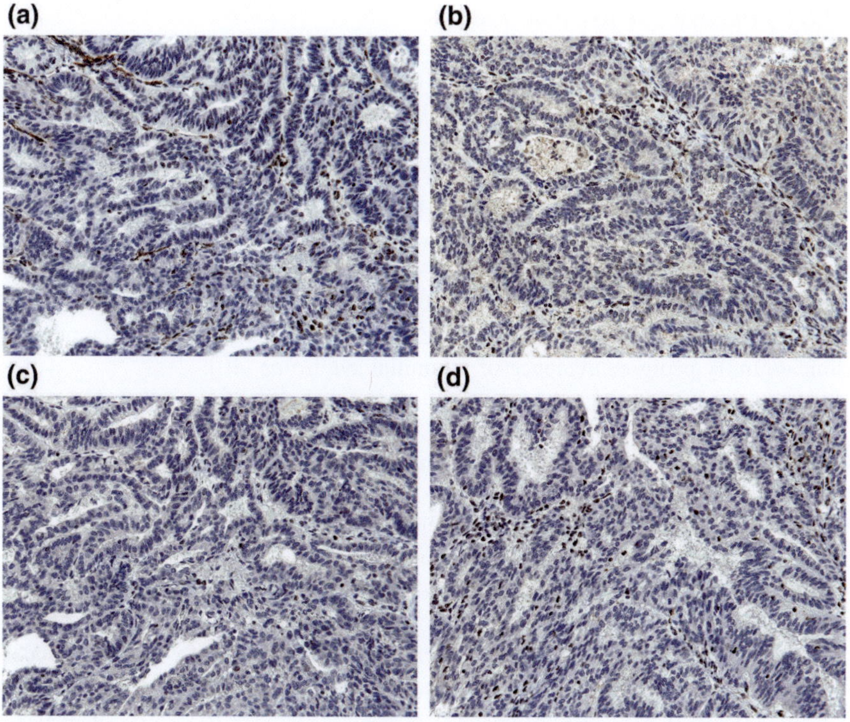

Fig. 9.6 Endometrial carcinoma with loss of all 4 mismatch repair proteins: **a** MLH1; **b** MSH2; **c** MSH6; and **d** PMS2. In many cases this is due to mutation in *MSH2* with epigenetic methylation of *MLH1*

(most commonly BAT25, BAT26, NR21, NR24, and NR27) and compares normal and tumoral tissue. Instability at two or more of these loci is classified as MSI-high, instability at a single locus is MSI-low, and an absence of instability is considered MS-stable [44].

Although not favored as a preliminary screen due to its inaccessibility at many centers, high cost, and inability to direct germline sequencing efforts, MSI testing can play an important role in the Lynch syndrome work-up in several situations. First, MSI testing can be enlisted in cases with equivocal immunohistochemistry results. Second, MSI has utility in resolving the differential for Lynch-like cancers as high level MSI supports the presence of a true mismatch repair defect (and argues against false immunohistochemistry results). Finally, MSI testing can be enlisted in patients with a negative MMR immunohistochemistry screen, but a strong clinical suspicion for a hereditary syndrome. Although MMR immunohistochemistry is more sensitive than MSI testing (particularly for *MSH6* and *PMS2* mutations, where MSI may fail to detect more than a quarter of cases), it has been reported that up to 10% of endometrial cancers with underlying MMR mutations and MSI may be missed by immunohistochemical screening [35].

MLH1 Promoter Methylation Analysis

Because immunohistochemical loss of MLH1 and PMS2 is most often attributable to sporadic methylation, PCR-based hypermethylation testing represents an important next step for endometrial cancers demonstrating this pattern, in order to prevent the perpetuation of unwarranted concern and further work-up for Lynch syndrome. In the colon and rectum *BRAF* testing is a reliable surrogate for the presence of *MLH1* hypermethylation; however, this is not the case in the uterus [11, 12, 19, 45]. *MLH1* hypermethylation demonstrates a heritable pattern in an exceedingly small minority of patients, therefore demonstration of hypermethylation effectively excludes Lynch syndrome in the absence of compelling clinical/family pedigree evidence of a familial syndrome [10].

DNA Mismatch Repair Gene Mutation Analysis

When mismatch repair protein loss and methylation data suggest a heritable syndrome, confirmatory germline sequencing is required for a diagnosis of Lynch syndrome. Because the mutations that underlie Lynch syndrome vary considerably, this requires whole genome sequencing of the suspected gene.

There is some variability in commercially available germline testing protocols and capabilities. Not all platforms have included *EPCAM* sequencing, although that is now performed with increasing frequency when relevant (e.g., loss of MSH2/6 without detection of mutations in either gene). Many assays are also unable to detect cryptic *MSH2* gene inversions, which can account for a falsely "normal" germline result in patients with loss of MLH1/PMS2 and no evidence of *MLH1* promoter hypermethylation [46, 47].

Somatic Gene Mutational Analysis

Historically, loss of mismatch repair protein expression (and the absence of *MLH1* hypermethylation for those showing MLH1/PMS2 dual loss) was considered tantamount to a Lynch syndrome diagnosis. We now know that a considerable portion (up to 50%) of such immunohistochemically deficient cases will fail to show mutations on directed sequencing [48–50]. The possible underlying etiologies of these "Lynch like" tumors include: (1) somatic alterations (including loss of heterozygosity and biallelic somatic mutations); (2) inaccurate immunohistochemistries; and (3) undetected germline mutations. In discordant cases that prove MSI-high on MSI testing, direct tumor testing can be performed to ascertain whether somatic mutations and/or loss of heterozygosity account for the observed mismatch repair dysfunction. Demonstration of a tumor-specific mutation that is not observed on adequate germline sequencing effectively eliminates a germline cancer predisposition syndrome.

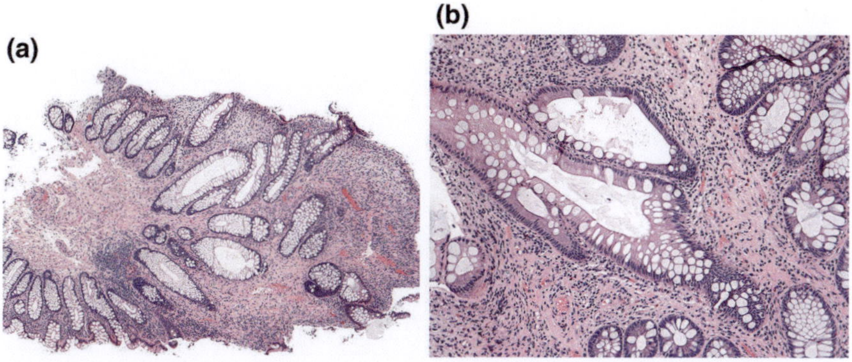

Fig. 9.7 Colon polyps in Cowden syndrome are typically small and sessile. **a** They exhibit an expanded and fibrotic lamina propria with **b** mild gland distortion and lymphoid follicles with some degree of smooth muscle proliferation and chronic inflammation. Ganglion cells, nerve fibers, and adipocytes within the lamina propria may also be seen

Cowden Syndrome

This autosomal dominant syndrome is extremely rare (affecting approximately 1 in 200,000) and accounts for a far smaller proportion of endometrial carcinomas than does Lynch syndrome [51–54]. Patients with Cowden syndrome are characterized by macrocephaly and a predilection for the development of multiple hamartomas involving the gastrointestinal tract (Fig. 9.7) and skin (facial trichilemmomas, acral keratoses, mucosal/cutaneous papillomatoses) [55]. In addition to endometrial carcinomas, Cowden syndrome patients are vulnerable to breast, thyroid, ovary, uterine cervix, colon, urinary bladder and renal malignancies [52, 53, 56, 57]. As with Lynch syndrome, endometrial cancers that arise in patients with Cowden syndrome present, on average, a decade prior to their mutation-negative counterparts.

Pathologic Features

Endometrial carcinomas associated with Cowden syndrome are classically of the endometrioid subtype (Fig. 9.8) [58–60]. However, recent evidence suggests that uterine serous carcinomas, clear cell carcinomas, mucinous carcinomas, and carcinosarcomas are also diagnosed in these patients [61].

Molecular Basis

Germline mutations in the *phosphatase and tensin homolog* (*PTEN*) gene, a tumor suppressor, located on 10q23.3 underlie Cowden syndrome. However, the identification of a *PTEN* mutation has virtually no specificity for Cowden syndrome

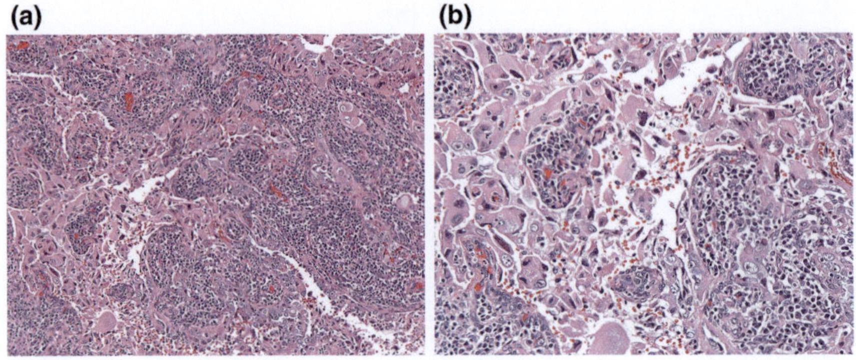

Fig. 9.8 a, b High grade endometrioid endometrial adenocarcinoma in patient with Cowden syndrome. Despite the high grade appearance, this tumor does not harbor a *p53* mutation

because between 77 and 94% of all endometrial cancers display this mutation [62]. This is true across the molecularly identified endometrial subtypes with the exception of high copy number (serous) tumors: the other three types [polymerase (ultramutated), microsatellite-unstable (hypermutated), and low copy number (endometrioid)] all show *PTEN* mutations in the majority of cases [62]. Futhermore, *PTEN* mutations can be found in a variety of hyperplastic and non-neoplastic endometria including normally cycling glands [63].

Confirmatory Testing

Combined with the extremely low prevalence of Cowden syndrome, the frequency of *PTEN* mutations in sporadic endometrial carcinomas and in non-neoplastic endometria obviates any utility of PTEN immunohistochemistry in Cowden syndrome screening and severely limits the utility of somatic tumor testing. Clinical screening criteria therefore play an important role in directing patients toward germline testing, with the recently released *PTEN* Cleveland Clinic risk assessment tool showing promise as a triage device [57]. Ultimate confirmation of a Cowden syndrome diagnosis relies on the identification of a germline mutation by sequencing.

Related Syndromes

Cowden-like syndromes have been identified in patients with mutations in *succinate dehydrogenase* genes (*SDH-B*, *SDH-C*, and *SDHB-D*) as well as *killen* (*KLLN*) genes [61, 64, 65]. In addition to endometrial carcinomas, patients with *SDHB-D* mutations are prone to paragangliomas, pheochromocytomas, thyroid carcinomas, renal carcinomas, gastrointestinal stromal tumors, and perhaps breast cancers

[65]. Germline promoter methylation of *KLLN*, which shares a transcriptional start site with *PTEN*, has been described in patients with a clinical impression of Cowden syndrome but no identifiable *PTEN* mutations [64]. Testing for *SDHB-D* and *KLLN* mutations may therefore be indicated in patients with a clinical scenario highly suspicious for Cowden syndrome whose germline testing fails to identify alterations in *PTEN*.

Familial Breast Ovarian Cancer Syndromes (*BRCA* Mutations)

Germline mutations in the *BRCA1* and *BRCA2* genes are notoriously linked to increased risk of ovarian and breast carcinoma. There is ongoing debate, however, as to whether or not inherited *BRCA* mutations also increase the risk of endometrial carcinoma. Initial work has suggested that *BRCA* mutations carriers are at no increased risk for endometrial carcinoma, while several subsequent studies have shown that risk is increased, but appears to be commensurate with and attributable to tamoxifen exposure [66–68]. However, recent data suggest that although the overall risk for uterine cancer after risk reducing salpingo-oophorectomy is not increased, the risk for serous or serous-like endometrial carcinoma is increased in women with germline *BRCA1* mutations [69]. When evaluating individual patients, it is important to keep in mind that increased somatic tumor testing is likely to identify a growing number of somatic *BRCA* mutations within endometrial carcinomas, and such results should not be interpreted as indicative of an inherited *BRCA* mutation in the absence of confirmatory germline testing.

Polymerase Proofreading-(*POLD1*) Associated Syndrome

Women with germline mutations in *POLD1* exonuclease are at risk for endometrial carcinoma (57.1% of female carriers), in addition to attenuated colorectal polyposis (>60% *POLD1* mutation carriers have $\geq$2 adenomas; on average, 16 adenomas), colorectal carcinoma (60–64% of carriers), and brain tumors (5.8%). Although the incidence is still under investigation, *POLD1* exonuclease mutations appear to account for 1% of MMR-proficient familial and/or early-onset nonpolyposis colorectal carcinomas [70].

Li-Fraumeni Syndrome

Li-Fraumeni syndrome (LFS) is a cancer predisposition syndrome associated with the development of soft tissue sarcoma, osteosarcoma, pre-menopausal breast cancer, brain tumors, adrenocortical carcinoma, and leukemias [70]. A variety of other neoplasms may occur, including ovarian and endometrial cancer. Affected patients harbor a germline mutation in *TP53*. Intensive surveillance programs for the core cancers associated with the syndrome are instituted at an early age; affected patients should avoid exposure to radiation therapy, whenever possible, to reduce the risk of secondary radiation-induced malignancies [1, 7].

References

1. Aarnio M, Sankila R, Pukkala E, Salovaara R, Aaltonen LA, de la Chapelle A, et al. Cancer risk in mutation carriers of DNA-mismatch-repair genes. Int J Cancer J Int Cancer. 1999;81 (2):214–8 (Epub 03 Apr 1999).
2. Barrow E, Hill J, Evans DG. Cancer risk in Lynch syndrome. Fam Cancer. 2013;12(2): 229–40 (Epub 23 Apr 2013).
3. Barrow E, Robinson L, Alduaij W, Shenton A, Clancy T, Lalloo F, et al. Cumulative lifetime incidence of extracolonic cancers in Lynch syndrome: a report of 121 families with proven mutations. Clin Genet. 2009;75(2):141–9 (Epub 14 Feb 2009).
4. Lynch HT, Lynch PM, Lanspa SJ, Snyder CL, Lynch JF, Boland CR. Review of the Lynch syndrome: history, molecular genetics, screening, differential diagnosis, and medicolegal ramifications. Clin Genet. 2009;76(1):1–18 (Epub 08 Aug 2009).
5. Quehenberger F, Vasen HF, van Houwelingen HC. Risk of colorectal and endometrial cancer for carriers of mutations of the hMLH1 and hMSH2 gene: correction for ascertainment. J Med Genet. 2005;42(6):491–6 (Epub 07 June 2005).
6. ten Broeke SW, Brohet RM, Tops CM, van der Klift HM, Velthuizen ME, Bernstein I, et al. Lynch syndrome caused by germline PMS2 mutations: delineating the cancer risk. J Clin Oncol: Off J Am Soc Clin Oncol. 2015;33(4):319–25 (Epub 17 Dec 2014).
7. Kempers MJ, Kuiper RP, Ockeloen CW, Chappuis PO, Hutter P, Rahner N, et al. Risk of colorectal and endometrial cancers in EPCAM deletion-positive Lynch syndrome: a cohort study. Lancet Oncol. 2011;12(1):49–55 (Epub 15 Dec 2010).
8. Ligtenberg MJ, Kuiper RP, Geurts van Kessel A, Hoogerbrugge N. EPCAM deletion carriers constitute a unique subgroup of Lynch syndrome patients. Fam Cancer. 2013;12(2):169–74 (Epub 25 Dec 2012).
9. Rumilla K, Schowalter KV, Lindor NM, Thomas BC, Mensink KA, Gallinger S, et al. Frequency of deletions of EPCAM (TACSTD1) in MSH2-associated Lynch syndrome cases. J Mol Diagn (JMD). 2011;13(1):93–9 (Epub 14 Jan 2011).
10. Niessen RC, Hofstra RM, Westers H, Ligtenberg MJ, Kooi K, Jager PO, et al. Germline hypermethylation of MLH1 and EPCAM deletions are a frequent cause of Lynch syndrome. Genes Chromosom Cancer. 2009;48(8):737–44 (Epub 21 May 2009).
11. Newton K, Jorgensen NM, Wallace AJ, Buchanan DD, Lalloo F, McMahon RF, et al. Tumour MLH1 promoter region methylation testing is an effective prescreen for Lynch Syndrome (HNPCC). J Med Genet. 2014;51(12):789–96 (Epub 05 Oct 2014).
12. Peterson LM, Kipp BR, Halling KC, Kerr SE, Smith DI, Distad TJ, et al. Molecular characterization of endometrial cancer: a correlative study assessing microsatellite instability, MLH1 hypermethylation, DNA mismatch repair protein expression, and PTEN, PIK3CA, KRAS, and BRAF mutation analysis. Int J Gynecol Pathol: Off J Int Soc Gynecol Pathol. 2012;31(3):195–205 (Epub 14 Apr 2012).
13. Bonadona V, Bonaiti B, Olschwang S, Grandjouan S, Huiart L, Longy M, et al. Cancer risks associated with germline mutations in MLH1, MSH2, and MSH6 genes in Lynch syndrome. JAMA. 2011;305(22):2304–10 (Epub 07 June 2011).

14. Hampel H, Frankel W, Panescu J, Lockman J, Sotamaa K, Fix D, et al. Screening for Lynch syndrome (hereditary nonpolyposis colorectal cancer) among endometrial cancer patients. Can Res. 2006;66(15):7810–7 (Epub 04 Aug 2006).
15. Hampel H, Frankel WL, Martin E, Arnold M, Khanduja K, Kuebler P, et al. Screening for the Lynch syndrome (hereditary nonpolyposis colorectal cancer). N Engl J Medicine. 2005;352 (18):1851–60 (Epub 06 May 2005).
16. Hampel H, Stephens JA, Pukkala E, Sankila R, Aaltonen LA, Mecklin JP, et al. Cancer risk in hereditary nonpolyposis colorectal cancer syndrome: later age of onset. Gastroenterology. 2005;129(2):415–21 (Epub 09 Aug 2005).
17. Watson P, Lynch HT. Extracolonic cancer in hereditary nonpolyposis colorectal cancer. Cancer. 1993;71(3):677–85 (Epub 01 Feb 1993.
18. Ferguson SE, Aronson M, Pollett A, Eiriksson LR, Oza AM, Gallinger S, et al. Performance characteristics of screening strategies for Lynch syndrome in unselected women with newly diagnosed endometrial cancer who have undergone universal germline mutation testing. Cancer. 2014;120(24):3932–9 (Epub 02 Aug 2014).
19. Mills AM, Liou S, Ford JM, Berek JS, Pai RK, Longacre TA. Lynch syndrome screening should be considered for all patients with newly diagnosed endometrial cancer. Am J Surg Pathol. 2014;38(11):1501–9 (Epub 18 Sep 2014).
20. Clarke BA, Cooper K. Identifying Lynch syndrome in patients with endometrial carcinoma: shortcomings of morphologic and clinical schemas. Adv Anat Pathol. 2012;19(4):231–8 (Epub 14 June 2012).
21. Hampel H, Frankel WL, Martin E, Arnold M, Khanduja K, Kuebler P, et al. Feasibility of screening for Lynch syndrome among patients with colorectal cancer. J Clin Oncol: Off J Am Soc Clin Oncol. 2008;26(35):5783–8 (Epub 24 Sep 2008).
22. Mills AM, Longacre TA. Lynch syndrome screening in the gynecologic tract: current state of the art. Am J Surg Pathol. 2016;40(4):e35–44 (Epub 13 Feb 2016).
23. Garg K, Leitao MM Jr, Kauff ND, Hansen J, Kosarin K, Shia J, et al. Selection of endometrial carcinomas for DNA mismatch repair protein immunohistochemistry using patient age and tumor morphology enhances detection of mismatch repair abnormalities. Am J Surg Pathol. 2009;33(6):925–33 (Epub 25 Feb 2009).
24. Mills A, Sloan E, Thomas M, et al. Clinicopathologic comparison of lynch syndrome-associated and lynch-like endometrial carcinomas identified on universal screening. Am J Surg Pathol. 2015 (In Press).
25. Rabban JT, Calkins SM, Karnezis AN, Grenert JP, Blanco A, Crawford B, et al. Association of tumor morphology with mismatch-repair protein status in older endometrial cancer patients: implications for universal versus selective screening strategies for Lynch syndrome. Am J Surg Pathol. 2014;38(6):793–800 (Epub 08 Feb 2014).
26. Broaddus RR, Lynch HT, Chen LM, Daniels MS, Conrad P, Munsell MF, et al. Pathologic features of endometrial carcinoma associated with HNPCC: a comparison with sporadic endometrial carcinoma. Cancer. 2006;106(1):87–94 (Epub 03 Dec 2005).
27. Carcangiu ML, Radice P, Casalini P, Bertario L, Merola M, Sala P. Lynch syndrome-related endometrial carcinomas show a high frequency of nonendometrioid types and of high FIGO grade endometrioid types. Int J Surg Pathol. 2010;18(1):21–6 (Epub 16 May 2009).
28. Honore LH, Hanson J, Andrew SE. Microsatellite instability in endometrioid endometrial carcinoma: correlation with clinically relevant pathologic variables. Int J Gynecol Cancer: Off J Int Gynecol Cancer Soc. 2006;16(3):1386–92 (Epub 29 June 2006).
29. Shia J, Black D, Hummer AJ, Boyd J, Soslow RA. Routinely assessed morphological features correlate with microsatellite instability status in endometrial cancer. Hum Pathol. 2008;39 (1):116–25 (Epub 24 Oct 2007).
30. Tafe LJ, Garg K, Chew I, Tornos C, Soslow RA. Endometrial and ovarian carcinomas with undifferentiated components: clinically aggressive and frequently underrecognized neoplasms. Mod Pathol: Off J US Can Acad Pathol Inc. 2010;23(6):781–9 (Epub 23 Mar 2010)
31. Mills AM, Sloan EA, Thomas M, Modesitt SC, Stoler MH, Atkins KA, et al. Clinicopathologic comparison of Lynch syndrome-associated and "Lynch-like" endometrial

carcinomas identified on universal screening using mismatch repair protein immunohistochemistry. Am J Surg Pathol. 2016;40(2):155–65 (Epub 03 Nov 2015).
32. Garg K, Soslow RA. Lynch syndrome (hereditary non-polyposis colorectal cancer) and endometrial carcinoma. J Clin Pathol. 2009;62(8):679–84 (Epub 30 July 2009).
33. de Leeuw WJ, Dierssen J, Vasen HF, Wijnen JT, Kenter GG, Meijers-Heijboer H, et al. Prediction of a mismatch repair gene defect by microsatellite instability and immunohistochemical analysis in endometrial tumours from HNPCC patients. J Pathol. 2000;192(3): 328–35 (Epub 31 Oct 2000).
34. McConechy MK, Talhouk A, Li-Chang HH, Leung S, Huntsman DG, Gilks CB, et al. Detection of DNA mismatch repair (MMR) deficiencies by immunohistochemistry can effectively diagnose the microsatellite instability (MSI) phenotype in endometrial carcinomas. Gynecol Oncol. 2015;137(2):306–10 (Epub 01 Feb 2015).
35. Modica I, Soslow RA, Black D, Tornos C, Kauff N, Shia J. Utility of immunohistochemistry in predicting microsatellite instability in endometrial carcinoma. Am J Surg Pathol. 2007;31 (5):744–51 (Epub 27 Apr 2007).
36. Ryan P, Mulligan AM, Aronson M, Ferguson SE, Bapat B, Semotiuk K, et al. Comparison of clinical schemas and morphologic features in predicting Lynch syndrome in mutation-positive patients with endometrial cancer encountered in the context of familial gastrointestinal cancer registries. Cancer. 2012;118(3):681–8 (Epub 02 July 2011).
37. Mills AM, Longacre TA. Lynch syndrome: female genital tract cancer diagnosis and screening. Surg Pathol Clin. 2016;9(2):201–14 (Epub 01 June 2016).
38. Mojtahed A, Schrijver I, Ford JM, Longacre TA, Pai RK. A two-antibody mismatch repair protein immunohistochemistry screening approach for colorectal carcinomas, skin sebaceous tumors, and gynecologic tract carcinomas. Mod Pathol: Off J US Can Acad Pathol Inc. 2011;24(7):1004–14 (Epub 19 Apr 2011)
39. Shia J, Tang LH, Vakiani E, Guillem JG, Stadler ZK, Soslow RA, et al. Immunohistochemistry as first-line screening for detecting colorectal cancer patients at risk for hereditary nonpolyposis colorectal cancer syndrome: a 2-antibody panel may be as predictive as a 4-antibody panel. Am J Surg Pathol. 2009;33(11):1639–45 (Epub 25 Aug 2009).
40. Hagen CE, Lefferts J, Hornick JL, Srivastava A. “Null pattern” of immunoreactivity in a Lynch syndrome-associated colon cancer due to germline MSH2 mutation and somatic MLH1 hypermethylation. Am J Surg Pathol. 2011;35(12):1902–5 (Epub 10 Nov 2011).
41. Dudley B, Brand RE, Thull D, Bahary N, Nikiforova MN, Pai RK. Germline MLH1 mutations are frequently identified in Lynch syndrome patients with colorectal and endometrial carcinoma demonstrating isolated loss of PMS2 immunohistochemical expression. Am J Surg Pathol. 2015;39(8):1114–20 (Epub 15 Apr 2015).
42. Pai RK, Plesec TP, Abdul-Karim FW, Yang B, Marquard J, Shadrach B, et al. Abrupt loss of MLH1 and PMS2 expression in endometrial carcinoma: molecular and morphologic analysis of 6 cases. Am J Surg Pathol. 2015;39(7):993–9 (Epub 19 Mar 2015).
43. Kato A, Sato N, Sugawara T, Takahashi K, Kito M, Makino K, et al. Isolated Loss of PMS2 immunohistochemical expression is frequently caused by heterogenous MLH1 promoter hypermethylation in lynch syndrome screening for endometrial cancer patients. Am J Surg Pathol. 2016;40(6):770–6 (Epub 06 Feb 2016).
44. Boland CR, Thibodeau SN, Hamilton SR, Sidransky D, Eshleman JR, Burt RW, et al. A national cancer institute workshop on microsatellite instability for cancer detection and familial predisposition: development of international criteria for the determination of microsatellite instability in colorectal cancer. Can Res. 1998;58(22):5248–57 (Epub 21 Nov 1998).
45. Parsons MT, Buchanan DD, Thompson B, Young JP, Spurdle AB. Correlation of tumour BRAF mutations and MLH1 methylation with germline mismatch repair (MMR) gene mutation status: a literature review assessing utility of tumour features for MMR variant classification. J Med Genet. 2012;49(3):151–7 (Epub 01 Mar 2012).

46. Liu Q, Hesson LB, Nunez AC, Packham D, Williams R, Ward RL, et al. A cryptic paracentric inversion of MSH2 exons 2-6 causes Lynch syndrome. Carcinogenesis. 2016;37(1):10–7 (Epub 27 Oct 2015).
47. Rhees J, Arnold M, Boland CR. Inversion of exons 1-7 of the MSH2 gene is a frequent cause of unexplained Lynch syndrome in one local population. Fam Cancer. 2014;13(2):219–25 (Epub 12 Oct 2013).
48. Buchanan DD, Rosty C, Clendenning M, Spurdle AB, Win AK. Clinical problems of colorectal cancer and endometrial cancer cases with unknown cause of tumor mismatch repair deficiency (suspected Lynch syndrome). Appl Clin Genet. 2014;7:183–93 (Epub 21 Oct 2014).
49. Haraldsdottir S, Hampel H, Tomsic J, Frankel WL, Pearlman R, de la Chapelle A, et al. Colon and endometrial cancers with mismatch repair deficiency can arise from somatic, rather than germline, mutations. Gastroenterology. 2014;147(6):1308–16.e1 (Epub 10 Sep 2014)
50. Mensenkamp AR, Vogelaar IP, van Zelst-Stams WA, Goossens M, Ouchene H, Hendriks-Cornelissen SJ, et al. Somatic mutations in MLH1 and MSH2 are a frequent cause of mismatch-repair deficiency in Lynch syndrome-like tumors. Gastroenterology. 2014;146(3):643–6.e8 (Epub 18 Dec 2013)
51. Eng C. Will the real Cowden syndrome please stand up: revised diagnostic criteria. J Med Genet. 2000;37(11):828–30 (Epub 10 Nov 2000).
52. Haibach H, Burns TW, Carlson HE, Burman KD, Deftos LJ. Multiple hamartoma syndrome (Cowden's disease) associated with renal cell carcinoma and primary neuroendocrine carcinoma of the skin (Merkel cell carcinoma). Am J Clin Pathol. 1992;97(5):705–12 (Epub 01 May 1992).
53. Schrager CA, Schneider D, Gruener AC, Tsou HC, Peacocke M. Clinical and pathological features of breast disease in Cowden's syndrome: an underrecognized syndrome with an increased risk of breast cancer. Hum Pathol. 1998;29(1):47–53 (Epub 28 Jan 1998).
54. Stadler ZK, Robson ME. Inherited predisposition to endometrial cancer: moving beyond Lynch syndrome. Cancer. 2015;121(5):644–7 (Epub 08 Nov 2014).
55. Shaco-Levy R, Jasperson KW, Martin K, Samadder NJ, Burt RW, Ying J, et al. Morphologic characterization of hamartomatous gastrointestinal polyps in Cowden syndrome, Peutz-Jeghers syndrome, and juvenile polyposis syndrome. Hum Pathol. 2016;49:39–48 (Epub 31 Jan 2016).
56. Pilarski R, Eng C. Will the real Cowden syndrome please stand up (again)? Expanding mutational and clinical spectra of the PTEN hamartoma tumour syndrome. J Med Genet. 2004;41(5):323–6 (Epub 04 May 2004).
57. Tan MH, Mester JL, Ngeow J, Rybicki LA, Orloff MS, Eng C. Lifetime cancer risks in individuals with germline PTEN mutations. Clin Cancer Res: Off J Am Assoc Cancer Res. 2012;18(2):400–7 (Epub 19 Jan 2012).
58. Liaw D, Marsh DJ, Li J, Dahia PL, Wang SI, Zheng Z, et al. Germline mutations of the PTEN gene in Cowden disease, an inherited breast and thyroid cancer syndrome. Nat Genet. 1997;16(1):64–7 (Epub 01 May 1997).
59. Nelen MR, Padberg GW, Peeters EA, Lin AY, van den Helm B, Frants RR, et al. Localization of the gene for Cowden disease to chromosome 10q22-23. Nat Genet. 1996;13(1):114–6 (Epub 01 May 1996).
60. Nelen MR, van Staveren WC, Peeters EA, Hassel MB, Gorlin RJ, Hamm H, et al. Germline mutations in the PTEN/MMAC1 gene in patients with Cowden disease. Hum Mol Genet. 1997;6(8):1383–7 (Epub 01 Aug 1997).
61. Mahdi H, Mester JL, Nizialek EA, Ngeow J, Michener C, Eng C. Germline PTEN, SDHB-D, and KLLN alterations in endometrial cancer patients with Cowden and Cowden-like syndromes: an international, multicenter, prospective study. Cancer. 2015;121(5):688–96 (Epub 08 Nov 2014).
62. Murali R, Soslow RA, Weigelt B. Classification of endometrial carcinoma: more than two types. Lancet Oncol. 2014;15(7):e268–78 (Epub 30 May 2014).

63. Mutter GL, Monte NM, Neuberg D, Ferenczy A, Eng C. Emergence, involution, and progression to carcinoma of mutant clones in normal endometrial tissues. Can Res. 2014;74 (10):2796–802 (Epub 26 Mar 2014).
64. Bennett KL, Mester J, Eng C. Germline epigenetic regulation of KILLIN in Cowden and Cowden-like syndrome. JAMA. 2010;304(24):2724–31 (Epub 24 Dec 2010).
65. Ni Y, Zbuk KM, Sadler T, Patocs A, Lobo G, Edelman E, et al. Germline mutations and variants in the succinate dehydrogenase genes in Cowden and Cowden-like syndromes. Am J Hum Genet. 2008;83(2):261–8 (Epub 06 Aug 2008).
66. Beiner ME, Finch A, Rosen B, Lubinski J, Moller P, Ghadirian P, et al. The risk of endometrial cancer in women with BRCA1 and BRCA2 mutations prospective study. Gynecol Oncol. 2007;104(1):7–10 Epub 12 Sep 2006).
67. Levine DA, Lin O, Barakat RR, Robson ME, McDermott D, Cohen L, et al. Risk of endometrial carcinoma associated with BRCA mutation. Gynecol Oncol. 2001;80(3):395–8 (Epub 27 Mar 2001).
68. Segev Y, Iqbal J, Lubinski J, Gronwald J, Lynch HT, Moller P, et al. The incidence of endometrial cancer in women with BRCA1 and BRCA2 mutations: an international prospective cohort study. Gynecol Oncol. 2013;130(1):127–31 (Epub 09 Apr 2013).
69. Su CA, Pike MC, Jotwani AR, Friebel TM, Soslow RA, Levine DA, et al. Uterine cancer after risk-reducing salpingo-oophorectomy without hysterectomy in women with *BRCA* mutations. JAMA Oncol. 2016;2(11):1434–1440.
70. Bellido F, Pineda M, Aiza G, Valdes-Mas R, Navarro M, Puente DA, et al. POLE and POLD1 mutations in 529 kindred with familial colorectal cancer and/or polyposis: review of reported cases and recommendations for genetic testing and surveillance. Genet Med 2015; 18(4):325–332.
71. Schneider K, Zelley K, Nichols KE, Garber J. Li-Fraumeni syndrome. In: Pagon RA, Adam MP, Ardinger HH, Wallace SE, Amemiya A, Bean LJH, et al., editors. GeneReviews®; 1993. Seattle, WA.

Chapter 10
Targeted Therapy and Prevention of Endometrial Cancer

Takaya Shiozaki and Shannon N. Westin

Introduction

Endometrial (uterine) cancer is a molecularly aberrant disease with over 80% demonstrating a molecular alteration. Primarily, these are in the phosphatidylinositol-3 kinase/protein kinase B (PI3K/AKT) signaling pathway. Given the number of abnormalities present, endometrial cancer has great potential to derive benefit from targeted therapy. However, there are significant unmet needs to maximize the development of targeted therapy in endometrial cancer, including prioritization of agents and pathways and identification and validation of candidate biomarkers to determine mechanisms of response and resistance. Further, as a tumor with a clear precursor lesion and a genetic cause, prevention of endometrial cancer has been explored, although success has been modest. This chapter will review pathways of interest and targeted therapy development in endometrial cancer as well as the current state of endometrial cancer prevention.

Introduction to Targeted Therapy for Endometrial Cancer

In contrary to the reduction observed in many other cancer types, the incidence of endometrial cancer has been increasing over the last five years, and mortality has been rising an average of 1.0% each year [178]. The majority of patients with

T. Shiozaki
Department of Obstetrics and Gynecology, Kinan Hospital, Minamimurogun, Mie, Japan
e-mail: shiozaki-takaya@mtf.biglobe.ne.jp

S.N. Westin (✉)
Department of Gynecologic Oncology and Reproductive Medicine,
The University of Texas M. D. Anderson Cancer Center, Houston, TX, USA
e-mail: swestin@mdanderson.org

M.T. Deavers and D.M. Coffey (eds.), *Precision Molecular Pathology of Uterine Cancer*, Molecular Pathology Library,
DOI 10.1007/978-3-319-57985-6_10

endometrial cancer are diagnosed at an early stage and are cured of disease by surgery, with or without adjuvant radiotherapy. However, there is a growing population of patients with advanced stage or recurrent endometrial cancer for whom treatment options are limited. Approximately 25% of early stage and more than 50% of advanced stage cancers recur [5]. Further, median survival for patients with advanced or recurrent disease is only 12–38 months and the 5-year survival for patients who have recurred is less than 15% [124, 138]. Currently, only hormonal therapy is FDA-approved for the treatment of metastatic/recurrent endometrial cancer. There is a great need for the development of novel approaches for treatment.

Over 80% of endometrial cancers have at least one aberration identified on molecular testing, including mutation, loss of protein expression, amplification, or copy number alteration [85, 104]. Efforts such as the Cancer Genome Atlas (TCGA) have shed light on the molecular landscape of endometrial tumors and helped to direct clinical research in this arena. However, similar to observations in other solid tumors, as clinical results have been reported, it has become clear that the efficacy of a given targeted agent is dependent upon several factors that must be considered besides the presence of a molecular abnormality.

As described in the next section, the molecular aberrations present in endometrial cancer vary based upon the histologic type. Indeed, it appears that the histology and tissue of origin may impact the sensitivity of the tumor to a given targeted agent [96, 109]. Additionally, not all mutations are created equal in regard to impact on treatment response and resistance, and it is not always clear which mutations are "drivers" that may impact clinical outcomes, and which are "passengers" that have an unclear clinical impact. Moreover, the presence of concurrent mutations may significantly change tumor sensitivity to targeted agents. For example, KRAS mutation is associated with non-response to targeted agents in several solid tumors [115]. The context in which mutations occur also matters (i.e., metabolic context, obesity, and hormonal milieu) and must be considered in the identification and validation of potential biomarkers [205]. Finally, there is tumor heterogeneity, either within a tumor or between the primary and metastasis. This can result in discordance in the mutations observed, and the impact of this discordance on response to therapy is unknown. These myriad issues must be clarified in the development of targeted therapies and in the validation of biomarkers to predict response and resistance to those therapies.

Molecular Landscape of Endometrial Cancer

Endometrioid adenocarcinoma is the most common histologic type of endometrial cancer (80%), compared to non-endometrioid carcinomas (20%), including serous and clear cell carcinomas, as well as carcinosarcoma [5]. Table 10.1 summarizes the known molecular changes in the histologic types of endometrial carcinoma. Briefly, endometrioid tumors are characterized by the loss of PTEN protein expression and mutations in key members of the PI3K/AKT pathway, such as

PTEN, *PIK3CA*, *PIK3R1*, *ARID1A* and *AKT*. *KRAS*, *beta-catenin,* and *FGRF-2* mutations are also relatively common. Conversely, non-endometrioid tumors have a higher frequency of mutations in *p53, HER2/neu, p16*, and *E-cadherin*, and a lower frequency of PI3K pathway mutations [85, 204]. An exception to this is clear cell carcinoma, which has a moderate frequency of PI3K abnormalities. Homologous recombination (HR) defects are also common in endometrial cancer, with nearly 50% harboring an abnormality in this pathway [22, 85, 104, 174].

As our understanding of endometrial cancer grows, so does the identification of potential pathways for therapeutic targeting. Among a myriad of molecular pathways, the PI3K/AKT pathway, which plays a central role in cell survival [67], and the Ras/Raf pathway, which plays a central role in cell proliferation [126], are arguably the most important for carcinogenesis in endometrial cancer. Figure 10.1 is a simplified schematic of the pathways in endometrial cancer and is meant to emphasize the extensive cross talk and interaction between the PI3K/AKT pathway and the other pathways of importance, including the Ras/Raf pathway, AMP protein kinase (AMPK) pathway, and hormones. Understanding these interactions is essential for anticipating and targeting resistance mechanisms and maximizing clinical activity.

Table 10.1 Molecular aberrations of interest across the histology types of endometrial cancer

Alteration	Endometrioid (%)	Non-endometrioid (%)
PI3K/AKT/mTOR pathway		
PTEN protein loss	75–80	5–43
PTEN mutation	30–40	0–11
PIK3CA mutation	30–40	20–38
PIK3R1 mutation	21–43	12–17
ARID1A mutation	34	0
AKT mutation	2–3	0
RAF/MEK/ERK pathway		
KRAS mutation	10–30	0–10
BRAF mutation	23	11
RTKs		
IGFIR overexpression	78	Rare
FGFR2 mutation	12–16	1
EGFR overexpression	46	34
EGFR mutation	Unknown	0
HER-2 overexpression	3–10	32
HER-2 amplification	1	17
Others		
beta-catenin mutation	15–50	0
p53 mutation	7–50 (dependent on grade)	54–90
BRCA1/2 mutation	13	0
Microsatellite instability	15–25	0–5

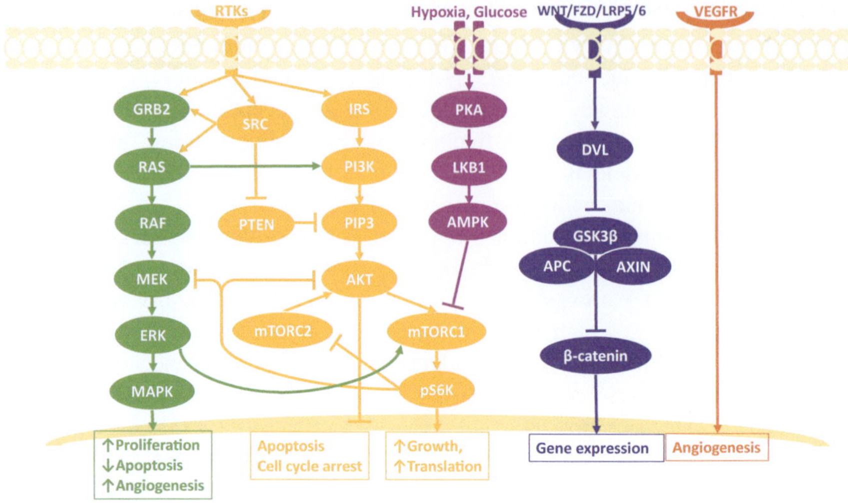

Fig. 10.1 Druggable signaling pathways in endometrial cancer. *Arrows* indicate activation while *blunt-headed arrows* indicate inhibition. Abbreviations: *RTKs* receptor tyrosine kineses; *GRB2* growth factor receptor-bound protein 2; *RAS* rat sarcoma gene; *RAF* V-raf-1 murine leukemia viral oncogene homolog 1; *MEK* mitogen-activated protein kinase kinase; *ERK* mitogen-activated protein kinase; *MAPK* mitogen-activated protein kinase; *SRC* V-src sarcoma (Schmidt-Ruppin A-2) viral oncogene homolog; *PTEN* phosphatase and tensin homolog deleted on chromosome 10; *IRS* insulin receptor substrate; *PI3K* phosphatidylinositol 3 kinase; *PIP3* phosphatidylinositol (3,4,5)-triphosphate; *AKT* v-akt murine thymoma viral oncogene homolog 1; *mTORC* mammalian target of rapamycin complex; *pS6K* protein S6 kinase; *PKA* protein kinase A; *LKB1* liver kinase B1; *AMPK* adenosine monophosphate kinase; *FZD* frizzled receptor; *LRP* low-density lipoprotein receptor; *DVL* disheveled protein; *GSK3β* glycogen synthase kinase 3β; *APC* adenomatous polyposis coli gene; *VEGFR* vascular endothelial growth factor receptor

Pathways of Interest in Endometrial Cancer

PI3K/AKT Pathway

The PI3K/AKT pathway is well-known to play a central role in growth, cell survival, and avoidance of apoptosis in many different cancer types [67]. Stimulation of this pathway occurs through receptor tyrosine kinases (RTKs), including epidermal growth factor receptor (EGFR), insulin-like growth factor I receptor (IGFIR), and fibroblast growth factor receptor 2 (FGFR2). Activated PI3K phosphorylates phosphatidylinositol 4,5-bisphosphate (PIP2) and converts it to phosphatidylinositol (3,4,5)-triphosphate (PIP3). PIP3 subsequently causes AKT phosphorylation. Phosphatase and tensin homolog deleted from chromosome 10 (PTEN) is a major negative regulator of the pathway and inhibits AKT activation through de-phosphorylation of PIP3 to PIP2 [189]. Activation of AKT leads to cellular proliferation and survival through various downstream targets, including mammalian target of rapamycin (mTOR). mTOR is composed of two complexes, mTORC1 and mTORC2, each with its own unique downstream effectors [200]. This pathway has negative feedback loops that must be considered when implementing targeted therapy. For example, mTORC1 up-regulation through AKT leads to subsequent activation of the protein S6 kinase (pS6K) that regulates protein translation, cell survival, and cell cycle progression from the G1 to S-phase. pS6K also has a negative feedback loop to suppress activation of AKT, MEK, and mTORC2 [145] (Fig. 10.1).

Given the frequency of abnormalities in the PI3K/AKT pathway, its members arguably represent the most promising targets for endometrial cancer. As noted in Table 10.1, up to 80% of endometrioid adenocarcinomas have an aberration in the PI3K/AKT pathway. Furthermore, alterations in the RTKs that activate the PI3K/AKT pathway are frequent in endometrial cancer including amplification/overexpression of HER2 [130, 182], mutation of FGFR2 [39, 151], overexpression of EGFR [88, 106], and overexpression of IGFIR [117]. Mutations in *PI3KCA* (30–40%) and *PTEN* (30–50%), as well as loss of PTEN protein expression (30–80%), are the most common causes of constitutive activation of this pathway in endometrial cancer [64, 93, 132, 139, 163]. Although AKT mutations are reported in only 2% of endometrioid adenocarcinoma, activating AKT1 mutations lead to constitutive activation of PI3K pathway signaling and may play a role in the pathogenesis of endometrial cancer [40, 177]. PTEN is also involved in maintaining genomic stability, and *PTEN* mutations may lead to defects in HR (responsible for repairing double-stranded DNA breaks) [119]. To date, several different PI3K/AKT pathway nodes have been targeted in endometrial cancer (Table 10.2). The drugs have included AKT inhibitors, mTORC1 inhibitors, mTORC1/2 inhibitors, pan-PI3K inhibitors, isoform-specific PI3K inhibitors, and dual PI3K/mTOR inhibitors. Other agents, such as metformin (discussed later), may also work via mTOR inhibition through the activation of AMPK.

AKT inhibition. AKT, a serine/threonine protein kinase with three isoforms, AKT1, AKT2, and AKT3, is a key node along the PI3K/AKT pathway. Activation of AKT leads to cellular proliferation and survival through various downstream targets, including mTOR. In vitro and in vivo studies of AKT inhibitors have demonstrated activity against endometrial cancer [42]. There are numerous small molecule inhibitors of AKT currently in development for endometrial cancer and solid tumors. Uprosertib (GSK2141795) is a novel member of the N-alkyl pyrazole class of orally available kinase inhibitors and has been shown to be a potent, ATP competitive, and pan-AKT inhibitor [61]. Common toxicities of uprosertib are gastrointestinal-related (diarrhea, nausea, and vomiting) and fatigue. MK-2206 is an allosteric AKT inhibitor that has shown anti-tumor activity in preclinical investigations [72]. A subsequent phase II trial that was stratified by PI3KCA mutation revealed only modest response, regardless of mutation status [133]. Several patients with uterine serous cancer had clinical benefit; however, a subsequent evaluation of MK-2206 in this population did not achieve meaningful clinical activity [94]. AZD5363 is a selective AKT kinase inhibitor that has been evaluated in a phase I trial of gynecologic malignancies with AKT mutations. Although the trial is

Table 10.2 Clinical trials of agents targeting the PI3K/AKT pathway

Target	Inhibitor	*n*	CR (%)	PR (%)	SD (%)	6-month PFS (%)	Median PFS (months)
PI3K	Buparlisib (BKM-120)	24	0	0		(2 month)	4.5
	High-grade strata	10	0	0		70	3.8
	Low-grade strata	14	0	0		57	8.3
	Pilaralisib (XL147)	67	3	3	37	11.9	–
Dual PI3K/mTOR	GDC-0980	56	0	9	–	20	3.5
	Gedatolisib (PKI-587)	40					
	Stathmin low		0	16	37		
	Stathmin high		0	16	11	–	–
AKT	MK2206						
	PI3KCA wt	27	0	3.7		11	
	PI3KCA mut	9	0	11	–	11	–
	MK2206 (serous only)	14	0	0	2	7	–
mTORC1	Everolimus	28	0	0	43	–	4.5
	Everolimus	44	0	9	27	–	2.8
	Ridaforolimus	45	0	11	18	18	–
	Ridaforolimus	31	0	8.8	53	–	–
	Ridaforolimus	64	0	0	35		3.6
	Temsirolimus						
	Prior chemo	25	0	4	48		
	Chemonaive	29	0	14	69	–	7.3
	Temsirolimus	50	6	16	52	–	–
Combination agents							
VEGFR/mTOR	Bevacizumab/Temsirolimus	49	2	22	47		5.6
MEK/AKT	Trametinib/GSK2141795	26	0	3.8	42.3	19	–
mTOR/Hormone	Everolimus/Letrozole	35	25.7	5.7	–	42	3.0

ongoing, preliminary results suggest promising activity with a tolerable safety profile [76].

mTOR inhibition. The protein kinase mTOR is a downstream effector of the PI3K/AKT pathway and holds a central position in cell growth regulation. Other than PI3K/AKT signaling, multiple cues modulate mTOR activity, including growth factors, stress, energy status, and amino acids [200]. As noted above, mTOR is composed of two complexes, mTORC1 and mTORC2, each with different downstream effectors, making inhibition of the PI3K/AKT pathway through mTOR inhibition challenging. For example, inhibition of mTORC1 can activate AKT by preventing a negative feedback loop mediated by the mTORC1-S6K1-induced phosphorylation of insulin receptor substrate 1 (IRS1) and growth factor receptor-bound protein 10 (GRB10) [145, 176]. Furthermore, mTORC1 inhibition results in the loss of inactivation of mTORC2, which leads to AKT activation (Fig. 10.1).

Thus far, the majority of studies on advanced and recurrent endometrial cancer have focused on rapalogs, which primarily inhibit mTORC1. mTORC1 inhibitors include everolimus (Afinitor, RAD001), ridaforolimus (AP23573), and temsirolimus (Torisel, CCI-77). Detailed results of clinical trials incorporating these agents in the treatment of endometrial cancer are listed in Table 10.2. Generally, the clinical effects of mTORC1 inhibitors have been modest, with response rates ranging from 0 to 22%, and the most frequent result being stable disease [26, 50, 141, 142, 143, 155, 183, 195]. These agents are fairly well tolerated, with predominant adverse events consisting of fatigue, hyperglycemia, mucositis, and rash.

There are data to indicate that resistance to hormonal agents in endometrial cancer (i.e., progesterone agents) may be secondary to activity of the PI3K/AKT pathway. Thus, combinations of anti-hormone options and rapalogs have been explored. Slomovitz and colleagues achieved significant objective response of 32% (9 CR) with the combination of everolimus and letrozole in recurrent endometrial cancer with 1–2 prior therapies [181]. Unfortunately, in the study by Fleming and colleagues, temsirolimus and megestrol acetate alternating with tamoxifen could not be combined safely due to extensive thrombotic events [50].

PI3K inhibition. If the PI3K pathway is considered a pyramid, with PI3K at the apex and multiple signaling branches downstream to mediate effects, the direct inhibition of PI3K holds the potential to have the strongest blockade for PI3K pathway signaling. A number of PI3K inhibitors have been developed, and many of them have been evaluated in clinical trials for endometrial cancer. Pan-PI3K inhibitors target all four isoforms of class I PI3K (α, β, γ, and δ). Buparlisib (BKM120) [69, 112], pictilisib (GDC-0941), and pilaralisib (XL147) [53, 173] are oral, pan-PI3K small molecule inhibitors that are undergoing evaluation in endometrial cancer (Table 10.2). Frequent adverse events for these agents include nausea, fatigue, rash, and hyperglycemia. As a single agent in recurrent endometrial cancer, pilaralisib had minimal clinical activity (RR 6%, 6-month PFS 12%) [116]. Although the results have not yet been reported, this agent was subsequently combined with paclitaxel and carboplatin in the same setting. In an attempt to decrease adverse effects, isoform-specific PI3K inhibitors have been developed, including NVP-BYL719 (PI3K-alpha selective inhibitor) [57], MLN1117 (PI3K-alpha selective inhibitor), and GSK2636771 (PI3K-beta selective inhibitor). They are currently in early-phase clinical trials. Decreasing adverse events can also be accomplished by varying the mode of administration of these agents. Copanlisib is an intravenous pan-PI3K inhibitor that has demonstrated promising activity and lower levels of adverse events in early-phase trials [149]. A phase II trial of copanlisib in *PI3KCA* mutant recurrent endometrial cancer is planned.

Dual inhibitors: Dual inhibitor agents include PI3K/mTOR inhibitors and mTORC1/2 inhibitors. Dual inhibition is intended to overcome existing resistance mechanisms and feedback loops, thereby providing greater activity. Dual PI3K/mTOR inhibitors are ATP competitive and have been developed using the sequence homology of the catalytic sites of PI3K and both mTOR complexes. These agents include GDC-0980 [197], PF04691502, gedatolisib (PF05212384), and XL-765 (SAR245409). A phase II trial of GDC-0980 in endometrial cancer recently reported preliminary results. Among 56 women treated with the agent, 9% had objective response and 20% were progression-free at 6 months [113]. A similar trial of both PF04691502 and gedatolisib in recurrent endometrial cancer was performed, stratified by stathmin expression. The PF04691502 (oral) arm was closed secondary to excessive toxicity including pneumonitis. The gedatolisib (intravenous) arm yielded modest activity in both the stathmin high (16% RR, 11% SD) and stathmin low (16% RR, 37% SD) expression cohorts [32]. mTORC-inhibiting agents that target both complexes, mTORC1 and mTORC2, include AZD2014, MLN0128, and OSI-027. The majority of these agents are still in early-phase trials, and results are eagerly anticipated.

Ideally, the success of agents targeting the PI3K/AKT pathway could be predicted by the known baseline molecular status of the tumor. Primary candidates for biomarkers of response include mutations in *PIK3CA*, *PTEN*, *AKT*, as well as overexpression of phosphorylated pathway members such as mTOR (pmTOR) and AKT (pAKT). Preclinical studies have suggested that *PIK3CA* mutations could predict response to PI3K and mTOR inhibitors, while mutations in the MAPK pathway (*KRAS, NRAS, BRAF*) might mediate resistance [33, 43, 78]. However, to date, markers including expression of PTEN and stathmin, as well as mutations *PIK3CA* and *KRAS,* have not correlated with response to therapy [110, 122, 194]. Interestingly, in a small study of patients treated with everolimus, the combination of KRAS mutation and expression of phosphorylated s6 protein was predictive of non-response [122]. Certainly, further analysis will be necessary to elucidate appropriate predictive markers to maximize benefit from these treatments.

Ras/Raf Pathway

The Ras/Raf pathway plays a critical role in multiple cellular functions including proliferation, growth, and senescence [126]. Activation of this pathway can result from activation/mutation of the upstream RTKs and RAS, or up-regulation/mutations in Raf and MEK (MAP2K). Upon activation, Raf acts as the MAP kinase kinase kinase (MAP3K) and activates MEK1 and MEK2 (MEK1/2), which act as the MAP kinase kinase (MAP2K). MEK1/2 in turn catalyzes activation of the effector ERK1 and ERK2 (ERK1/2) kinases. Once activated, ERK1/2 translocates into the nucleus and phosphorylates a number of effector proteins and transcriptional factors that regulate cell proliferation, motility, differentiation, and survival [126] (Fig. 10.1). ERK activation can also induce overexpression of EGFR ligands important for tumor growth [37]. The Ras/Raf pathway is a major mediator of Ras-induced carcinogenesis, but recent data have shown that Ras can activate and interact with other signaling pathways including PI3K/AKT [44].

In addition to aberrations in the RTKs that activate the Ras/Raf pathway, mutations in key pathway nodes including MEK, Ras, and Raf can stimulate constitutive pathway activation. There is a relatively high prevalence of *KRAS* mutation in endometrial cancer, especially among endometrioid adenocarcinomas [95, 165, 171], which makes this pathway an attractive target for treatment. Thus far, MEK inhibitors are the most clinically developed agents targeting this pathway [55]. Further, combined inhibition of the Ras/Raf and PI3K/AKT pathways has been suggested as a therapeutic strategy, although success has been limited by excessive toxicity [9, 13, 43, 65, 74, 81, 154, 192, 206].

MEK inhibition. MEK serves as a downstream effector of the Ras/Raf pathway, causing phosphorylation of MAPK and subsequent activation of proteins including s6 kinase [120]. Agents that inhibit MEK have been quite successful in a number of solid tumors, including melanoma and thyroid cancer [49, 102]. In endometrial cancer, MEK inhibitors that have been studied alone and in combination with AKT inhibitors include selumetinib (AZD6244) and trametinib (GSK1120212). In a phase II study of recurrent endometrial cancer performed by the GOG, selumetinib achieved an objective response in 6% of patients, with 12% of patients progression-free at 6 months [25]. The combination of the AKT inhibitor uprosertib with trametinib in a population of recurrent endometrial cancer patients stratified by KRAS mutation had minimal activity in the setting of significant adverse events [206].

Prediction of response and resistance to MEK inhibition based on biomarker expression has been limited in endometrial cancer. It may be inferred from experience in other solid tumors that the presence of a *BRAF* mutation yields sensitivity to MEK inhibition [38, 148]. Since *BRAF* mutations are rare in endometrial cancer [86, 162], this may be why there have been low response rates thus far in trials. Certainly, KRAS mutation is also of interest, although no data have been reported in endometrial cancer. There are transcriptional signatures that are of interest from preclinical studies on the prediction of response to MEK inhibition; however, these have not yet been reported as part of a clinical trial [35].

Angiogenesis

Angiogenesis (new blood vessel formation) includes the recruitment of vasculature, circulating endothelial cells, and pro-angiogenic mediators [208]. It is a complicated process that occurs through the balance of a number of stimulatory and inhibitory factors. The vascular endothelial growth factor (VEGF) family ligands include VEGF-A, VEGF-B, VEGF-C, VEGF-D, VEGF-E, placental growth factor (PLGF)-1, and PLGF-2. These ligands interact with a variety of receptors including VEGF receptor (VEGFR)-1, VEGFR-2, and VEGFR-3. VEGFR-1 and VEGFR-2 are RTKs expressed specifically on endothelial cells, to which VEGF-A binds [70]. VEGFR-2 mainly transmits signals into the cytoplasm through activation of phospholipase C (PLC)-γ, which then activates downstream pathways such as Ras/Raf. Angiogenesis has been shown to play an important role in the growth and metastatic potential of many tumors, including endometrial cancer [70]. In endometrial cancer, higher tumor microvessel density (MVD) levels are associated with nodal metastases, advanced stage, and poor survival [73, 84]. Similarly, high tumor VEGF levels are associated with higher grade tumors, deep myometrial invasion, nodal metastases, and more advanced stage disease [98]. These findings have made angiogenesis an attractive target for endometrial cancer.

VEGF Inhibition. Options for targeting VEGF include monoclonal antibodies, small molecule inhibitors, and decoy receptors that trap VEGF. Bevacizumab (Avastin), a monoclonal antibody to VEGF, has had promising single-agent activity in endometrial cancer, with 13.5% of patients achieving an objective response (1 CR, 6 PR) and 40% of patients surviving progression-free at 6 months [3]. Bevacizumab was combined with standard of care chemotherapy, paclitaxel and carboplatin, in a multi-arm trial for chemonaive advanced stage and recurrent endometrial cancer. The combination demonstrated response rates and progression-free survival similar to historical controls; however, there was an apparent overall survival benefit, although it was unclear if this was simply related to a difference in patient populations [2]. Interestingly, when combined with paclitaxel and carboplatin for recurrent disease previously treated with chemotherapy, bevacizumab significantly improved response rates and progression-free survival [107]. This combination is under further evaluation to fully elucidate its role in advanced stage and recurrent endometrial cancer. A combination of bevacizumab with temsirolimus yielded an increased response rate of 29%, although there was no difference in the proportion of patients surviving progression-free at 6 months compared to bevacizumab alone, despite increased toxicity [4]. Aflibercept, a decoy receptor to VEGF, demonstrated less single-agent activity in recurrent endometrial cancer compared to bevacizumab. It yielded a 7% partial response rate with frequent severe toxicity, including cardiovascular, metabolic, hemorrhagic complications, and pain [24].

VEGFR Inhibition. There are a number of small molecule inhibitors that target VEGFR in addition to other relevant targets. Cediranib (AZD2171) inhibits VEGFR-2, c-kit, and platelet-derived growth factor receptor (PDGFR). This agent achieved a response rate of 12% in recurrent endometrial cancer, with 30% of patients surviving progression-free at 6 months [14]. Sorafenib is another multi-kinase inhibitor that targets Raf as well as VEGFR and PDGFR. This agent yielded only a 5% partial response among 40 patients with recurrent endometrial cancer, although 42.5% of patients achieved stable disease [135]. Sunitinib, an inhibitor of VEGFR, PDGFR, EGF, and Kit, has also undergone evaluation in this population. Thirty percent of women had disease control for 6 months (n = 34), with 18% having a PR after treatment with this agent [27].

Fibroblast growth factor (FGF) Inhibition. FGFs are a family of 22 ligands that may bind to four FGF receptors (FGFRs). FGF ligand binding causes activation of an intracellular tyrosine kinase that leads to mitogenic and angiogenic activities implicated in a variety of biological process including embryogenesis, wound healing, and tumor growth [63]. The activation cascade includes growth factor receptor bound 2 (Grb2), and thereby the Ras/Raf pathway (Fig. 10.1). Oncogenic activating mutations of *FGFR2* have been identified in 12–16% of endometrioid endometrial adenocarcinomas [151] (Table 10.1). Thus, a phase II trial of dovitinib, an inhibitor of FGFR as well as VEGFR, c-kit, and PDGFR, was performed in patients with recurrent endometrial cancer, with stratification based on the presence of a *FGFR2* mutation. There was insufficient activity to warrant further exploration of this agent, and, surprisingly, activity was not associated with the presence of an activating *FGFR2* mutation [91]. A single-agent trial of brivanib, a dual inhibitor of FGFR and VEGFR2, in recurrent endometrial cancer yielded a 19% response rate, with one complete response and 30% progression-free survival at 6 months [152]. Conversely, nintedanib (BIBF-1120), which targets VEGFR, PDGFR, and FGFR, had only a 9% response rate among 32 patients with endometrial cancer [34]. These findings indicate some benefit for agents targeting these receptors, although it is clear that further clarification regarding patient selection will be necessary to achieve maximum impact.

Overall, prediction of response to anti-angiogenic agents in endometrial cancer has undergone limited study. In a phase II trial of thalidomide, which has anti-angiogenic properties by an unknown mechanism of action, the authors studied a number of relevant markers including VEGF, basic FGF, and soluble endometrial protein C receptor. Among 24 patients, 12.5% had PR and only 8.3% were progression-free at 6 months. There was no association between biomarker expression and response to thalidomide therapy; however, VEGF was associated with poor prognosis independent of thalidomide treatment [118].

Poly ADP-Ribose Polymerase (PARP) Pathway

The cell has a myriad of mechanisms to repair DNA damage, including direct repair, base-excision repair, mismatch repair, and nucleotide excision repair. Resistance to cytotoxic chemotherapy may be found in cancer cells with a high activity of DNA damage repair pathways. PARP 1 and 2 are enzymes involved in base-excision repair of single-strand DNA breaks (SSBs) [31, 59, 169, 201]. Inhibition of PARP leads to unrepaired SSBs, which result in double-strand breaks (DSBs) following DNA replication. HR is the mechanism involved in the repair of these DSBs after the process of replication. The combination of PARP inhibition with defective HR leads to enhanced cell death, a concept termed "synthetic lethality" [59]. Thus, PARP inhibition has been developed for use in therapy in patients with impaired DNA repair mechanisms, such as breast and ovarian cancer patients with BRCA mutation [31, 52, 111]. In addition to activity through direct inhibition of PARP enzymes, PARP inhibitors also appear to act by trapping PARP enzymes and through promotion of DNA repair by non-homologous end joining, which is fraught with errors. Given these numerous mechanisms of activity, the use of PARP inhibitors holds great promise in endometrial cancer. Endometrial cancer has known deficiencies in HR based on defects in HR genes such as ATM, ATR, and ARID1A [22, 104, 174]. Interestingly, PTEN loss, which is common in endometrial cancer, may also lead to defects in HR by impairing repair of DSBs, creating cellular susceptibility to PARP inhibition [119].

In vitro studies of endometrial cancer cell lines have demonstrated cellular growth inhibition and apoptosis after treatment with a PARP inhibitor. These intriguing findings, coupled with case reports indicating that endometrial cancer with aberrations in PTEN may benefit from treatment with PARP inhibitors, have led to the development of several trials of PARP inhibitors, alone or in combination with other targeted therapies, for the treatment of endometrial cancer. To date, no results have been reported.

Epidermal Growth Factor Receptor (EGFR) Pathway

The EGFR family is made up of RTKs which work as mitogens for important downstream pathways such as PI3K/AKT and Ras/Raf. There are four receptors that make up this group, EGFR (HER-1, ERBB1), HER-2 (ERBB2), HER-3 (ERBB3), and HER-4 (ERBB4) [23, 30, 134, 136]. Mutation and overexpression of these members are known to impact tumorigenesis in a variety of solid tumors. EGFR is overexpressed in a large proportion of endometrial cancer, up to 46% of endometrioid adenocarcinomas and 34% of non-endometrioid carcinomas [88] (Table 10.1). EGFR overexpression has been reported to be associated with poor overall survival in endometrial cancer [92]. On the other hand, rates of *EGFR* mutation are quite low. Data in multiple tumors have indicated that EGFR overexpression is not sufficient to predict response to therapy and that *EGFR* mutation is more closely correlated with response [21], thus further study is indicated to determine the relevance of these agents for endometrial cancer. HER-2 is another potentially relevant target in endometrial cancer, with approximately 30% of non-endometrioid tumors exhibiting HER-2 overexpression. Overexpression of HER-2 is associated with poor prognosis, especially among serous tumors [60, 164, 182].

EGFR Inhibition. Clinical trials targeting EGFR have demonstrated only modest success in the treatment of endometrial cancer, with response rates ranging between 3–12% and little improvement in progression-free survival [99, 144, 184]. Certainly, the aforementioned data that EGFR overexpression is not sufficient to predict response to therapy may be relevant in endometrial cancer as well. In a study of gefitinib as a single agent, there was no association between response and expression of relevant biomarkers including phosphorylated EGFR, phosphorylated ERK, *EGFR* mutation, or EGFR protein expression [99].

HER-2 Inhibition. Trastuzumab, a humanized monoclonal antibody to HER-2, was evaluated in a phase II trial for advanced and recurrent endometrial cancers with overexpression or amplification of HER-2. Unfortunately, there were no clinical responses, and only 12 of 30 patients had SD [51]. An ongoing trial in uterine serous cancer is comparing treatment with paclitaxel/carboplatin with or without herceptin among patients with tumor expression of HER-2/neu by immunohistochemistry and *HER-2/neu* gene amplification documented by FISH.

Dual Inhibition. A dual tyrosine kinase inhibitor of EGFR and HER-2, lapatinib, was also studied in recurrent endometrial cancers with one to two prior therapies; however, clinical activity was low [100]. There are few plans to further evaluate the role of anti-EGFR agents in endometrial cancer at this point.

Other Agents and Targets of Interest

Metformin

Metformin (N′-N′ dimethylguanide) is an oral biguanide widely used for the treatment of type 2 diabetes and has been demonstrated to reduce cancer risk and provide anti-tumor activity in a variety of cancers [45, 103]. Theoretical mechanisms for the anticancer activity of metformin are twofold, including direct and indirect models [12, 209]. The direct model proposes that metformin acts through activation of AMPK, phosphorylation of TSC-2, and subsequent inhibition of the downstream target mTOR. In the indirect model, metformin acts through increase of insulin sensitivity, decrease in circulating insulin, increase of glucose uptake into the cell, and decrease of gluconeogenesis. Ultimately, this agent has been shown to induce cell cycle arrest and apoptosis [18], as well as induce progesterone receptor expression and reverse progesterone resistance in endometrial cancer cell lines [207, 212]. Interestingly, metformin may be an effective agent in tumors with activating mutations of *KRAS*. The proposed mechanism is inhibition of *KRAS* signaling through mislocalization of *KRAS* from the plasma membrane into the cytoplasm [77]. Two window of opportunity studies of metformin in primary endometrial cancer patients prior to surgical resection have revealed the potential activity of this agent based on pharmacodynamic markers. Metformin demonstrated down-regulation of the PI3K/AKT and Ras/Raf pathways based on reduction in phosphorylated AKT and MAPK, as well as reduction in downstream regulators including ps6, and p4EBP-1 [168]. Interestingly, in a study by Soliman and colleagues, there was no change in phosphorylated ACC, indicating a lack of direct action by metformin on AMPK [188].

These findings have led to several studies of metformin for primary and recurrent tumors, including evaluation in the conservative treatment of primary endometrial cancer. In addition, the NRG Oncology—Gynecologic Oncology Group (GOG) is assessing the impact of the addition of metformin to standard of care chemotherapy with paclitaxel and carboplatin in chemonaive advanced stage and recurrent endometrial cancer.

Dasatinib

Dasatinib is a multi-kinase inhibitor of Src and EphA2, as well as bcr-abl, c-kit, and PDGF [6]. There is great interest in this agent, given the importance of several of these targets in endometrial cancer. The proto-oncogenec-Src (Src) family of protein kinases regulates multiple tumorigenic activities across solid tumors [191]. Further, the ephrin ligands, including EphA2, are involved in a number of key cellular processes including angiogenesis and cellular migration [20, 71, 89, 123]. Elevated EphA2 has been demonstrated to correlate with poor prognosis in endometrial cancer [83]. Early-phase trials of Dasatinib as a single agent and in combination with paclitaxel and carboplatin were well tolerated with promising activity [6, 90, 170]. A pilot study of dasatinib in combination with paclitaxel and carboplatin in advanced stage and recurrent endometrial cancer has been completed, and the results are anticipated.

Angiopoietin (Ang)/Tie-2

Alternative angiogenic pathways are under exploration for the treatment of endometrial cancer. The interaction between angiopoietins, Ang-1 and Ang-2, and their receptor, Tie-2, stimulates proliferation of endothelial cells, in addition to promoting survival and motility. Ang-1 and Ang-2 support vascular maturation through the recruitment of pericytes [66, 161]. Trebananib (AMG-386) is a peptide fusion protein that binds the angiopoietins and blocks interaction with their receptor [125]. Although early-phase trials demonstrated reasonable safety and promising efficacy across gynecologic malignancies, trebaninib as a single agent in recurrent endometrial yielded only one objective response out of 32 patients [128].

P53

P53 has long been a target of great interest in a number of advanced solid tumors, and endometrial cancer is no exception. Uterine serous tumors have a high frequency of *p53* mutation, and this target is also common in grade 3 endometrioid tumors and in carcinosarcoma [85]. There are a number of agents in development that may have a role in the treatment of endometrial cancer, including Wee1 inhibitors and agents that restore p53 function [198]. P53 serves as a regulator of the cell cycle at G1, and loss of its function creates dependency on the G2 cell cycle checkpoint. This checkpoint is regulated by Wee1, with inhibition of Wee1 leading to cell death after failure of DNA damage repair [146, 153]. The most developed Wee1 inhibitor is AZD1775, which has been evaluated in ovarian cancer. Early-phase trials of p53 agents, including in endometrial cancer, are ongoing.

Immune Therapy

Harnessing the immune system to target cancer cells has been difficult until recent years. As our understanding of the mechanisms of tumor immune system evasion has grown, so have the number of successful immune therapy agents [185, 193]. Although initial efforts had focused on immune driven cancers, the activity of immune therapy has recently been associated with molecular aberrations common to endometrial cancer, including microsatellite instability (MSI) and the presence of mutations in POLE [11, 75, 196]. Thus, the use of agents including avelumab, nivolumab, and pembrolizumab is under exploration in recurrent endometrial cancer. A recent phase Ib study of pembrolizumab in microsatellite unstable solid tumors, including endometrial cancer, reported a 71% response rate (n = 7) [97]. Further, in a separate study of unselected endometrial cancers, pembrolizumab achieved 13% PR and 19% progression-free survival at 6 months [140]. These promising results have led to the implementation of numerous phase II studies in microsatellite unstable and unselected recurrent endometrial cancer.

Prevention of Endometrial Cancer

To understand the prevention of cancer, knowledge of risk factors is paramount. This defines the population for prevention efforts and guides the development of strategies. For prevention, it is important to understand if a risk factor is modifiable or actionable, as this will provide an opportunity for intervention. Fortunately, endometrioid endometrial adenocarcinoma has a number of well-defined risk factors, including hormonal, metabolic, lifestyle, and hereditary factors [5, 82] (Table 10.3). Risk factors for non-endometrioid endometrial cancer have not been well defined, in part due to their relative infrequency. However, a meta-analysis by Setiawan et al. [172] revealed that non-endometrioid endometrial cancer shares many etiologic factors with the endometrioid type, including high body mass index (BMI), low parity, low age at menarche, and diabetes. The closing section of this chapter will discuss modifiable risk factors for endometrial cancer and potential interventions for endometrial cancer prevention. Other populations of interest for endometrial cancer prevention will also be reviewed.

Modifiable Risk Factors

Unopposed estrogen exposure. A strong association between estrogen exposure and endometrioid endometrial adenocarcinoma has been demonstrated. Risk factors related to increased estrogen can come from exogenous as well as endogenous sources, including hormone replacement therapy (HRT), polycystic ovary

Table 10.3 Endometrial cancer risk factors and protective factors

	Relative risk	Modifiable
Hormonal factors		
HRT		Yes
Continuous combined therapy	0.71×	
Cyclic combined therapy	1.05×	
Estrogen alone	1.45×	
Contraceptives		
OC	0.5×	Yes
Non-hormonal IUD	0.54×	
LNG-IUS	0.5×	
Other agents		Yes
Tamoxifen	2.53×	
Aromatase inhibitors	1×	
Obesity		Yes
BMI 18.5–24.9	1×	
BMI 25.0–29.9	1.5×	
BMI 30.0–34.9	2.53×	
BMI 35.0–39.9	2.77×	
BMI 40.0–	6.25×	
PCOS		Possible
PCOS	4×	
Parity		No
Nulliparity	1×	
1 birth	0.9×	
2 births	0.8×	
3 or more births	0.7×	
Menstruation		No
Early menarche	2.4×	
Late menopause	1.7×	
Factors related to endocrine metabolic disease and lifestyle		
Diabetes, hypertension, and dyslipidemia		Possible
Type 1 diabetes	2.7×	
Type 2 diabetes	1.5×	
Hypertension	1.44×	
Low HDL (<50 mg/dl)	1.06×	
High TG (≥ 150 mg/dl)	1.19×	
Alcohol intake		Yes
0 g/day	1×	
>0 to <12 g/day	0.91×	
12 to <24 g/day	0.89×	
≥ 24 g/day	1.59×	

(continued)

Table 10.3 (continued)

	Relative risk	Modifiable
Cigarette smoking		Yes
In premenopausal women	1.06×	
In postmenopausal women	0.71×	
Physical activity		Yes
Regular exercise	0.67–0.78×	
Diet		Yes
Increased caloric intake	1.7×	
Cholesterol	2.1×	
Saturated fatty acids	1.3×	
Fiber	0.6×	
Hereditary factors		
HNPCC	40–60% lifetime risk	
Cowden syndrome	28% lifetime risk	

syndrome (PCOS), nulliparity, early age of menarche, and late age of menopause [41, 82]. The majority of these factors are not modifiable, although the use of HRT can be optimized to avoid the risk of endometrial cancer. Representative relative risks of each category of HRT are shown in Table 10.3. Certainly, HRT with unopposed estrogen increases the risk of endometrial cancer, while HRT containing progestin does not increase the risk and, in some cases, may be protective [15].

Tamoxifen, which is used to treat or prevent breast cancer due to an anti-estrogenic effect on the mammary gland, is known to have a modest estrogenic effect on endometrium. Postmenopausal women treated with tamoxifen have an increased risk of endometrial cancer [48]. Therefore, these women should be monitored for early detection of endometrial cancer based on symptoms. There is no recommendation for routine endometrial cancer screening through endometrial biopsy or transvaginal ultrasound in this patient population. Of note, aromatase inhibitors, which can be effective for breast cancer prevention and treatment in some situations, do not increase the risk of endometrial cancer [36].

Obesity. Obesity is a known risk factor for incidence and cancer-related death in a variety of solid tumors [8, 156]; however, the impact of obesity is greatest among patients with endometrial cancer [17]. There is a step-wise association of endometrial cancer risk and mortality based on incremental increase in BMI [157]. The role of obesity in the etiology of endometrial cancer is multifactorial. First, there is an association between increased BMI and circulating estrogens due to aromatization of androgen to estrogens in adipose tissue [19, 179]. Further, obesity is associated with decreased serum hormone-binding globulins (SHBG), which allows for increased free estrogen in the obese patient [129]. Obese women are often noted to have progesterone deficiency secondary to anovulation, which further promotes the proliferation of the endometrium and subsequent development of endometrial neoplasia [82]. Finally, insulin resistance and hyperinsulinemia are tightly related to obesity and have been suggested to act as a further risk factor for endometrial cancer. This is in part due to insulin's direct effect as a mitogen-stimulating tumorigenic pathway such as PI3K/AKT[114]. In addition, insulin is an anti-apoptotic growth factor in the endometrium and can increase levels of free estrogen through down-regulation of SHBG [28]. Arguably, obese women are the group that stands to benefit most from prevention strategies. Based on the strong association of increased BMI and endometrial cancer risk, there is a significant opportunity to prevent endometrial cancer through promotion of weight loss and use of treatments to counteract insulin resistance.

Physical activity. As part of a prospective study of cancer incidence and prevention, the American Cancer Society found that any level of physical activity and the avoidance of a sedentary lifestyle were significantly associated with a reduction in endometrial cancer risk [147]. Moore and colleagues performed a meta-analysis of nine prospective cohort studies that revealed a 30% reduction in risk of endometrial cancer among active women compared to inactive women. The activities covered a wide range from mild exercise, such as walking or cycling, to intense exercise such as running [127]. Of note, it appears that body weight modifies the association of physical activity and endometrial cancer risk, so it is important to address all aspects of health in order to reduce the risk of endometrial cancer [147, 167].

Diet. Although not thoroughly evaluated, it appears that specific diet components play a role in the development of endometrial cancer. Levi and colleagues reported in 1993 that after controlling for high caloric intake, food type had an impact on endometrial cancer risk. Specifically, high fat and sugar intake were associated with increased risk of endometrial cancer [101]. Further studies have indicated that a diet high in red meat, fat, and cholesterol are associated with increased endometrial cancer risk. Conversely, the intake of fresh fruit, vegetables, and whole grains significantly reduces this risk [16, 101, 160].

Alcohol intake. Ethanol has traditionally been thought to increase the risk of endometrial cancer through an increase in estrogen levels [58, 62, 158]. However, moderate alcohol intake is known to decrease insulin levels and increase overall sensitivity to insulin, which could reduce endometrial cancer risk [29]. There have been many conflicting clinical studies regarding the true impact. A thorough meta-analysis has demonstrated an apparent dose–response relationship between alcohol and endometrial cancer risk. Specifically, compared to nondrinkers, women who drank 0.5–1 drink per day have a lower risk of endometrial cancer. However, in women who drink more than 2 drinks a day or more than 2.5 drinks a day, the risk of endometrial cancer increases 14 and 25%, respectively [54]. This risk is further increased in women who drink more than 2.5 drinks a day. Certainly, counseling patients to avoid significant intake of alcohol in order to reduce endometrial cancer risk is reasonable.

Tobacco intake. It is important to note that there is a significant protective effect of cigarette smoking on the risk of endometrial cancer among postmenopausal women [213]. However, the increased risk of lung cancer as well as other hazardous effects on the respiratory and cardiovascular systems eclipses the potential advantage of smoking, and it is never recommended.

Potentially Modifiable Risk Factors

Diabetes, hypertension, and dyslipidemia. Type 1 and type 2 diabetes, hypertension, and dyslipidemia are frequently comorbid with endometrial cancer; however, epidemiologic studies have demonstrated them to be independent risk factors for the development of endometrial cancer after controlling for age and body weight [56, 186, 202, 210]. Therefore, appropriate treatments such as lifestyle counseling and medical treatments of these diseases may also reduce the risk of endometrial cancer.

PCOS. In women less than 50 years of age those with PCOS had a fourfold increased risk of endometrial cancer compared to those without PCOS [46]. Elevated endogenous estrogen, lack of progesterone, as well as obesity, and insulin resistance in PCOS may contribute to the increased risk for endometrial cancer. Further investigation will be required to determine whether treatment of this condition yields a decreased risk of endometrial cancer.

Interventions

Contraceptives. In many studies, oral contraceptives (OCP) have been demonstrated to prevent the development of endometrial cancer, with increasing effects seen with longer duration of use. OCP use reduces the risk of endometrial cancer by 50% in women at no increased risk for the disease [87, 203]. Stanford and colleagues demonstrated that women who used OCPs for <1 year, 1–2 years, 3–4 years, 5–9 years, and 10 and more years gained a risk reduction of 0.7, 0.3, 0.3, 0.7, and 0.2, respectively, compared to nonusers [190]. A meta-analysis demonstrated that this protective effect persisted for 20 years after discontinuation (RR 0.33, 0.41, and 0.51 for 5, 10, 20 years after OC cessation, respectively, compared to nonusers) [131]. Lu and colleagues assessed the pathologic impact of a 3-month course of hormonal contraceptives (depomedroxyprogesterone acetate or OCPs) on the endometrium of women with Lynch syndrome. They found a significant reduction in endometrial proliferation with evidence of progesterone effect based on pathologic examination and expression of estrogen-induced transcripts [108]. It appears that the use of hormonal contraceptives should be considered for further study for the prevention of endometrial cancer in this high-risk patient population.

Interestingly, non-hormonal intrauterine devices also provide a protective effect (RR 0.54) against endometrial cancer, although the exact mechanism is not clear. The protective effect increased with the duration of use and was still observed after cessation of use (RR 0.91 in 5 years) [10]. Finally, the levonorgestrel-releasing intrauterine system has been reported to have a risk-reducing effect for endometrial cancer (RR 0.5) [47]. This agent was assessed for the prevention endometrial pathology in women treated with tamoxifen, yielding a significant reduction of endometrial polyps (RR 0.22) and endometrial hyperplasia (RR 0.13); however, further study is needed before this is incorporated into clinical practice [175].

Metformin. As noted above, metformin is an oral medication for type 2 diabetes mellitus that has been demonstrated to have an intriguing association with reduction in endometrial cancer risk [80]. Preclinical studies in a rat model revealed a reduction in estrogen-mediated endometrial proliferation after treatment with metformin [211]. This agent is currently undergoing evaluation in a prospective chemoprevention study for obese women at risk for the development of endometrial cancer.

Surgery. In addition to adjustments in diet and increasing physical activity, bariatric surgery is an option for weight loss reduction. Large cohort studies have revealed that overall cancer risk is reduced among patients who achieve weight loss after bariatric surgery [1, 7, 180]. Ward et al. [199] reported that any bariatric surgery was associated with a 71% reduced risk for uterine malignancy among obese women. This risk reduction was even greater among women who had successful bariatric surgery and were obese at the time of the study. Bariatric surgery would appear to be a reasonable option for the prevention of endometrial cancer, although ideally this should be evaluated in a prospective fashion.

Education. Given the number of potentially modifiable risk factors for the development of endometrial cancer, there is a significant opportunity for education intervention as a prevention technique. A survey of 1545 women, 68% of whom were overweight or obese, revealed that the majority (58%) were not aware that endometrial cancer risk was associated with obesity [187]. This lack of knowledge was higher among black women. A similar study among 93 obese women under consideration for bariatric surgery found that although 50% of women realized that obesity increased their risk of uterine cancer, they did not think that they were personally at risk [68]. These findings suggest that educational interventions may have a significant impact on women for reduction of endometrial cancer risk.

Other Populations for Prevention Strategies

Hereditary cancer syndromes. Although the majority of endometrial cancer is sporadic in nature, hereditary causes account for 2–5% of these tumors [121]. Lynch syndrome is an autosomal dominant disease caused by germ line mutations in the DNA mismatch repair (MMR) gene family, *MLH1*, *MSH2 MSH6*, and *PMS2*. Mutations in MMR genes result in MSI and genetic susceptibility to some types of malignancies including endometrial (lifetime risk 40–60%, compared with 2.6% in general population), colorectal (lifetime risk 60%), and ovarian cancer (lifetime risk 9–12%). Please see Chap. 9 in this textbook for full detail. Annual endometrial sampling and transvaginal ultrasound of the uterus and ovaries beginning at age 30–35 are recommended for women with Lynch syndrome [105]. Upon completion of childbearing, prophylactic hysterectomy has been demonstrated to eliminate the risk of endometrial cancer in this patient population [166].

Cowden syndrome is an autosomal dominant disease associated with PTEN mutation, predisposing affected individuals to a variety of malignancies including breast (lifetime risk 85%), thyroid (lifetime risk 35%), and endometrial cancer (lifetime risk 28%). The average age at diagnosis is 40–59 years, and annual screening recommendations are the same as for patients with Lynch syndrome [150]. It is unclear if hysterectomy offers the same benefit to patients with Cowden syndrome as it does to those patients with Lynch syndrome, although it is reasonable to consider in the absence of specific studies, given the rare nature of this condition.

Conclusion

Molecular abnormalities make endometrial cancer an attractive option for the use of targeted therapy. Success has been limited, but incremental changes have been made. With increased understanding of molecular mechanisms, there is no doubt that future clinical trials will have a greater impact on clinical outcomes. Novel combination agents and clinical trials that combine a number of agents across different pathways will be necessary. Certainly, understanding which patients may benefit from a given agent and, conversely, which patients may harbor resistance is essential to future developments in this field. Ultimately, the goal of prevention of endometrial cancer should take precedence. As knowledge of the metabolic and molecular mechanisms of endometrial cancer development grows, it will be essential to consider novel therapeutics as well as lifestyle changes to prevent this disease.

References

1. Adams TD, Stroup AM, Gress RE, Adams KF, Calle EE, Smith SC, Halverson RC, Simper SC, Hopkins PN, Hunt SC. Cancer incidence and mortality after gastric bypass surgery. Obesity (Silver Spring). 2009;17(4):796–802. doi:10.1038/oby.2008.610.
2. Aghajanian C, Filiaci VL, Dizon DS, Carlson JW, Powell MA, Secord AA, Tewari KS, Bender D, O'Malley DM, Stuckey A, Rotmensch J, Levine DA, Lankes HA, Moore KN. A randomized phase II study of paclitaxel/carboplatin/bevacizumab, paclitaxel/carboplatin/temsirolimus and ixabepilone/carboplatin/bevacizumab as initial therapy for measurable stage III or IVA, stage IVB or recurrent endometrial cancer, GOG-86P. J Clin Oncol. 2015;33(suppl; abstr 5500).
3. Aghajanian C, Sill MW, Darcy KM, Greer B, McMeekin DS, Rose PG, Rotmensch J, Barnes MN, Hanjani P, Leslie KK. Phase II trial of bevacizumab in recurrent or persistent endometrial cancer: a gynecologic oncology group study. J Clin Oncol. 2011;29 (16):2259–65. doi:10.1200/JCO.2010.32.6397 (JCO.2010.32.6397 [pii]).

4. Alvarez EA, Brady WE, Walker JL, Rotmensch J, Zhou XC, Kendrick JE, Yamada SD, Schilder JM, Cohn DE, Harrison CR, Moore KN, Aghajanian C. Phase II trial of combination bevacizumab and temsirolimus in the treatment of recurrent or persistent endometrial carcinoma: a Gynecologic Oncology Group study. Gynecol Oncol. 2013;129 (1):22–7. doi:10.1016/j.ygyno.2012.12.022.
5. Amant F, Moerman P, Neven P, Timmerman D, Van Limbergen E, Vergote I. Endometrial cancer. Lancet. 2005;366(9484):491–505. doi:S0140–6736(05)67063-8 [pii] 10.1016/S0140-6736(05)67063-8.
6. Araujo J, Logothetis C. Dasatinib: a potent SRC inhibitor in clinical development for the treatment of solid tumors. Cancer Treat Rev. 2010;36(6):492–500. doi:10.1016/j.ctrv.2010.02.015 (S0305-7372(10)00035-6 [pii]).
7. Ashrafian H, Ahmed K, Rowland SP, Patel VM, Gooderham NJ, Holmes E, Darzi A, Athanasiou T. Metabolic surgery and cancer: protective effects of bariatric procedures. Cancer. 2011;117(9):1788–99. doi:10.1002/cncr.25738.
8. Ballard-Barbash R, Swanson CA. Body weight: estimation of risk for breast and endometrial cancers. Am J Clin Nutr. 1996;63(3 Suppl):437S–41S.
9. Bedard PL, Tabernero J, Janku F, Wainberg ZA, Paz-Ares L, Vansteenkiste J, Van Cutsem E, Perez-Garcia J, Stathis A, Britten CD, Le N, Carter K, Demanse D, Csonka D, Peters M, Zubel A, Nauwelaerts H, Sessa C. A phase Ib dose-escalation study of the oral pan-PI3K inhibitor buparlisib (BKM120) in combination with the oral MEK1/2 inhibitor trametinib (GSK1120212) in patients with selected advanced solid tumors. Clin Cancer Res. 2015;21(4):730–8. doi:10.1158/1078-0432.CCR-14-1814.
10. Beining RM, Dennis LK, Smith EM, Dokras A. Meta-analysis of intrauterine device use and risk of endometrial cancer. Ann Epidemiol. 2008;18(6):492–9. doi:10.1016/j.annepidem.2007.11.011.
11. Bellone S, Centritto F, Black J, Schwab C, English D, Cocco E, Lopez S, Bonazzoli E, Predolini F, Ferrari F, Silasi DA, Ratner E, Azodi M, Schwartz PE, Santin AD. Polymerase epsilon (POLE) ultra-mutated tumors induce robust tumor-specific CD4+ T cell responses in endometrial cancer patients. Gynecol Oncol. 2015;138(1):11–7. doi:10.1016/j.ygyno.2015.04.027.
12. Ben Sahra I, Le Marchand-Brustel Y, Tanti JF, Bost F. Metformin in cancer therapy: a new perspective for an old antidiabetic drug? Mol Cancer Ther. 2010;9(5):1092–99. doi:10.1158/1535-7163.MCT-09-1186 (1535-7163.MCT-09-1186 [pii]).
13. Bendell J, LoRusso P, Kwak E, Pandya S, Musib L, Jones C, De Crespigny A, Belvin M, McKenzie M, Gates MR, Chan I, Sharpiro G. Clinical combination of the MEK inhibitor GDC-0973 and the PI3K inhibitor GSC-0941: a first-in-human phase Ib study in patients with advanced solid tumors. 2011. AACR meeting abstracts abstract LB-89.
14. Bender D, Sill MW, Lankes HA, Reyes HD, Darus CJ, Delmore JE, Rotmensch J, Gray HJ, Mannel RS, Schilder JM, Hunter MI, McCourt CK, Samuelson MI, Leslie KK. A phase II evaluation of cediranib in the treatment of recurrent or persistent endometrial cancer: an NRG Oncology/Gynecologic Oncology Group study. Gynecol Oncol. 2015;138(3):507–12. doi:10.1016/j.ygyno.2015.07.018.
15. Beral V, Bull D, Reeves G, Million Women Study C. Endometrial cancer and hormone-replacement therapy in the million women study. Lancet. 2005;365(9470):1543–51. doi:10.1016/S0140-6736(05)66455-0.
16. Bravi F, Scotti L, Bosetti C, Zucchetto A, Talamini R, Montella M, Greggi S, Pelucchi C, Negri E, Franceschi S, La Vecchia C. Food groups and endometrial cancer risk: a case-control study from Italy. Am J Obstet Gynecol. 2009;200(3):293 e291–7. doi:10.1016/j.ajog.2008.09.015.
17. Calle EE, Rodriguez C, Walker-Thurmond K, Thun MJ. Overweight, obesity, and mortality from cancer in a prospectively studied cohort of U.S. adults. N Engl J Med. 2003;348 (17):1625–38. doi:10.1056/NEJMoa021423.

18. Cantrell LA, Zhou C, Mendivil A, Malloy KM, Gehrig PA, Bae-Jump VL. Metformin is a potent inhibitor of endometrial cancer cell proliferation–implications for a novel treatment strategy. Gynecol Oncol. 2016;116(1):92–8. doi:10.1016/j.ygyno.2009.09.024 (S0090-8258(09)00723-9 [pii]).
19. Cauley JA, Gutai JP, Kuller LH, LeDonne D, Powell JG. The epidemiology of serum sex hormones in postmenopausal women. Am J Epidemiol. 1989;129(6):1120–31.
20. Cheng N, Brantley DM, Chen J. The ephrins and Eph receptors in angiogenesis. Cytokine Growth Factor Rev. 2002;13(1):75–85.
21. Cheng L, Zhang S, Alexander R, Yao Y, MacLennan GT, Pan CX, Huang J, Wang M, Montironi R, Lopez-Beltran A. The landscape of EGFR pathways and personalized management of non-small-cell lung cancer. Future Oncol. 2011;7(4):519–41. doi:10.2217/fon.11.25.
22. Cheung LW, Hennessy BT, Li J, Yu S, Myers AP, Djordjevic B, Lu Y, Stemke-Hale K, Zhang F, Ju Z, Cantley LC, Scherer SE, Liang H, Lu KH, Broaddus RR, Mills GB. High frequency of PIK3R1 and PIK3R2 mutations in endometrial cancer elucidates a novel mechanism for regulation of PTEN protein stability. Cancer Discov. 2011;1(2):170–85. doi:10.1158/2159-8290.CD-11-0039.
23. Ciardiello F, Tortora G. EGFR antagonists in cancer treatment. N Engl J Med. 2008;358(11):1160–74. doi:10.1056/NEJMra0707704 (358/11/1160 [pii]).
24. Coleman RL, Sill MW, Lankes HA, Fader AN, Finkler NJ, Hoffman JS, Rose PG, Sutton GP, Drescher CW, McMeekin DS, Hu W, Deavers M, Godwin AK, Alpaugh RK, Sood AK. A phase II evaluation of aflibercept in the treatment of recurrent or persistent endometrial cancer: a Gynecologic Oncology Group study. Gynecol Oncol. 2012;127(3):538–43. doi:10.1016/j.ygyno.2012.08.020.
25. Coleman R, Sill M, Thaker PH, De Geest K, Street D, McGuire W, Rotmensch J. A phase II evaluation of AZD6244, a selective MEK-1/2 inhibitor in the treatment of recurrent or persistent endometrial cancer: a Gynecologic Oncology Group study. Gynecol Oncol. 2013;130(1):e12–3.
26. Colombo N, McMeekin DS, Schwartz PE, Sessa C, Gehrig PA, Holloway R, Braly P, Matei D, Morosky A, Dodion PF, Einstein MH, Haluska F. Ridaforolimus as a single agent in advanced endometrial cancer: results of a single-arm, phase 2 trial. Br J Cancer. 2013;108(5):1021–6. doi:10.1038/bjc.2013.59.
27. Correa R, Mackay H, Hirte HW, Morgan R, Welch S, Fleming GF, Wang L, Blattler C, Ivey SP, Oza AM. A phase II study of sunitinib in recurrent or metastastic endometrial carcinoma: a trial of the Princess Margaret Hospital, The University of Chicago, and California Cancer Phase II Consortia. J Clin Oncol. 2010;28:15s(suppl; abstr 5038).
28. Cust AE, Allen NE, Rinaldi S, Dossus L, Friedenreich C, Olsen A, Tjönneland A, Overvad K, Clavel-Chapelon F, Boutron-Ruault MC, Linseisen J, Chang-Claude J, Boeing H, Schulz M, Benetou V, Trichopoulou A, Trichopoulos D, Palli D, Berrino F, Tumino R, Mattiello A, Vineis P, Quiros JR, Agudo A, Sanchez MJ, Larranaga N, Navarro C, Ardanaz E, Bueno-de-Mesquita HB, Peeters PH, van Gils CH, Bingham S, Khaw KT, Key T, Slimani N, Riboli E, Kaaks R. Serum levels of C-peptide, IGFBP-1 and IGFBP-2 and endometrial cancer risk; results from the European prospective investigation into cancer and nutrition. Int J Cancer. 2007;120(12):2656–64. doi:10.1002/ijc.22578.
29. Davies MJ, Baer DJ, Judd JT, Brown ED, Campbell WS, Taylor PR. Effects of moderate alcohol intake on fasting insulin and glucose concentrations and insulin sensitivity in postmenopausal women: a randomized controlled trial. JAMA. 2002;287(19):2559–62.
30. De Luca A, Carotenuto A, Rachiglio A, Gallo M, Maiello MR, Aldinucci D, Pinto A, Normanno N. The role of the EGFR signaling in tumor microenvironment. J Cell Physiol. 2008;214(3):559–67. doi:10.1002/jcp.21260.
31. Dedes KJ, Wilkerson PM, Wetterskog D, Weigelt B, Ashworth A, Reis-Filho JS. Synthetic lethality of PARP inhibition in cancers lacking BRCA1 and BRCA2 mutations. Cell Cycle. 2011;10(8):1192–9. doi:10.4161/cc.10.8.15273 ([pii]).

32. Del Campo JM, Birrer M, Davis C, Fujiwara K, Gollerkeri A, Gore M, Houk B, Lau S, Poveda A, Gonzalez-Martin A, Muller C, Muro K, Pierce K, Suzuki M, Vermette J, Oza A. A randomized phase II non-comparative study of PF-04691502 and gedatolisib (PF-05212384) in patients with recurrent endometrial cancer. Gynecol Oncol. 2016;142 (1):62–9. doi:10.1016/j.ygyno.2016.04.019.
33. Di Nicolantonio F, Arena S, Tabernero J, Grosso S, Molinari F, Macarulla T, Russo M, Cancelliere C, Zecchin D, Mazzucchelli L, Sasazuki T, Shirasawa S, Geuna M, Frattini M, Baselga J, Gallicchio M, Biffo S, Bardelli A. Deregulation of the PI3K and KRAS signaling pathways in human cancer cells determines their response to everolimus. J Clin Invest. 2010;120(8):2858–66. doi:10.1172/JCI37539 (37539 [pii]).
34. Dizon DS, Sill MW, Schilder JM, McGonigle KF, Rahman Z, Miller DS, Mutch DG, Leslie KK. A phase II evaluation of nintedanib (BIBF-1120) in the treatment of recurrent or persistent endometrial cancer: an NRG Oncology/Gynecologic Oncology Group Study. Gynecol Oncol. 2014;135(3):441–5. doi:10.1016/j.ygyno.2014.10.001.
35. Dry JR, Pavey S, Pratilas CA, Harbron C, Runswick S, Hodgson D, Chresta C, McCormack R, Byrne N, Cockerill M, Graham A, Beran G, Cassidy A, Haggerty C, Brown H, Ellison G, Dering J, Taylor BS, Stark M, Bonazzi V, Ravishankar S, Packer L, Xing F, Solit DB, Finn RS, Rosen N, Hayward NK, French T, Smith PD. Transcriptional pathway signatures predict MEK addiction and response to selumetinib (AZD6244). Cancer Res. 2010;70(6):2264–73. doi:10.1158/0008-5472.CAN-09-1577.
36. Duffy SR, Distler W, Howell A, Cuzick J, Baum M. A lower incidence of gynecologic adverse events and interventions with anastrozole than with tamoxifen in the ATAC trial. Am J Obstet Gynecol. 2009;200(1):80 e81–7. doi:10.1016/j.ajog.2008.07.062.
37. Duggan BD, Felix JC, Muderspach LI, Tsao JL, Shibata DK. Early mutational activation of the c-Ki-ras oncogene in endometrial carcinoma. Cancer Res. 1994;54(6):1604–7.
38. Dummer R, Robert C, Chapman PB, Sosman JA, Middleton M, Bastholt L, Kemsley K, Cantarini MV, Morris C, Kirkwood JM. AZD6244 (ARRY-142886) vs temozolomide (TMZ) in patients (pts) with advanced melanoma: an open-label, randomized, multicenter, phase II study. J Clin Oncol. 2008;26:Suppl; abstr 9033.
39. Dutt A, Salvesen HB, Chen TH, Ramos AH, Onofrio RC, Hatton C, Nicoletti R, Winckler W, Grewal R, Hanna M, Wyhs N, Ziaugra L, Richter DJ, Trovik J, Engelsen IB, Stefansson IM, Fennell T, Cibulskis K, Zody MC, Akslen LA, Gabriel S, Wong KK, Sellers WR, Meyerson M, Greulich H. Drug-sensitive FGFR2 mutations in endometrial carcinoma. Proc Natl Acad Sci U S A. 2008;105(25):8713–7. doi:10.1073/pnas.0803379105 (0803379105 [pii]).
40. Dutt A, Salvesen HB, Greulich H, Sellers WR, Beroukhim R, Meyerson M. Somatic mutations are present in all members of the AKT family in endometrial carcinoma. Br J Cancer. 2009;101(7):1218–9 (author reply 1220–11). doi:10.1038/sj.bjc.6605301 (6605301 [pii]).
41. Elwood JM, Cole P, Rothman KJ, Kaplan SD. Epidemiology of endometrial cancer. J Natl Cancer Inst. 1977;59(4):1055–60.
42. Engel JB, Honig A, Schonhals T, Weidler C, Hausler S, Krockenberger M, Grunewald TG, Dombrowski Y, Rieger L, Dietl J, Wischhusen J. Perifosine inhibits growth of human experimental endometrial cancers by blockade of AKT phosphorylation. Eur J Obstet Gynecol Reprod Biol. 2008;141(1):64–9. doi:10.1016/j.ejogrb.2008.06.007.
43. Engelman JA, Chen L, Tan X, Crosby K, Guimaraes AR, Upadhyay R, Maira M, McNamara K, Perera SA, Song Y, Chirieac LR, Kaur R, Lightbown A, Simendinger J, Li T, Padera RF, Garcia-Echeverria C, Weissleder R, Mahmood U, Cantley LC, Wong KK. Effective use of PI3K and MEK inhibitors to treat mutant Kras G12D and PIK3CA H1047R murine lung cancers. Nat Med. 2008;14(12):1351–6. doi:10.1038/nm.1890.
44. Engelman JA, Janne PA. Mechanisms of acquired resistance to epidermal growth factor receptor tyrosine kinase inhibitors in non-small cell lung cancer. Clin Cancer Res. 2008;14 (10):2895–9. doi:10.1158/1078-0432.CCR-07-2248 (14/10/2895 [pii]).

45. Evans JM, Donnelly LA, Emslie-Smith AM, Alessi DR, Morris AD. Metformin and reduced risk of cancer in diabetic patients. BMJ. 2005;330(7503):1304–5. doi:10.1136/bmj.38415.708634.F7 (bmj.38415.708634.F7 [pii]).
46. Fearnley EJ, Marquart L, Spurdle AB, Weinstein P, Webb PM, Australian Ovarian Cancer Study G, Australian National Endometrial Cancer Study Group. Polycystic ovary syndrome increases the risk of endometrial cancer in women aged less than 50 years: an Australian case-control study. Cancer Causes Control: CCC. 2010;21(12):2303–8. doi:10.1007/s10552-010-9658-7.
47. Felix AS, Gaudet MM, La Vecchia C, Nagle CM, Shu XO, Weiderpass E, Adami HO, Beresford S, Bernstein L, Chen C, Cook LS, De Vivo I, Doherty JA, Friedenreich CM, Gapstur SM, Hill D, Horn-Ross PL, Lacey JV, Levi F, Liang X, Lu L, Magliocco A, McCann SE, Negri E, Olson SH, Palmer JR, Patel AV, Petruzella S, Prescott J, Risch HA, Rosenberg L, Sherman ME, Spurdle AB, Webb PM, Wise LA, Xiang YB, Xu W, Yang HP, Yu H, Zeleniuch-Jacquotte A, Brinton LA. Intrauterine devices and endometrial cancer risk: a pooled analysis of the Epidemiology of Endometrial Cancer Consortium. Int J Cancer. 2015;136(5):E410–22. doi:10.1002/ijc.29229.
48. Fisher B, Costantino JP, Wickerham DL, Redmond CK, Kavanah M, Cronin WM, Vogel V, Robidoux A, Dimitrov N, Atkins J, Daly M, Wieand S, Tan-Chiu E, Ford L, Wolmark N. Tamoxifen for prevention of breast cancer: report of the National Surgical Adjuvant Breast and Bowel Project P-1 Study. J Natl Cancer Inst. 1998;90(18):1371–88.
49. Flaherty KT, Robert C, Hersey P, Nathan P, Garbe C, Milhem M, Demidov LV, Hassel JC, Rutkowski P, Mohr P, Dummer R, Trefzer U, Larkin JM, Utikal J, Dreno B, Nyakas M, Middleton MR, Becker JC, Casey M, Sherman LJ, Wu FS, Ouellet D, Martin AM, Patel K, Schadendorf D. Improved survival with MEK inhibition in BRAF-mutated melanoma. N Engl J Med. 2012;367(2):107–14. doi:10.1056/NEJMoa1203421.
50. Fleming GF, Filiaci VL, Marzullo B, Zaino RJ, Davidson SA, Pearl M, Makker V, Burke JJ 2nd, Zweizig SL, Van Le L, Hanjani P, Downey G, Walker JL, Reyes HD, Leslie KK. Temsirolimus with or without megestrol acetate and tamoxifen for endometrial cancer: a gynecologic oncology group study. Gynecol Oncol. 2014;132(3):585–92. doi:10.1016/j.ygyno.2014.01.015.
51. Fleming GF, Sill MW, Darcy KM, McMeekin DS, Thigpen JT, Adler LM, Berek JS, Chapman JA, DiSilvestro PA, Horowitz IR, Fiorica JV. Phase II trial of trastuzumab in women with advanced or recurrent, HER2-positive endometrial carcinoma: a Gynecologic Oncology Group study. Gynecol Oncol. 2009;116(1):15–20. doi:10.1016/j.ygyno.2009.09.025 (S0090-8258(09)00724-0 [pii]).
52. Fong PC, Boss DS, Yap TA, Tutt A, Wu P, Mergui-Roelvink M, Mortimer P, Swaisland H, Lau A, O'Connor MJ, Ashworth A, Carmichael J, Kaye SB, Schellens JH, de Bono JS. Inhibition of poly(ADP-ribose) polymerase in tumors from BRCA mutation carriers. N Engl J Med. 2009;361(2):123–34. doi:10.1056/NEJMoa0900212 (NEJMoa0900212 [pii]).
53. Foster P, Yamaguchi K, Hsu PP, Qian F, Du X, Wu J, Won KA, Yu P, Jaeger CT, Zhang W, Marlowe CK, Keast P, Abulafia W, Chen J, Young J, Plonowski A, Yakes FM, Chu F, Engell K, Bentzien F, Lam ST, Dale S, Yturralde O, Matthews DJ, Lamb P, Laird AD. The selective PI3K inhibitor XL147 (SAR245408) inhibits tumor growth and survival and potentiates the activity of chemotherapeutic agents in preclinical tumor models. Mol Cancer Ther. 2015;14(4):931–40. doi:10.1158/1535-7163.MCT-14-0833.
54. Friberg E, Orsini N, Mantzoros CS, Wolk A. Alcohol intake and endometrial cancer risk: a meta-analysis of prospective studies. Br J Cancer. 2010;103(1):127–31. doi:10.1038/sj.bjc.6605698.
55. Friday BB, Adjei AA. Advances in targeting the Ras/Raf/MEK/Erk mitogen-activated protein kinase cascade with MEK inhibitors for cancer therapy. Clin Cancer Res. 2008;14(2):342–6. doi:10.1158/1078-0432.CCR-07-4790 (14/2/342 [pii]).

56. Friedenreich CM, Biel RK, Lau DC, Csizmadi I, Courneya KS, Magliocco AM, Yasui Y, Cook LS. Case-control study of the metabolic syndrome and metabolic risk factors for endometrial cancer. Cancer Epidemiol Biomarkers Prev. 2011;20(11):2384–95. doi:10.1158/1055-9965.EPI-11-0715.
57. Fritsch C, Huang A, Chatenay-Rivauday C, Schnell C, Reddy A, Liu M, Kauffmann A, Guthy D, Erdmann D, De Pover A, Furet P, Gao H, Ferretti S, Wang Y, Trappe J, Brachmann SM, Maira SM, Wilson C, Boehm M, Garcia-Echeverria C, Chene P, Wiesmann M, Cozens R, Lehar J, Schlegel R, Caravatti G, Hofmann F, Sellers WR. Characterization of the novel and specific PI3Kalpha inhibitor NVP-BYL719 and development of the patient stratification strategy for clinical trials. Mol Cancer Ther. 2014;13(5):1117–29. doi:10.1158/1535-7163.MCT-13-0865.
58. Gavaler JS, Van Thiel DH. Hormonal status of postmenopausal women with alcohol-induced cirrhosis: further findings and a review of the literature. Hepatology. 1992;16(2):312–9.
59. Gien LT, Mackay HJ. The emerging role of PARP inhibitors in the treatment of epithelial ovarian cancer. J Oncol. 2010. doi:10.1155/2010/151750 (ID 151750).
60. Grushko TA, Filiaci VL, Mundt AJ, Ridderstrale K, Olopade OI, Fleming GF. An exploratory analysis of HER-2 amplification and overexpression in advanced endometrial carcinoma: a Gynecologic Oncology Group study. Gynecol Oncol. 2008;108(1):3–9. doi:10.1016/j.ygyno.2007.09.007 (S0090-8258(07)00727-5 [pii]).
61. Gungor H, Saleem A, Babar S, Dina R, El-Bahrawy MA, Curry E, Rama N, Chen M, Pickford E, Agarwal R, Blagden S, Carme S, Salinas C, Madison S, Krachey E, Santiago-Walker A, Smith DA, Morris SR, Stronach EA, Gabra H. Dose-finding quantitative 18F-FDG PET imaging study with the oral pan-AKT inhibitor GSK2141795 in patients with gynecologic malignancies. J Nucl Med. 2015;56(12):1828–35. doi:10.2967/jnumed.115.156505.
62. Hankinson SE, Willett WC, Manson JE, Hunter DJ, Colditz GA, Stampfer MJ, Longcope C, Speizer FE. Alcohol, height, and adiposity in relation to estrogen and prolactin levels in postmenopausal women. J Natl Cancer Inst. 1995;87(17):1297–302.
63. Haugsten EM, Wiedlocha A, Olsnes S, Wesche J. Roles of fibroblast growth factor receptors in carcinogenesis. Mol Cancer Res. 2010;8(11):1439–52. doi:10.1158/1541-7786.MCR-10-0168.
64. Hayes MP, Wang H, Espinal-Witter R, Douglas W, Solomon GJ, Baker SJ, Ellenson LH. PIK3CA and PTEN mutations in uterine endometrioid carcinoma and complex atypical hyperplasia. Clin Cancer Res. 2006;12(20 Pt 1):5932–5. doi:10.1158/1078-0432.CCR-06-1375 (12/20/5932 [pii]).
65. Heist RS, Gandhi L, Shapiro G, Rizvi NA, Burris HA, Bendell JC, Baselga J, Yerganian SB, Hsu K, Ogden J, Vincent L, von Richter O, Locatelli G, Asatiani E, Infante JR. Combination of a MEK inhibitor, pimasertib (MSC1936369B), and a PI3K/mTOR inhibitor, SAR245409, in patients with advanced solid tumors: results of a phase Ib dose-escalation trial. J Clin Oncol. 2013;31(suppl; abstr 2530).
66. Hellstrom M, Phng LK, Gerhardt H. VEGF and Notch signaling: the yin and yang of angiogenic sprouting. Cell Adh Migr. 2007;1(3):133–6. doi:4978 ([pii]).
67. Hennessy BT, Smith DL, Ram PT, Lu Y, Mills GB. Exploiting the PI3K/AKT pathway for cancer drug discovery. Nat Rev Drug Discov. 2005;4(12):988–1004. doi:10.1038/nrd1902 (nrd1902 [pii]).
68. Henretta MS, Copeland AR, Kelley SL, Hallowell PT, Modesitt SC. Perceptions of obesity and cancer risk in female bariatric surgery candidates: highlighting the need for physician action for unsuspectingly obese and high risk patients. Gynecol Oncol. 2014;133(1):73–7. doi:10.1016/j.ygyno.2014.01.016.
69. Heudel P-E, Fabbro M, Roemer-Becuwe C, Treilleux I, Kaminsky M-C, Arnaud A, Joly F, Forestier SR, Herve R, Ray-Coquard I. Phase II study of the PI3K inhibitor BKM120 monotherapy in patients with advanced or recurrent endometrial carcinoma: ENDOPIK, GINECO Study. J Clin Oncol. 2015;33(Suppl; abstr 5588).

70. Hicklin DJ, Ellis LM. Role of the vascular endothelial growth factor pathway in tumor growth and angiogenesis. J Clin Oncol. 2005;23(5):1011–27. doi:10.1200/JCO.2005.06.081 (JCO.2005.06.081 [pii]).
71. Himanen JP, Goldgur Y, Miao H, Myshkin E, Guo H, Buck M, Nguyen M, Rajashankar KR, Wang B, Nikolov DB. Ligand recognition by A-class Eph receptors: crystal structures of the EphA2 ligand-binding domain and the EphA2/ephrin-A1 complex. EMBO Rep. 2009;10(7):722–8. doi:10.1038/embor.2009.91.
72. Hirai H, Sootome H, Nakatsuru Y, Miyama K, Taguchi S, Tsujioka K, Ueno Y, Hatch H, Majumder PK, Pan BS, Kotani H. MK-2206, an allosteric Akt inhibitor, enhances antitumor efficacy by standard chemotherapeutic agents or molecular targeted drugs in vitro and in vivo. Mol Cancer Ther. 2010;9(7):1956–67. doi:10.1158/1535-7163.MCT-09-1012.
73. Hirai M, Nakagawara A, Oosaki T, Hayashi Y, Hirono M, Yoshihara T. Expression of vascular endothelial growth factors (VEGF-A/VEGF-1 and VEGF-C/VEGF-2) in postmenopausal uterine endometrial carcinoma. Gynecol Oncol. 2001;80(2):181–8. doi:10.1006/gyno.2000.6056S0090-8258(00)96056-6 ([pii]).
74. Hoeflich KP, O'Brien C, Boyd Z, Cavet G, Guerrero S, Jung K, Januario T, Savage H, Punnoose E, Truong T, Zhou W, Berry L, Murray L, Amler L, Belvin M, Friedman LS, Lackner MR. In vivo antitumor activity of MEK and phosphatidylinositol 3-kinase inhibitors in basal-like breast cancer models. Clin Cancer Res. 2009;15(14):4649–64. doi:10.1158/1078-0432.CCR-09-0317.
75. Howitt BE, Sholl LM, Ritterhouse L, Watkins JC, Rodig SJ, Strickland K, D'Andrea AD, Matulonis U, Konstantinopoulos P. Association of POLE-mutated and MSI endometrial cancers with an elevated number of tumor-infiltrating and peritumoral lymphocytes and higher expression of PD-L1. J Clin Oncol. 2015;33(suppl; abstr 5511).
76. Hyman DM, Smyth L, Bedard PL, Oza A, Dean E, Armstrong A, Lima J, Bando H, Kabos P, Perez-Fidalgo JA, Moore KM, Westin SN, You B, Chandarlapaty S, Alland L, Ambrose H, Foxley A, Lindemann J, Pass M, Rugman P, Salim S, Schiavon G, Tamura K, Baselga J, Banerji U. AZD5363, a catalytic pan-Akt inhibitor, in Akt1 D17K mutation positive advanced solid tumors. In: AACR-NCI-EORTC International conference molecular targets and cancer therapeutics, Boston, MA; 2016.
77. Iglesias DA, Yates MS, van der Hoeven D, Rodkey TL, Zhang Q, Co NN, Burzawa J, Chigurupati S, Celestino J, Bowser J, Broaddus R, Hancock JF, Schmandt R, Lu KH. Another surprise from metformin: novel mechanism of action via K-Ras influences endometrial cancer response to therapy. Mol Cancer Ther. 2013;12(12):2847–56. doi:10.1158/1535-7163.MCT-13-0439.
78. Ihle NT, Lemos R Jr, Wipf P, Yacoub A, Mitchell C, Siwak D, Mills GB, Dent P, Kirkpatrick DL, Powis G. Mutations in the phosphatidylinositol-3-kinase pathway predict for antitumor activity of the inhibitor PX-866 whereas oncogenic Ras is a dominant predictor for resistance. Cancer Res. 2009;69(1):143–50. doi:10.1158/0008-5472.CAN-07-6656.
79. Jackman DM, Miller VA, Cioffredi LA, Yeap BY, Janne PA, Riely GJ, Ruiz MG, Giaccone G, Sequist LV, Johnson BE. Impact of epidermal growth factor receptor and KRAS mutations on clinical outcomes in previously untreated non-small cell lung cancer patients: results of an online tumor registry of clinical trials. Clin Cancer Res. 2009;15(16):5267–73. doi:10.1158/1078-0432.CCR-09-0888 (1078-0432.CCR-09-0888 [pii]).
80. Jalving M, Gietema JA, Lefrandt JD, de Jong S, Reyners AK, Gans RO, de Vries EG. Metformin: taking away the candy for cancer? Eur J Cancer. 2010;46(13):2369–80. doi:10.1016/j.ejca.2010.06.012.
81. Juric D, Soria JC, Sharma S, Banerji U, Azaro A, Desai J, Ringeisen FP, Kaag A, Radhakrishnan R, Hourcade-Potelleret F, Maacke H, Ahnert JR. A phase 1b dose-escalation study of BYL719 plus binimetinib (MEK162) in patients with selected advanced solid tumors. J Clin Oncol. 2014;32:5s (suppl; abstr 9051).

82. Kaaks R, Lukanova A, Kurzer MS. Obesity, endogenous hormones, and endometrial cancer risk: a synthetic review. Cancer Epidemiol Biomarkers Prev. 2002;11(12):1531–43.
83. Kamat AA, Coffey D, Merritt WM, Nugent E, Urbauer D, Lin YG, Edwards C, Broaddus R, Coleman RL, Sood AK. EphA2 overexpression is associated with lack of hormone receptor expression and poor outcome in endometrial cancer. Cancer. 2009;115(12):2684–92. doi:10.1002/cncr.24335.
84. Kamat AA, Merritt WM, Coffey D, Lin YG, Patel PR, Broaddus R, Nugent E, Han LY, Landen CN Jr, Spannuth WA, Lu C, Coleman RL, Gershenson DM, Sood AK. Clinical and biological significance of vascular endothelial growth factor in endometrial cancer. Clin Cancer Res. 2007;13(24):7487–95. doi:10.1158/1078-0432.CCR-07-1017 (13/24/7487 [pii]).
85. Kandoth C, Schultz N, Cherniack AD, Akbani R, Liu Y, Shen H, Robertson AG, Pashtan I, Shen R, Benz CC, Yau C, Laird PW, Ding L, Zhang W, Mills GB, Kucherlapati R, Mardis ER, Levine DA. Integrated genomic characterization of endometrial carcinoma. Nature. 2013;497 (7447):67–73. doi:10.1038/nature12113.
86. Kang S, Lee JM, Jeon ES, Lee S, Kim H, Kim HS, Seo SS, Park SY, Sidransky D, Dong SM. RASSF1A hypermethylation and its inverse correlation with BRAF and/or KRAS mutations in MSI-associated endometrial carcinoma. Int J Cancer. 2006;119(6):1316–21. doi:10.1002/ijc.21991.
87. Kaufman DW, Shapiro S, Slone D, Rosenberg L, Miettinen OS, Stolley PD, Knapp RC, Leavitt T Jr, Watring WG, Rosenshein NB, Lewis JL Jr, Schottenfeld D, Engle RL Jr. Decreased risk of endometrial cancer among oral-contraceptive users. N Engl J Med. 1980;303(18):1045–7. doi:10.1056/NEJM198010303031807.
88. Khalifa MA, Mannel RS, Haraway SD, Walker J, Min KW. Expression of EGFR, HER-2/neu, P53, and PCNA in endometrioid, serous papillary, and clear cell endometrial adenocarcinomas. Gynecol Oncol. 1994;53(1):84–92. doi:10.1006/gyno.1994.1092 (S0090-8258(84)71092-4 [pii]).
89. Kikawa KD, Vidale DR, Van Etten RL, Kinch MS. Regulation of the EphA2 kinase by the low molecular weight tyrosine phosphatase induces transformation. J Biol Chem. 2002;277 (42):39274–9. doi:10.1074/jbc.M207127200.
90. Kim LC, Rix U, Haura EB. Dasatinib in solid tumors. Expert Opin Investig Drugs. 2010;19 (3):415–25. doi:10.1517/13543781003592097.
91. Konecny GE, Finkler N, Garcia AA, Lorusso D, Lee PS, Rocconi RP, Fong PC, Squires M, Mishra K, Upalawanna A, Wang Y, Kristeleit R. Second-line dovitinib (TKI258) in patients with FGFR2-mutated or FGFR2-non-mutated advanced or metastatic endometrial cancer: a non-randomised, open-label, two-group, two-stage, phase 2 study. Lancet Oncol. 2015;16 (6):686–94. doi:10.1016/S1470-2045(15)70159-2.
92. Konecny GE, Meng YG, Untch M, Wang HJ, Bauerfeind I, Epstein M, Stieber P, Vernes JM, Gutierrez J, Hong K, Beryt M, Hepp H, Slamon DJ, Pegram MD. Association between HER-2/neu and vascular endothelial growth factor expression predicts clinical outcome in primary breast cancer patients. Clin Cancer Res. 2004;10(5):1706–16.
93. Kong D, Suzuki A, Zou TT, Sakurada A, Kemp LW, Wakatsuki S, Yokoyama T, Yamakawa H, Furukawa T, Sato M, Ohuchi N, Sato S, Yin J, Wang S, Abraham JM, Souza RF, Smolinski KN, Meltzer SJ, Horii A. PTEN1 is frequently mutated in primary endometrial carcinomas. Nat Genet. 1997;17(2):143–4. doi:10.1038/ng1097-143.
94. Konstantinopoulos P, Makker V, Barry WT, Liu J, Horowitz NS, Birrer MJ, Doyle LA, Berlin ST, Whalen C, Van Hummelen P, Coleman RL, Aghajanian C, Mills GB, Matulonis U, Westin SN, Myers AP. Phase II, single stage, cohort expansion study of MK-2206 in recurrent endometrial serous cancer. J Clin Oncol. 2014;32:5s (suppl; abstr 5515).
95. Koul A, Willen R, Bendahl PO, Nilbert M, Borg A. Distinct sets of gene alterations in endometrial carcinoma implicate alternate modes of tumorigenesis. Cancer. 2002;94(9):2369–79. doi:10.1002/cncr.10498.

96. Kris MG, Natale RB, Herbst RS, Lynch TJ Jr, Prager D, Belani CP, Schiller JH, Kelly K, Spiridonidis H, Sandler A, Albain KS, Cella D, Wolf MK, Averbuch SD, Ochs JJ, Kay AC. Efficacy of gefitinib, an inhibitor of the epidermal growth factor receptor tyrosine kinase, in symptomatic patients with non-small cell lung cancer: a randomized trial. JAMA. 2003;290 (16):2149–58. doi:10.1001/jama.290.16.2149290/16/2149 [pii].
97. Le DT, Uram JN, Wang H, Bartlett BR, Kemberling H, Eyring AD, Skora AD, Luber BS, Azad NS, Laheru D, Biedrzycki B, Donehower RC, Zaheer A, Fisher GA, Crocenzi TS, Lee JJ, Duffy SM, Goldberg RM, de la Chapelle A, Koshiji M, Bhaijee F, Huebner T, Hruban RH, Wood LD, Cuka N, Pardoll DM, Papadopoulos N, Kinzler KW, Zhou S, Cornish TC, Taube JM, Anders RA, Eshleman JR, Vogelstein B, Diaz LA Jr. PD-1 blockade in tumors with mismatch-repair deficiency. N Engl J Med. 2015;372(26):2509–20. doi:10.1056/NEJMoa1500596.
98. Lee CN, Cheng WF, Chen CA, Chu JS, Hsieh CY, Hsieh FJ. Angiogenesis of endometrial carcinomas assessed by measurement of intratumoral blood flow, microvessel density, and vascular endothelial growth factor levels. Obstet Gynecol. 2000;96(4):615–21.
99. Leslie KK, Sill MW, Fischer E, Darcy KM, Mannel RS, Tewari KS, Hanjani P, Wilken JA, Baron AT, Godwin AK, Schilder RJ, Singh M, Maihle NJ. A phase II evaluation of gefitinib in the treatment of persistent or recurrent endometrial cancer: a Gynecologic Oncology Group study. Gynecol Oncol. 2013;129(3):486–94. doi:10.1016/j.ygyno.2013.02.019.
100. Leslie KK, Sill MW, Lankes HA, Fischer EG, Godwin AK, Gray H, Schilder RJ, Walker JL, Tewari K, Hanjani P, Abulafia O, Rose PG. Lapatinib and potential prognostic value of EGFR mutations in a Gynecologic Oncology Group phase II trial of persistent or recurrent endometrial cancer. Gynecol Oncol. 2012;127(2):345–50. doi:10.1016/j.ygyno.2012.07.127.
101. Levi F, Franceschi S, Negri E, La Vecchia C. Dietary factors and the risk of endometrial cancer. Cancer. 1993;71(11):3575–81.
102. Li Y, Nakamura M, Kakudo K. Targeting of the BRAF gene in papillary thyroid carcinoma (review). Oncol Rep. 2009;22(4):671–81.
103. Li D. Metformin as an antitumor agent in cancer prevention and treatment. J Diabetes. 2011. doi:10.1111/j.1753-0407.2011.00119.x
104. Liang H, Cheung LW, Li J, Ju Z, Yu S, Stemke-Hale K, Dogruluk T, Lu Y, Liu X, Gu C, Guo W, Scherer SE, Carter H, Westin SN, Dyer MD, Verhaak RG, Zhang F, Karchin R, Liu CG, Lu KH, Broaddus RR, Scott KL, Hennessy BT, Mills GB. Whole-exome sequencing combined with functional genomics reveals novel candidate driver cancer genes in endometrial cancer. Genome Res. 2012;22(11):2120–9. doi:10.1101/gr.137596.112.
105. Lindor NM, Petersen GM, Hadley DW, Kinney AY, Miesfeldt S, Lu KH, Lynch P, Burke W, Press N. Recommendations for the care of individuals with an inherited predisposition to Lynch syndrome: a systematic review. JAMA. 2006;296(12):1507–17. doi:10.1001/jama.296.12.1507.
106. Livasy CA, Reading FC, Moore DT, Boggess JF, Lininger RA. EGFR expression and HER2/neu overexpression/amplification in endometrial carcinosarcoma. Gynecol Oncol. 2006;100(1):101–6. doi:10.1016/j.ygyno.2005.07.124.
107. Lorusso D, Ferrandina G, Colombo N, Pignata S, Salutari V, Maltese G, Pisano C, Lapresa M, Savarese A, Tagliaferri P, Sorio R, Cinieri S, Breda E, Sabbatini R, Lepori S, Conte C, Cecere SC, Raspagliesi F, Scambia G. Randomized phase II trial of carboplatin-paclitaxel (CP) compared to carboplatin-paclitaxel-bevacizumab (CP-B) in advanced (stage III-IV) or recurrent endometrial cancer: the MITO END-2 trial. J Clin Oncol. 2015;33(suppl; abstr 5502).
108. Lu Y, Wang SS, Sullivan-Halley J, Chang ET, Clarke CA, Henderson KD, Ma H, Duan L, Lacey JV Jr, Deapen D, Bernstein L. Oral contraceptives, menopausal hormone therapy use and risk of B-cell non-Hodgkin lymphoma in the California Teachers Study. Int J Cancer. 2011;129(4):974–82. doi:10.1002/ijc.25730.
109. Lynch TJ. The evolving story of the epidermal growth factor receptor as a target for non-small-cell lung cancer. Clin Adv Hematol Oncol. 2004;2(12):786–7.

110. Mackay HJ, Eisenhauer EA, Kamel-Reid S, Tsao M, Clarke B, Karakasis K, Werner HM, Trovik J, Akslen LA, Salvesen HB, Tu D, Oza AM. Molecular determinants of outcome with mammalian target of rapamycin inhibition in endometrial cancer. Cancer. 2013;. doi:10.1002/cncr.28414.
111. Madhusudan S, Middleton MR. The emerging role of DNA repair proteins as predictive, prognostic and therapeutic targets in cancer. Cancer Treat Rev. 2005;31(8):603–17. doi:10.1016/j.ctrv.2005.09.006 (S0305-7372(05)00174-X [pii]).
112. Maira SM, Pecchi S, Huang A, Burger M, Knapp M, Sterker D, Schnell C, Guthy D, Nagel T, Wiesmann M, Brachmann S, Fritsch C, Dorsch M, Chene P, Shoemaker K, De Pover A, Menezes D, Martiny-Baron G, Fabbro D, Wilson CJ, Schlegel R, Hofmann F, Garcia-Echeverria C, Sellers WR, Voliva CF. Identification and characterization of NVP-BKM120, an orally available pan-class I PI3-kinase inhibitor. Mol Cancer Ther. 2012;11(2):317–28. doi:10.1158/1535-7163.MCT-11-0474.
113. Makker V, Recio FO, Ma L, Matulonis U, Lauchle JO, Parmar H, Gilbert H, Wang Y, Koeppen H, Spoerke JM, Lackner M, Aghajanian C. Phase II trial of GDC-0980 (dual PI3K/mTOR inhibitor) in patients with advanced endometrial carcinoma: Final study results. J Clin Oncol. 2014;32:5s (suppl; abstr 5513).
114. Marino M, Galluzzo P, Ascenzi P. Estrogen signaling multiple pathways to impact gene transcription. Curr Genomics. 2006;7(8):497–508.
115. Massarelli E, Varella-Garcia M, Tang X, Xavier AC, Ozburn NC, Liu DD, Bekele BN, Herbst RS, Wistuba II. KRAS mutation is an important predictor of resistance to therapy with epidermal growth factor receptor tyrosine kinase inhibitors in non-small-cell lung cancer. Clin Cancer Res. 2007;13(10):2890–6. doi:10.1158/1078-0432.CCR-06-3043 (13/10/2890 [pii]).
116. Matulonis U, Vergote I, Backes F, Martin LP, McMeekin S, Birrer M, Campana F, Xu Y, Egile C, Ghamande S. Phase II study of the PI3K inhibitor pilaralisib (SAR245408; XL147) in patients with advanced or recurrent endometrial carcinoma. Gynecol Oncol. 2015;136(2):246–53. doi:10.1016/j.ygyno.2014.12.019.
117. McCampbell AS, Broaddus RR, Loose DS, Davies PJ. Overexpression of the insulin-like growth factor I receptor and activation of the AKT pathway in hyperplastic endometrium. Clin Cancer Res. 2006;12(21):6373–8. doi:10.1158/1078-0432.CCR-06-0912 (12/21/6373 [pii]).
118. McMeekin DS, Sill MW, Benbrook D, Darcy KM, Stearns-Kurosawa DJ, Eaton L, Yamada SD. A phase II trial of thalidomide in patients with refractory endometrial cancer and correlation with angiogenesis biomarkers: a Gynecologic Oncology Group study. Gynecol Oncol. 2007;105(2):508–16. doi:10.1016/j.ygyno.2007.01.019 (S0090-8258(07)00034-0 [pii]).
119. Mendes-Pereira AM, Martin SA, Brough R, McCarthy A, Taylor JR, Kim JS, Waldman T, Lord CJ, Ashworth A. Synthetic lethal targeting of PTEN mutant cells with PARP inhibitors. EMBO Mol Med. 2009;1(6–7):315–22. doi:10.1002/emmm.200900041.
120. Messersmith WA, Falchook GS, Fecher LA, Gordon MS, Vogelzang NJ, DeMarini DJ, Peddareddigari VG, Xu Y, Bendell JC, Infante JR. Clinical activity of the oral MEK1/MEK2 inhibitor GSK1120212. J Clin Oncol. 2011;29(suppl 4: abstr 246).
121. Meyer LA, Broaddus RR, Lu KH. Endometrial cancer and Lynch syndrome: clinical and pathologic considerations. Cancer Control. 2009;16(1):14–22.
122. Meyer LA, Slomovitz BM, Djordjevic B, Westin SN, Iglesias DA, Munsell MF, Jiang Y, Schmandt R, Broaddus RR, Coleman RL, Galbincea JM, Lu KH. The search continues: looking for predictive biomarkers for response to mammalian target of rapamycin inhibition in endometrial cancer. Int J Gynecol Cancer. 2014;24(4):713–7. doi:10.1097/IGC.0000000000000118.
123. Miao H, Li DQ, Mukherjee A, Guo H, Petty A, Cutter J, Basilion JP, Sedor J, Wu J, Danielpour D, Sloan AE, Cohen ML, Wang B. EphA2 mediates ligand-dependent inhibition and ligand-independent promotion of cell migration and invasion via a reciprocal regulatory loop with Akt. Cancer Cell. 2009;16(1):9–20. doi:10.1016/j.ccr.2009.04.009.

124. Miller DS, Filiaci VJ, Fleming G, Mannel R, Cohn DE, Matsumoto T, Tewari K, DiSilvestro PA, Pearl M, Zaino RJ. Randomized phase III noninferiority trial of first line chemotherapy for metastatic or recurrent endometrial carcinoma: a Gynecologic Oncology Group study. Gynecol Oncol. 2012;125:771.
125. Mita AC, Takimoto CH, Mita M, Tolcher A, Sankhala K, Sarantopoulos J, Valdivieso M, Wood L, Rasmussen E, Sun YN, Zhong ZD, Bass MB, Le N, LoRusso P. Phase 1 study of AMG 386, a selective angiopoietin 1/2-neutralizing peptibody, in combination with chemotherapy in adults with advanced solid tumors. Clin Cancer Res. 2010;16(11):3044–56. doi:10.1158/1078-0432.CCR-09-3368 (1078-0432.CCR-09-3368 [pii]).
126. Montagut C, Settleman J. Targeting the RAF-MEK-ERK pathway in cancer therapy. Cancer Lett. 2009;283(2):125–34. doi:10.1016/j.canlet.2009.01.022 (S0304-3835(09)00054-8 [pii]).
127. Moore SC, Gierach GL, Schatzkin A, Matthews CE. Physical activity, sedentary behaviours, and the prevention of endometrial cancer. Br J Cancer. 2010;103(7):933–8. doi:10.1038/sj.bjc.6605902.
128. Moore KN, Sill MW, Tenney ME, Darus CJ, Griffin D, Werner TL, Rose PG, Behrens R. A phase II trial of trebananib (AMG 386; IND#111071), a selective angiopoietin 1/2 neutralizing peptibody, in patients with persistent/recurrent carcinoma of the endometrium: an NRG/Gynecologic Oncology Group trial. Gynecol Oncol. 2015;138(3):513–8. doi:10.1016/j.ygyno.2015.07.006.
129. Morisset AS, Blouin K, Tchernof A. Impact of diet and adiposity on circulating levels of sex hormone-binding globulin and androgens. Nutr Rev. 2008;66(9):506–16. doi:10.1111/j.1753-4887.2008.00083.x.
130. Morrison C, Zanagnolo V, Ramirez N, Cohn DE, Kelbick N, Copeland L, Maxwell GL, Fowler JM. HER-2 is an independent prognostic factor in endometrial cancer: association with outcome in a large cohort of surgically staged patients. J Clin Oncol. 2006;24(15):2376–85. doi:10.1200/JCO.2005.03.4827.
131. Mueck AO, Seeger H, Rabe T. Hormonal contraception and risk of endometrial cancer: a systematic review. Endocr Relat Cancer. 2010;17(4):R263–71. doi:10.1677/ERC-10-0076.
132. Mutter GL, Lin MC, Fitzgerald JT, Kum JB, Baak JP, Lees JA, Weng LP, Eng C. Altered PTEN expression as a diagnostic marker for the earliest endometrial precancers. J Natl Cancer Inst. 2000;92(11):924–30.
133. Myers AP, Broaddus R, Makker V, Konstantinopoulos P, Drapkin R, Horowitz NS, Liu J, Van Hummelen P, Meric-Bernstam F, Birrer MJ, Doyle A, Coleman RL, Aghajanian C, Mills GB, Cantley L, Matulonis UA, Westin SN. Phase II, two-stage, two-arm, PIK3CA mutation stratified trial of MK-2206 in recurrent endometrial cancer. J Clin Oncol. 2013;31(suppl; abstr 5524).
134. Nicholson RI, Gee JM, Harper ME. EGFR and cancer prognosis. Eur J Cancer. 2001;37(Suppl 4):S9–15.
135. Nimeiri HS, Oza AM, Morgan RJ, Huo D, Elit L, Knost JA, Wade JL 3rd, Agamah E, Vokes EE, Fleming GF. A phase II study of sorafenib in advanced uterine carcinoma/carcinosarcoma: a trial of the Chicago, PMH, and California Phase II Consortia. Gynecol Oncol. 2010;117(1):37–40. doi:10.1016/j.ygyno.2010.01.013.
136. Normanno N, De Luca A, Bianco C, Strizzi L, Mancino M, Maiello MR, Carotenuto A, De Feo G, Caponigro F, Salomon DS. Epidermal growth factor receptor (EGFR) signaling in cancer. Gene. 2006;366(1):2–16. doi:10.1016/j.gene.2005.10.018 (S0378-1119(05)00634-7 [pii]).
137. Normanno N, Tejpar S, Morgillo F, De Luca A, Van Cutsem E, Ciardiello F. Implications for KRAS status and EGFR-targeted therapies in metastatic CRC. Nat Rev Clin Oncol. 2009;6(9):519–27. doi:10.1038/nrclinonc.2009.111 (nrclinonc.2009.111 [pii]).
138. Obel JC, Friberg G, Fleming GF. Chemotherapy in endometrial cancer. Clin Adv Hematol Oncol. 2006;4(6):459–68.
139. Oda K, Stokoe D, Taketani Y, McCormick F. High frequency of coexistent mutations of PIK3CA and PTEN genes in endometrial carcinoma. Cancer Res. 2005;65(23):10669–73. doi:10.1158/0008-5472.CAN-05-2620 (65/23/10669 [pii]).

140. Ott PA, Bang Y-J, Berton-Rigaud D, Elez E, Pishvaian MJ, Rugo HS, Puzanov I, Morgan MA, Mehnert JM, Aung KL, Carrigan M, Saraf S, Chen M, Soria J-C. Pembrolizumab in advanced endometrial cancer: Preliminary results from the phase Ib KEYNOTE-028 study. J Clin Oncol. 2016;34(suppl; abstr 5581).
141. Oza AM, Elit L, Biagi J, Chapman W, Tsao M, Hedley D, Hansen C, Dancey J, Eisenhauer E. Molecular correlates associated with a phase II study of temsirolimus (CCI-779) in patients with metastatic or recurrent endometrial cancer–NCIC IND 160. J Clin Oncol. 2006;24(18S):3003.
142. Oza AM, Elit L, Tsao MS, Kamel-Reid S, Biagi J, Provencher DM, Gotlieb WH, Hoskins PJ, Ghatage P, Tonkin KS, Mackay HJ, Mazurka J, Sederias J, Ivy P, Dancey JE, Eisenhauer EA. Phase II study of temsirolimus in women with recurrent or metastatic endometrial cancer: a trial of the NCIC Clinical Trials Group. J Clin Oncol. 2011;29 (24):3278–85. doi:10.1200/JCO.2010.34.1578.
143. Oza AM, Pignata S, Poveda A, McCormack M, Clamp A, Schwartz B, Cheng J, Li X, Campbell K, Dodion P, Haluska FG. Randomized phase ii trial of ridaforolimus in advanced endometrial carcinoma. J Clin Oncol. 2015;33(31):3576–82. doi:10.1200/JCO.2014.58.8871 .
144. Oza AM, Eisenhauer EA, Elit L, Cutz JC, Sakurada A, Tsao MS, Hoskins PJ, Biagi J, Ghatage P, Mazurka J, Provencher D, Dore N, Dancey J, Fyles A. Phase II study of erlotinib in recurrent or metastatic endometrial cancer: NCIC IND-148. J Clin Oncol. 2008;26(26):4319–25. doi:10.1200/JCO.2007.15.8808 (JCO.2007.15.8808 [pii]).
145. O'Reilly KE, Rojo F, She QB, Solit D, Mills GB, Smith D, Lane H, Hofmann F, Hicklin DJ, Ludwig DL, Baselga J, Rosen N. mTOR inhibition induces upstream receptor tyrosine kinase signaling and activates Akt. Cancer Res. 2006;66(3):1500–8. doi:10.1158/0008-5472. CAN-05-2925 (66/3/1500 [pii]).
146. Parker LL, Piwnica-Worms H. Inactivation of the p34cdc2-cyclin B complex by the human WEE1 tyrosine kinase. Science. 1992;257(5078):1955–7.
147. Patel AV, Feigelson HS, Talbot JT, McCullough ML, Rodriguez C, Patel RC, Thun MJ, Calle EE. The role of body weight in the relationship between physical activity and endometrial cancer: results from a large cohort of US women. Int J Cancer. 2008;123 (8):1877–82. doi:10.1002/ijc.23716.
148. Patel SP, Lazar AJ, Mahoney S, Vaughn C, Gonzalez N, Papadopoulos NE, Liu P, Infante JR, LoRusso P, Kim KB. Clinical responses to AZD6244 (ARRY-142886)-based combination therapy stratified by gene mutations in patients with metastatic melanoma. In: 2010 ASCO molecular markers. 2010.
149. Pena CE, Jeffers M, Genvresse I, Appleman LJ, Ramanathan RK, Patnaik A. Biomarker analysis from a Phase I study of copanlisib with expansion cohorts in solid tumors with and without PIK3CA mutations and NHL. J Clin Oncol. 2016;33(Suppl; abstr 2548).
150. Pilarski R, Burt R, Kohlman W, Pho L, Shannon KM, Swisher E. Cowden syndrome and the PTEN hamartoma tumor syndrome: systematic review and revised diagnostic criteria. J Natl Cancer Inst. 2013;105(21):1607–16. doi:10.1093/jnci/djt277.
151. Pollock PM, Gartside MG, Dejeza LC, Powell MA, Mallon MA, Davies H, Mohammadi M, Futreal PA, Stratton MR, Trent JM, Goodfellow PJ. Frequent activating FGFR2 mutations in endometrial carcinomas parallel germline mutations associated with craniosynostosis and skeletal dysplasia syndromes. Oncogene. 2007;26(50):7158–62. doi:10.1038/sj.onc. 1210529 (1210529 [pii]).
152. Powell MA, Sill MW, Goodfellow PJ, Benbrook DM, Lankes HA, Leslie KK, Jeske Y, Mannel RS, Spillman MA, Lee PS, Hoffman JS, McMeekin DS, Pollock PM. A phase II trial of brivanib in recurrent or persistent endometrial cancer: an NRG Oncology/Gynecologic Oncology Group Study. Gynecol Oncol. 2014;135(1):38–43. doi:10.1016/j.ygyno.2014.07. 083.
153. Qi W, Xie C, Li C, Caldwell JT, Edwards H, Taub JW, Wang Y, Lin H, Ge Y. CHK1 plays a critical role in the anti-leukemic activity of the wee1 inhibitor MK-1775 in acute myeloid leukemia cells. J Hematol Oncol. 2014;7:53. doi:10.1186/s13045-014-0053-9.

154. Ramanathan RK, Von Hoff DD, Eskens F, Blumenschein GR, Richards DA, Renshaw FG, Rajogopaian P, Kelly A, Pena CE, Mross KB. A phase 1b trial of PI3K inhibitor copanlisib (BAY 80–6946) combined with the allosteric-MEK inhibitor refametinib (BAY 86-9766) in patients with advanced cancer. J Clin Oncol. 2014;32:5s (suppl; abstr 2588).
155. Ray-Coquard I, Favier L, Weber B, Roemer-Becuwe C, Bougnoux P, Fabbro M, Floquet A, Joly F, Plantade A, Paraiso D, Pujade-Lauraine E. Everolimus as second- or third-line treatment of advanced endometrial cancer: ENDORAD, a phase II trial of GINECO. Br J Cancer. 2013;108(9):1771–7. doi:10.1038/bjc.2013.183.
156. Reeves GK, Pirie K, Beral V, Green J, Spencer E, Bull D, Million Women Study Collaboration. Cancer incidence and mortality in relation to body mass index in the Million Women Study: cohort study. BMJ. 2007;335(7630):1134. doi:10.1136/bmj.39367.495995.AE.
157. Renehan AG, Tyson M, Egger M, Heller RF, Zwahlen M. Body-mass index and incidence of cancer: a systematic review and meta-analysis of prospective observational studies. Lancet. 2008;371(9612):569–78. doi:10.1016/S0140-6736(08)60269-X.
158. Rinaldi S, Peeters PH, Bezemer ID, Dossus L, Biessy C, Sacerdote C, Berrino F, Panico S, Palli D, Tumino R, Khaw KT, Bingham S, Allen NE, Key T, Jensen MK, Overvad K, Olsen A, Tjonneland A, Amiano P, Ardanaz E, Agudo A, Martinez-Garcia C, Quiros JR, Tormo MJ, Nagel G, Linseisen J, Boeing H, Schulz M, Grobbee DE, Bueno-de-Mesquita HB, Koliva M, Kyriazi G, Thrichopoulou A, Boutron-Ruault MC, Clavel-Chapelon F, Ferrari P, Slimani N, Saracci R, Riboli E, Kaaks R. Relationship of alcohol intake and sex steroid concentrations in blood in pre- and post-menopausal women: the European Prospective Investigation into Cancer and Nutrition. Cancer Causes Control: CCC. 2006;17 (8):1033–43. doi:10.1007/s10552-006-0041-7.
159. Rizvi NA, Rusch V, Pao W, Chaft JE, Ladanyi M, Miller VA, Krug LM, Azzoli CG, Bains M, Downey R, Flores R, Park B, Singh B, Zakowski M, Heelan RT, Shen R, Kris MG. Molecular characteristics predict clinical outcomes: prospective trial correlating response to the EGFR tyrosine kinase inhibitor gefitinib with the presence of sensitizing mutations in the tyrosine binding domain of the EGFR gene. Clin Cancer Res. 2011;17 (10):3500–6. doi:10.1158/1078-0432.CCR-10-2102 (1078-0432.CCR-10-2102 [pii]).
160. Rock CL, Demark-Wahnefried W. Nutrition and survival after the diagnosis of breast cancer: a review of the evidence. J Clin Oncol. 2002;20(15):3302–16.
161. Sainson RC, Harris AL. Regulation of angiogenesis by homotypic and heterotypic notch signalling in endothelial cells and pericytes: from basic research to potential therapies. Angiogenesis. 2008;11(1):41–51. doi:10.1007/s10456-008-9098-0.
162. Salvesen HB, Kumar R, Stefansson I, Angelini S, MacDonald N, Smeds J, Jacobs IJ, Hemminki K, Das S, Akslen LA. Low frequency of BRAF and CDKN2A mutations in endometrial cancer. Int J Cancer. 2005;115(6):930–4. doi:10.1002/ijc.20702.
163. Samuels Y, Wang Z, Bardelli A, Silliman N, Ptak J, Szabo S, Yan H, Gazdar A, Powell SM, Riggins GJ, Willson JK, Markowitz S, Kinzler KW, Vogelstein B, Velculescu VE. High frequency of mutations of the PIK3CA gene in human cancers. Science. 2004;304 (5670):554. doi:10.1126/science.1096502 (1096502 [pii]).
164. Santin AD, Bellone S, Gokden M, Palmieri M, Dunn D, Agha J, Roman JJ, Hutchins L, Pecorelli S, O'Brien T, Cannon MJ, Parham GP. Overexpression of HER-2/neu in uterine serous papillary cancer. Clin Cancer Res. 2002;8(5):1271–9.
165. Sasaki H, Nishii H, Takahashi H, Tada A, Furusato M, Terashima Y, Siegal GP, Parker SL, Kohler MF, Berchuck A, et al. Mutation of the Ki-ras protooncogene in human endometrial hyperplasia and carcinoma. Cancer Res. 1993;53(8):1906–10.
166. Schmeler KM, Lynch HT, Chen LM, Munsell MF, Soliman PT, Clark MB, Daniels MS, White KG, Boyd-Rogers SG, Conrad PG, Yang KY, Rubin MM, Sun CC, Slomovitz BM, Gershenson DM, Lu KH. Prophylactic surgery to reduce the risk of gynecologic cancers in the Lynch syndrome. N Engl J Med. 2006;354(3):261–9. doi:10.1056/NEJMoa052627.
167. Schouten LJ, Goldbohm RA, van den Brandt PA. Anthropometry, physical activity, and endometrial cancer risk: results from the Netherlands Cohort Study. J Natl Cancer Inst. 2004;96(21):1635–8. doi:10.1093/jnci/djh291.

168. Schuler KM, Rambally BS, DiFurio MJ, Sampey BP, Gehrig PA, Makowski L, Bae-Jump VL. Antiproliferative and metabolic effects of metformin in a preoperative window clinical trial for endometrial cancer. Cancer Med. 2015;4(2):161–73. doi:10.1002/cam4.353.
169. Schultz N, Lopez E, Saleh-Gohari N, Helleday T. Poly(ADP-ribose) polymerase (PARP-1) has a controlling role in homologous recombination. Nucleic Acids Res. 2003;31(17):4959–64.
170. Secord AA, Teoh DK, Barry WT, Yu M, Broadwater G, Havrilesky LJ, Lee PS, Berchuck A, Lancaster J, Wenham RM. A phase I trial of dasatinib, an SRC-family kinase inhibitor, in combination with paclitaxel and carboplatin in patients with advanced or recurrent ovarian cancer. Clin Cancer Res. 2012;18(19):5489–98. doi:10.1158/1078-0432.CCR-12-0507.
171. Semczuk A, Berbec H, Kostuch M, Cybulski M, Wojcierowski J, Baranowski W. K-ras gene point mutations in human endometrial carcinomas: correlation with clinicopathological features and patients' outcome. J Cancer Res Clin Oncol. 1998;124(12):695–700.
172. Setiawan VW, Yang HP, Pike MC, McCann SE, Yu H, Xiang YB, Wolk A, Wentzensen N, Weiss NS, Webb PM, van den Brandt PA, van de Vijver K, Thompson PJ, Australian National Endometrial Cancer Study G, Strom BL, Spurdle AB, Soslow RA, Shu XO, Schairer C, Sacerdote C, Rohan TE, Robien K, Risch HA, Ricceri F, Rebbeck TR, Rastogi R, Prescott J, Polidoro S, Park Y, Olson SH, Moysich KB, Miller AB, McCullough ML, Matsuno RK, Magliocco AM, Lurie G, Lu L, Lissowska J, Liang X, Lacey JV Jr, Kolonel LN, Henderson BE, Hankinson SE, Hakansson N, Goodman MT, Gaudet MM, Garcia-Closas M, Friedenreich CM, Freudenheim JL, Doherty J, De Vivo I, Courneya KS, Cook LS, Chen C, Cerhan JR, Cai H, Brinton LA, Bernstein L, Anderson KE, Anton-Culver H, Schouten LJ, Horn-Ross PL. Type I and II endometrial cancers: have they different risk factors? J Clin Oncol. 2013;31(20):2607–18. doi:10.1200/JCO.2012.48.2596.
173. Shapiro GI, Rodon J, Bedell C, Kwak EL, Baselga J, Brana I, Pandya SS, Scheffold C, Laird AD, Nguyen LT, Xu Y, Egile C, Edelman G. Phase I safety, pharmacokinetic, and pharmacodynamic study of SAR245408 (XL147), an oral pan-class I PI3K inhibitor, in patients with advanced solid tumors. Clin Cancer Res. 2014;20(1):233–45. doi:10.1158/1078-0432.CCR-13-1777.
174. Shen J, Peng Y, Wei L, Zhang W, Yang L, Lan L, Kapoor P, Ju Z, Mo Q, Shih Ie M, Uray IP, Wu X, Brown PH, Shen X, Mills GB, Peng G. ARID1A deficiency impairs the DNA damage checkpoint and sensitizes cells to PARP inhibitors. Cancer Discov. 2015;5(7):752–67. doi:10.1158/2159-8290.CD-14-0849.
175. Shi Q, Li J, Li M, Wu J, Yao Q, Xing A. The role of levonorgestrel-releasing intrauterine system for endometrial protection in women with breast cancer taking tamoxifen. Eur J Gynaecol Oncol. 2014;35(5):492–8.
176. Shi Y, Yan H, Frost P, Gera J, Lichtenstein A. Mammalian target of rapamycin inhibitors activate the AKT kinase in multiple myeloma cells by up-regulating the insulin-like growth factor receptor/insulin receptor substrate-1/phosphatidylinositol 3-kinase cascade. Mol Cancer Ther. 2005;4(10):1533–40. doi:10.1158/1535-7163.MCT-05-0068.
177. Shoji K, Oda K, Nakagawa S, Hosokawa S, Nagae G, Uehara Y, Sone K, Miyamoto Y, Hiraike H, Hiraike-Wada O, Nei T, Kawana K, Kuramoto H, Aburatani H, Yano T, Taketani Y. The oncogenic mutation in the pleckstrin homology domain of AKT1 in endometrial carcinomas. Br J Cancer. 2009;101(1):145–8. doi:10.1038/sj.bjc.6605109 (6605109 [pii]).
178. Siegel RL, Miller KD, Jemal A (2016) Cancer statistics, 2016. CA Cancer J Clin 66 (1):7–30. doi:10.3322/caac.21332.
179. Simpson ER, Mendelson CR. Effect of aging and obesity on aromatase activity of human adipose cells. Am J Clin Nutr. 1987;45(1 Suppl):290–5.
180. Sjostrom L, Narbro K, Sjostrom CD, Karason K, Larsson B, Wedel H, Lystig T, Sullivan M, Bouchard C, Carlsson B, Bengtsson C, Dahlgren S, Gummesson A, Jacobson P, Karlsson J, Lindroos AK, Lonroth H, Naslund I, Olbers T, Stenlof K, Torgerson J, Agren G,

Carlsson LM, Swedish Obese Subjects S. Effects of bariatric surgery on mortality in Swedish obese subjects. N Engl J Med. 2007;357(8):741–52. doi:10.1056/NEJMoa066254.
181. Slomovitz BM, Jiang Y, Yates MS, Soliman PT, Johnston T, Nowakowski M, Levenback C, Zhang Q, Ring K, Munsell MF, Gershenson DM, Lu KH, Coleman RL. Phase II study of everolimus and letrozole in patients with recurrent endometrial carcinoma. J Clin Oncol. 2015;33(8):930–6. doi:10.1200/JCO.2014.58.3401.
182. Slomovitz BM, Broaddus RR, Burke TW, Sneige N, Soliman PT, Wu W, Sun CC, Munsell MF, Gershenson DM, Lu KH. Her-2/neu overexpression and amplification in uterine papillary serous carcinoma. J Clin Oncol. 2004;22(15):3126–32. doi:10.1200/JCO.2004.11.154 (22/15/3126 [pii]).
183. Slomovitz BM, Lu KH, Johnston T, Coleman RL, Munsell M, Broaddus RR, Walker C, Ramondetta LM, Burke TW, Gershenson DM, Wolf J. A phase 2 study of the oral mammalian target of rapamycin inhibitor, everolimus, in patients with recurrent endometrial carcinoma. Cancer. 2010a. doi:10.1002/cncr.25515
184. Slomovitz BM, Schmeler K, Miller DS, Lu K, Ramirez PT, Caputo T, Coleman R, Burke T, Gershenson DM, Wolf J. Phase II study of cetuximab (Erbitux) in patients with progressive or recurrent endometrial cancer. Gynecol Oncol. 2010b;166(suppl; abstr 13).
185. Smith EL, Zamarin D, Lesokhin AM. Harnessing the immune system for cancer therapy. Curr Opin Oncol. 2014;26(6):600–7. doi:10.1097/CCO.0000000000000128.
186. Soler M, Chatenoud L, Negri E, Parazzini F, Franceschi S, la Vecchia C. Hypertension and hormone-related neoplasms in women. Hypertension. 1999;34(2):320–5.
187. Soliman PT, Bassett RL Jr, Wilson EB, Boyd-Rogers S, Schmeler KM, Milam MR, Gershenson DM, Lu KH. Limited public knowledge of obesity and endometrial cancer risk: what women know. Obstet Gynecol. 2008;112(4):835–42. doi:10.1097/AOG.0b013e318187d022.
188. Soliman PT, Broaddus R, Westin SN, Iglesias DA, Burzawa JK, Zhang Q, Munsell MF, Schmandt R, Ramondetta LM, Lu KH. Prospective evaluation of the molecular effects of metformin on the endometrium in women with newly diagnosed endometrial cancer: a window of opportunity study. J Clin Oncol. 2014;32:5s (suppl; abstr 5510).
189. Song MS, Salmena L, Pandolfi PP. The functions and regulation of the PTEN tumour suppressor. Nat Rev Mol Cell Biol. 2012;13(5):283–96. doi:10.1038/nrm3330.
190. Stanford JL, Brinton LA, Berman ML, Mortel R, Twiggs LB, Barrett RJ, Wilbanks GD, Hoover RN. Oral contraceptives and endometrial cancer: do other risk factors modify the association? Int J Cancer. 1993;54(2):243–8.
191. Summy JM, Gallick GE. Treatment for advanced tumors: SRC reclaims center stage. Clin Cancer Res. 2006;12(5):1398–401. doi:10.1158/1078-0432.CCR-05-2692.
192. Tolcher AW, Khan K, Ong M, Banerji U, Papadimitrakopoulou V, Gandara DR, Patnaik A, Baird RD, Olmos D, Garrett CR, Skolnik JM, Rubin EH, Smith PD, Huang P, Learoyd M, Shannon KA, Morosky A, Tetteh E, Jou YM, Papadopoulos KP, Moreno V, Kaiser B, Yap TA, Yan L, de Bono JS. Antitumor activity in RAS-driven tumors by blocking AKT and MEK. Clin Cancer Res. 2015;21(4):739–48. doi:10.1158/1078-0432.CCR-14-1901.
193. Topalian SL, Hodi FS, Brahmer JR, Gettinger SN, Smith DC, McDermott DF, Powderly JD, Carvajal RD, Sosman JA, Atkins MB, Leming PD, Spigel DR, Antonia SJ, Horn L, Drake CG, Pardoll DM, Chen L, Sharfman WH, Anders RA, Taube JM, McMiller TL, Xu H, Korman AJ, Jure-Kunkel M, Agrawal S, McDonald D, Kollia GD, Gupta A, Wigginton JM, Sznol M. Safety, activity, and immune correlates of anti-PD-1 antibody in cancer. N Engl J Med. 2012;366(26):2443–54. doi:10.1056/NEJMoa1200690.
194. Tredan O, Treilleux I, Wang Q, Gane N, Pissaloux D, Bonnin N, Petit T, Cretin J, Bonichon-Lamichhane N, Priou F, Lavau-Denes S, Mari V, Freyer G, Lebrun D, Alexandre J, Ray-Coquard I. Predicting everolimus treatment efficacy in patients with advanced endometrial carcinoma: a GINECO group study. Target Oncol. 2013;8(4):243–51. doi:10.1007/s11523-012-0242-9.
195. Tsoref D, Welch S, Lau S, Biagi J, Tonkin K, Martin LA, Ellard S, Ghatage P, Elit L, Mackay HJ, Allo G, Tsao MS, Kamel-Reid S, Eisenhauer EA, Oza AM. Phase II study of

oral ridaforolimus in women with recurrent or metastatic endometrial cancer. Gynecol Oncol. 2014;135(2):184–9. doi:10.1016/j.ygyno.2014.06.033.

196. Van Gool IC, Eggink FA, Freeman-Mills L, Stelloo E, Marchi E, de Bruyn M, Palles C, Nout RA, de Kroon CD, Osse EM, Klenerman P, Creutzberg CL, Tomlinson IP, Smit VT, Nijman HW, Bosse T, Church DN. POLE proofreading mutations elicit an antitumor immune response in endometrial cancer. Clin Cancer Res. 2015;21(14):3347–55. doi:10.1158/1078-0432.CCR-15-0057.
197. Wallin JJ, Edgar KA, Guan J, Berry M, Prior WW, Lee L, Lesnick JD, Lewis C, Nonomiya J, Pang J, Salphati L, Olivero AG, Sutherlin DP, O'Brien C, Spoerke JM, Patel S, Lensun L, Kassees R, Ross L, Lackner MR, Sampath D, Belvin M, Friedman LS. GDC-0980 is a novel class I PI3K/mTOR kinase inhibitor with robust activity in cancer models driven by the PI3K pathway. Mol Cancer Ther. 2011;10(12):2426–36. doi:10.1158/1535-7163.MCT-11-0446.
198. Wang Z, Sun Y. Targeting p53 for novel anticancer therapy. Transl Oncol. 2010;3(1):1–12.
199. Ward KK, Roncancio AM, Shah NR, Davis MA, Saenz CC, McHale MT, Plaxe SC. Bariatric surgery decreases the risk of uterine malignancy. Gynecol Oncol. 2014;133(1):63–6. doi:10.1016/j.ygyno.2013.11.012.
200. Watanabe R, Wei L, Huang J. mTOR signaling, function, novel inhibitors, and therapeutic targets. J Nucl Med. 2011;52(4):497–500. doi:10.2967/jnumed.111.089623 (jnumed.111.089623 [pii]).
201. Weaver AN, Yang ES. Beyond DNA repair: additional functions of PARP-1 in cancer. Front Oncol. 2013;3:290. doi:10.3389/fonc.2013.00290.
202. Weiderpass E, Persson I, Adami HO, Magnusson C, Lindgren A, Baron JA. Body size in different periods of life, diabetes mellitus, hypertension, and risk of postmenopausal endometrial cancer (Sweden). Cancer Causes Control: CCC. 2000;11(2):185–92.
203. Weiss NS, Sayvetz TA. Incidence of endometrial cancer in relation to the use of oral contraceptives. N Engl J Med. 1980;302(10):551–4. doi:10.1056/NEJM198003063021004.
204. Westin SN, Broaddus RR. Personalized therapy in endometrial cancer: challenges and opportunities. Cancer Biol Ther. 2012;13(1):1–13. doi:10.4161/cbt.13.1.18438.
205. Westin SN, Ju Z, Broaddus RR, Krakstad C, Li J, Pal N, Lu KH, Coleman RL, Hennessy BT, Klempner SJ, Werner HM, Salvesen HB, Cantley LC, Mills GB, Myers AP. PTEN loss is a context-dependent outcome determinant in obese and non-obese endometrioid endometrial cancer patients. Mol Oncol. 2015. doi:10.1016/j.molonc.2015.04.014.
206. Westin SN, Sill M, Coleman RL, Waggoner SE, Moore KN, Mathews CA, Jain A, Modesitt SC, Schilder R, Aghajanian C. Limited access safety lead-in of the MEK inhibitor trametinib in combination with GSK2141795, an AKT inhibitor, in patients with recurrent or persistent endometrial cancer: a NRG Oncology Gynecologic Oncology Group study. In: Society of gynecologic oncology, San Diego, California. 2016.
207. Xie Y, Wang YL, Yu L, Hu Q, Ji L, Zhang Y, Liao QP. Metformin promotes progesterone receptor expression via inhibition of mammalian target of rapamycin (mTOR) in endometrial cancer cells. J Steroid Biochem Mol Biol. 2010. doi:10.1016/j.jsbmb.2010.12.006 (S0960-0760(10)00380-8 [pii]).
208. Yancopoulos GD, Davis S, Gale NW, Rudge JS, Wiegand SJ, Holash J. Vascular-specific growth factors and blood vessel formation. Nature. 2000;407(6801):242–8. doi:10.1038/35025215.
209. Zakikhani M, Dowling R, Fantus IG, Sonenberg N, Pollak M. Metformin is an AMP kinase-dependent growth inhibitor for breast cancer cells. Cancer Res. 2006;66(21):10269–73. doi:10.1158/0008-5472.CAN-06-1500 (0008-5472.CAN-06-1500 [pii]).
210. Zendehdel K, Nyren O, Ostenson CG, Adami HO, Ekbom A, Ye W. Cancer incidence in patients with type 1 diabetes mellitus: a population-based cohort study in Sweden. J Natl Cancer Inst. 2003;95(23):1797–800.

211. Zhang Q, Celestino J, Schmandt R, McCampbell AS, Urbauer DL, Meyer LA, Burzawa JK, Huang M, Yates MS, Iglesias D, Broaddus RR, Lu KH. Chemopreventive effects of metformin on obesity-associated endometrial proliferation. Am J Obstet Gynecol. 2013;209 (1):24 e21–24 e12. doi:10.1016/j.ajog.2013.03.008.
212. Zhang Z, Dong L, Sui L, Yang Y, Liu X, Yu Y, Zhu Y, Feng Y. Metformin reverses progestin resistance in endometrial cancer cells by downregulating GloI expression. Int J Gynecol Cancer. 2011;21(2):213–21. doi:10.1097/IGC.0b013e318207dac7 (00009577-201102000-00005 [pii]).
213. Zhou B, Yang L, Sun Q, Cong R, Gu H, Tang N, Zhu H, Wang B. Cigarette smoking and the risk of endometrial cancer: a meta-analysis. Am J Med. 2008;121(6):501–8 e503. doi:10.1016/j.amjmed.2008.01.044.

Part III
Uterine Mesenchymal Tumors

Chapter 11
Molecular Pathology of Uterine Mesenchymal Tumors

Brooke E. Howitt and Marisa R. Nucci

Smooth Muscle Tumors

Smooth muscle tumors are the most common neoplasms of the uterus and include benign leiomyoma and variants, intravenous leiomyomatosis, smooth muscle tumors of uncertain malignant potential (STUMP), and leiomyosarcoma (LMS). Most are characterized by spindled cells with eosinophilic cytoplasm in predominantly fascicular growth, with a smaller subset demonstrating epithelioid morphology or myxoid matrix. Immunohistochemically, they share expression of the smooth muscle markers desmin, caldesmon, and smooth muscle actin (SMA) (except in some poorly differentiated leiomyosarcomas) and are generally, but not always, negative for CD10. Smooth muscle tumors are broken down into both biologic and morphologic variants; while various molecular alterations are specific to certain types of smooth muscle tumors, there is some overlap.

Conventional Leiomyoma

Leiomyoma (Fig. 11.1) is the most common uterine tumor and is characterized by recurrent point mutations and small deletions, and characteristic chromosomal translocations. The most common gene mutated in leiomyoma is *MED12*, with heterozygous *MED12* mutations found in up to 70–80% of uterine leiomyomas [1–6]. The vast majority of these are located in exon 2 at the codon 44 position.

B.E. Howitt · M.R. Nucci (✉)
Department of Pathology, Harvard Medical School, Brigham and Women's Hospital, 75 Francis St, Boston, MA 02115, USA
e-mail: mnucci@partners.org

B.E. Howitt
e-mail: bhowitt@partners.org

M.T. Deavers and D.M. Coffey (eds.), *Precision Molecular Pathology of Uterine Cancer*, Molecular Pathology Library,
DOI 10.1007/978-3-319-57985-6_11

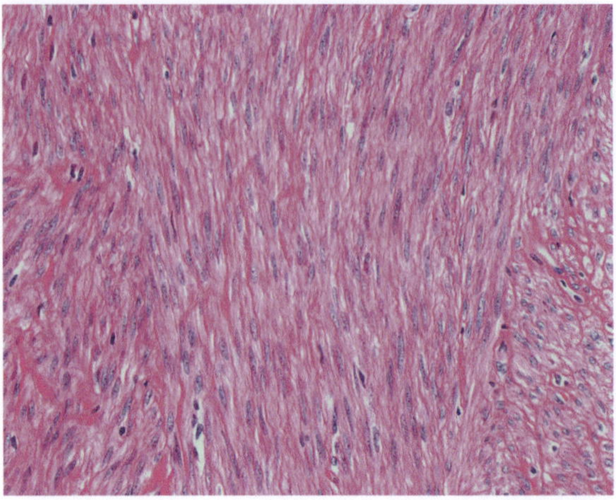

Fig. 11.1 Leiomyoma is characterized by intersecting fascicles of smooth muscle cells with eosinophilic cytoplasm and bland, *cigar-shaped* nuclei

There is no evidence to date that germline *MED12* mutations play a role in the development of leiomyoma.

HMGA1 or HMGA2 overexpression is common in leiomyoma, reflecting chromosomal translocations involving 6p21 (*HMGA1*) and 12q14 (*HMGA2*). HMGA2 overexpression is found in approximately 10% of uterine leiomyomas and tends to be mutually exclusive with *MED12* mutations [3]. When considering only those uterine leiomyomas lacking *MED12* mutation, HMGA2 overexpression is found in 40% of tumors. Other recurrent molecular aberrations in leiomyoma include *COL4A5/6* deletions, which are mutually exclusive with *MED12*, *HMGA2*, and *FH* alterations [7]. Leiomyomas lack *TP53* mutations [4, 7].

The karyotypes of leiomyoma are either normal (60%) or noncomplex with one or more chromosomal translocations (40%) [8, 9]. Recurrent chromosomal aberrations include those mentioned above involving *HMGA2* (up to 25% of leiomyomas; most commonly resulting in fusion with *RAD51B* on chromosome 14), *HMGA1* (6p21), 13q, 1p36, and 10q22 [10–12]. Other cytogenetic abnormalities frequently identified in conventional karyotype or array comparative genomic hybridization include 7q deletion [13, 14], trisomy 12 [10–12, 15, 16], 1p deletion [13] and less frequently, monosomy 22 [10]. Interestingly, 7q deletions have been identified in both *MED12* mutated and *HMGA2* mutated leiomyoma, suggesting that 7q may be important for progression rather than initiation of tumorigenesis. Mitotically active leiomyoma appears to have molecular features similar to conventional leiomyoma, with frequent *MED12* mutations [4].

Cellular Leiomyoma

Few studies have examined molecular alterations in cellular leiomyoma. They appear to lack *TP53* mutations [4], 6% have *PTEN* deletions, and only 9–14% have

MED12 mutations [4, 17], suggesting the pathogenesis of cellular leiomyoma may differ from conventional leiomyoma. 1p deletion was present in 23% of cellular leiomyomas in one study [18], and a subset have been reported to have 10q22 rearrangements which have also been described in conventional leiomyoma [19].

Atypical Leiomyoma

Atypical leiomyoma is characterized by significant cytologic atypia (readily seen from 4× objective) but lacks necrosis and significant mitotic activity [20]. It has been proposed that these be termed "leiomyoma with bizarre nuclei;" [21] however, many of the molecular alterations present in these tumors overlap with those found in leiomyosarcoma. Specifically, 12% have *TP53* mutations [4], 10% have *MED12* mutations [4], and 24% have *PTEN* deletion [4]. In one study, the miRNA profile of atypical leiomyoma was more similar to LMS/STUMP than to conventional leiomyoma or cellular leiomyoma [4].

Hereditary Leiomyomatosis and Renal Cell Carcinoma Syndrome

Hereditary leiomyomatosis and renal cell carcinoma syndrome (formerly known as "Reed syndrome") is characterized by numerous uterine leiomyomata, often presenting at a very young age [22]. Histologically, the leiomyomas are characterized by epithelioid nuclei with very prominent nucleoli (characteristically cherry red or "orangophilic") with perinucleolar clearing (Fig. 11.2), as well as intracellular and extracellular aggregates of eosinophilic material [23–25]; however, these features are not entirely specific or sensitive [26]. Patients with this syndrome have germline mutations in the fumarate hydratase gene, *FH*, located on 1q42.1. The tumors from patients with this syndrome accumulate a secondary somatic inactivation of *FH*, resulting in complete loss of protein function and expression that can be demonstrated with FH immunohistochemical staining (loss of staining in tumor cells) [23]. Rarely, loss of FH can be found in non-syndromic leiomyomata [27]. *FH* inactivation is thought to account for less than 2% of all uterine leiomyomas [27] and is mutually exclusive with *MED12* and *HMGA2* mutations.

Conventional Leiomyosarcoma

Conventional LMS is characterized histologically by atypical spindle tumor cells growing in fascicles. Tumor cell necrosis and abundant mitotic activity are usually

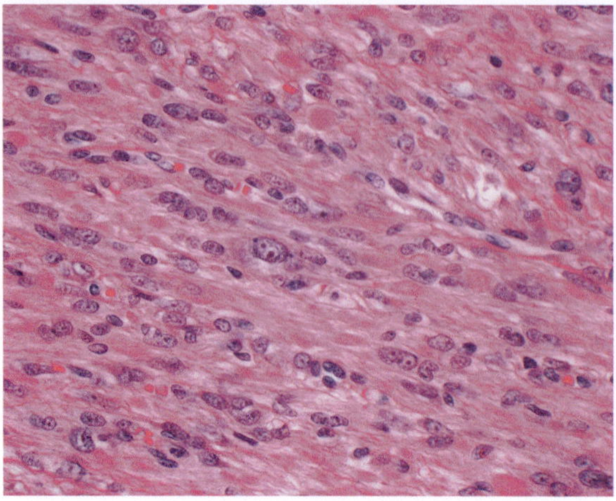

Fig. 11.2 HLRCC-associated leiomyoma is characterized by plump nuclei with large, *cherry red* nucleoli with perinucleolar clearing. Extracellular eosinophilic material may also be present

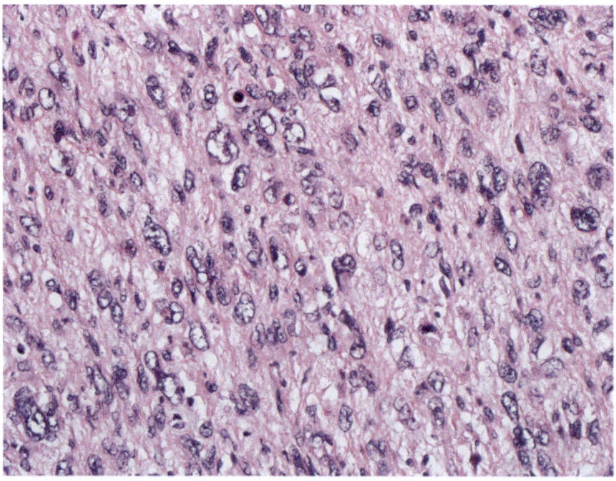

Fig. 11.3 Conventional leiomyosarcoma typically displays cytologic atypia, mitoses, and necrosis (not shown here)

present (Fig. 11.3). The degree of nuclear atypia varies, and no study has shown prognostic importance of morphologic grade. Immunohistochemically, they are usually positive for the smooth muscle markers SMA, desmin, and caldesmon; however, it is not unusual for there to be loss of expression of one or more of these, particularly in morphologically high-grade tumors. Most of the molecular alterations known about LMS are derived from studies of conventional or mixed morphologic types. No studies have specifically evaluated the molecular features of morphologic variants such as myxoid LMS, or epithelioid LMS. While LMS generally is considered to arise de novo, there is molecular evidence for LMS arising from a preexisting leiomyoma in at least a subset of cases [28, 29]. LMSs have markedly complex karyotypes, which make it difficult to identify alterations specific to LMS. Some of the recurring chromosome arm level alterations described in LMS include gains of 1q, 17p, and Xp, and loss of heterozygosity for 10q (containing *PTEN*) and 13q (containing *RB1*), which are present in >50% of LMS [13, 30–32].

TP53 mutations are common in LMS, reported in up to 52% of cases [4, 33]. *MED12* mutations are found in $\sim$10% of LMS [3, 4, 34], although reports range from 2 to 20% [5, 6, 34–37]; however, many of the *MED12* mutations present in LMS are not the typical hot spot mutations, but rather represent complex or truncating mutations [4]. HMGA2 overexpression is seen in $\sim$35% of LMSs and appears to be mutually exclusive with *MED12* mutation [3], similar to leiomyoma. *HMGA1* rearrangements have been described in only two LMS [38]. α-thalassemia/mental retardation syndrome X-linked (ATRX) or death domain-associated (DAXX) are two genes recently found to be frequently mutated in LMS, and are associated with an alternative lengthening of telomere (ALT) phenotype contributing to the pathogenesis of uterine leiomyosarcoma in up to 60% of cases [35, 39]. In addition, activated AKT/mTOR pathway proteins are highly expressed in uterine LMS, which has led to mTOR inhibition being proposed for therapy [40–42].

Unusual Smooth Muscle Neoplasms ("Quasi-malignant")

Some uterine smooth muscle tumors appear histologically benign, but have features that are suggestive of aggressive behavior, such as vascular invasion or spread beyond the uterus. Other tumors may have histologically indeterminate features of malignancy and are not easily categorized into benign or malignant categories.

Intravenous leiomyomatosis (IVL) is a condition in which a tumor morphologically indistinguishable from conventional leiomyoma (or variants) grows within vascular spaces, and in dramatic cases may extend through the vena cava into the right heart. Molecularly, these tumors appear to have cytogenetic alterations commonly seen in conventional leiomyoma, such as t(12;14) [43, 44]. Regional losses on chromosomes 22q and 1p, and gains on chromosomes 12q were the most common alterations in one study [45]. *MED12* mutations have not been documented in IVL [45, 46].

Benign metastasizing leiomyoma (BML) is a somewhat controversial entity characterized by bland appearing smooth muscle tumors in the lung or lymph nodes, and may represent "metastasis" from a histologically unremarkable uterine leiomyoma, a theory supported by molecular evidence of common origin [47, 48]. BML is rare and shares a genetic profile with approximately 3% of all uterine leiomyomas, specifically 19q and 22q terminal deletions [49]. Others have proposed a relationship between BML and IVL based on X inactivation studies [50]; however, the generally non-overlapping cytogenetic profiles of these tumors would suggest otherwise.

STUMP molecular features are not well-defined secondary to poor reproducibility of morphologic diagnosis, but with this caveat in mind, one study found that 11% of STUMPs harbor *MED12* mutations, similar in frequency to LMS [4]. Similarly, 33% of STUMPs have *PTEN* deletion [4].

PEComa

Perivascular epithelioid cell tumor (PEComa) is in the family of myomelanocytic tumors with its morphology and immunoprofile containing smooth muscle and melanocytic features. Histologically, it is characterized by plump epithelioid cells with abundant granular pale to eosinophilic cytoplasm (Fig. 11.4) that immunohistochemically express both smooth muscle (SMA and desmin) and melanocytic (HMB-45, MelanA and microphthalmia-associated transcription factor) markers. Occasionally, uterine PEComas display a predominant spindle cell morphology, but most often there is a combination of epithelioid and spindled cells. Diagnostic difficulty arises when trying to distinguish between PEComa and uterine smooth muscle tumors, particularly those with epithelioid morphology, as they may have overlapping immunoprofiles [51–57]. Most studies interrogating the molecular alterations in PEComa include tumors from various anatomic sites, including the uterus, so the molecular features discussed are not only specific to uterine PEComas, but rather PEComas of any anatomic site.

The most well-characterized alterations are those resulting in inactivation of *TSC2* (16p13.3) or less commonly *TSC1* (9q34), due to the association of PEC tumors (angiomyolipoma and lymphangioleiomyomatosis) with the genetic disease tuberous sclerosis complex. TSC1/2 are involved in many cell cycle regulatory pathways, including the mTOR pathway. Loss of *TSC1/2* results in increased activation of mTOR [58], thus many have proposed using mTOR inhibitors in these

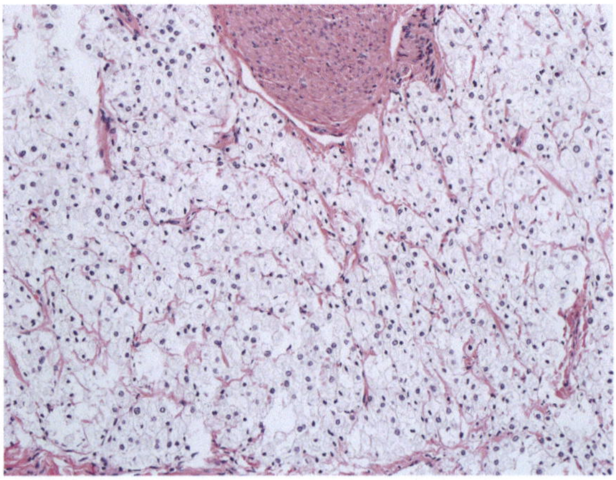

Fig. 11.4 PEComa is often composed of epithelioid cells with plump nuclei and clear to pale eosinophilic cytoplasm

tumors [59–62]. While any inactivating genetic hit in *TSC1/2* (mutation, deletion, copy number loss) may contribute to pathogenesis [60, 63], not all PEComas have inactivation of *TSC1/2*. One reported uterine PEComa lacked loss of heterozygosity at *TSC1* and *TSC2* [64]. As some PEComas lack inactivation of *TSC2* and activation of the mTOR pathway, some have suggested that mTOR pathway activation be confirmed before treating a PEComa patient with an mTOR inhibitor [65].

TFE3, a member of the MIT/TFE family of transcription factors, has been demonstrated to be rearranged in a subset of PEComas [66–68], including those occurring in the uterus. This likely represents a minority of uterine PEComas, as one of the largest studies showed no evidence of *TFE3* rearrangement in any case [69]. PEComas harboring *TFE3* rearrangements have a slightly different morphology, typically with purely epithelioid cells with cleared cytoplasm and nested architecture, and immunohistochemical lack of SMA and desmin expression [70]. Interestingly, *TFE3* rearranged PEComas lack *TSC2* inactivation, suggesting that this subset of PEComa has an alternate pathogenesis and may not be amenable to mTOR inhibition therapy [71, 72]. One PEComa was reported to have *TFE3* amplification rather than rearrangement [66]. The *TFE3* translocation partners documented in alveolar soft part sarcoma and Xp11 translocation renal cell carcinoma have not been found in PEComa to date. Recently, multiple groups have identified *PSF* as the most frequent translocation partner, resulting in a SFPQ/*PSF-TFE3* gene fusion [71, 73, 74], and one case harbored a *DVL2-TFE3* gene fusion [71].

RAD51B (14q24) translocations (resulting in *RAD51B-RRAGB* or *RAD51B-OPHN1* gene fusions) were identified in a small minority (8%) of uterine PEComas in one study [71]. In one of these cases, *TSC2* and *TP53* mutations were also identified, suggesting that these PEComas, unlike the *TFE3*-associated PEComas, likely have a shared pathogenesis with the *TSC2* inactivated PEComas. Interestingly, it was reported that the *RAD51B* translocation PEComas were initially diagnosed as leiomyosarcoma. Other translocations have also been recently reported in small numbers (one case each *HTR4-ST3GAL1* and *RASSF1-PDZRN3*) [71].

Array comparative genomic hybridization studies have identified a number of recurrent losses/gains, most notably loss of chromosomes 19, 16p, 17p, 1p, and 18p, and gains of X, 12q, 3q, 5, and 2q [63]. Of note, the *TSC2* gene is on 16p, suggesting a mechanism for TSC2 loss of function in PEComa. Similarly, *TP53* is on 17p and suggests a mechanism for biallelic inactivation in *TP53*-mutated tumors.

Endometrial Stromal Neoplasms

Endometrial stromal neoplasms include both stromal nodule and stromal sarcomas. Endometrial stromal sarcoma is further separated into low- and high-grade sarcoma. High-grade endometrial stromal sarcoma (HGESS) has recently been recognized as a distinct entity [21], largely due to its unique histology, clinical behavior, and underlying molecular alterations [21, 75]. Immunohistochemistry and molecular studies frequently serve as a useful adjunct in the diagnosis of endometrial stromal neoplasms.

Endometrial Stromal Nodule and Low-Grade Endometrial Stromal Sarcoma

Both endometrial stromal nodule (ESN) and low-grade endometrial stromal sarcoma (LGESS) resemble the non-neoplastic stroma of proliferative endometrium with ovoid to fusiform cells often encircling the frequent arteriole-like blood vessel component (Fig. 11.5). Similar to non-neoplastic endometrial stroma, ESN and LGESS are positive for CD10 by immunohistochemistry. The distinction between LGESS and ESN is made on histologic grounds; specifically, the interface with myometrium and the presence of LVI [21, 76, 77]. ESS typically exhibits prominent finger-like penetration of the myometrium and/or LVI; up to three foci of invasion measuring less than 3 mm (but without LVI) is allowed for the diagnosis of ESN [78]. Both ESN and ESS may demonstrate variant morphology, including smooth muscle differentiation and sex cord-like differentiation, making the diagnosis more difficult [77, 79, 80].

Recurrent Translocations/Gene Fusions

JAZF1–SUZ12 is the most common gene fusion in both low-grade ESS and ESN, found in greater than 50% of tumors (reported frequency ranges from 25 to >90% depending on the study design and tumor morphology) [81–88]. This gene fusion

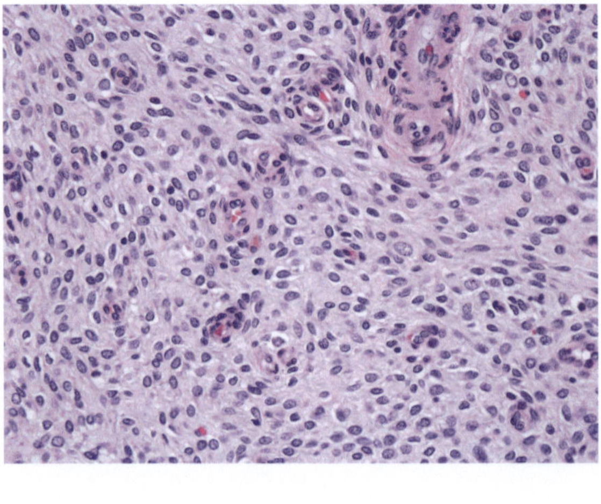

Fig. 11.5 Low-grade endometrial stromal tumors (endometrial stromal nodules and sarcomas) are characterized by cells with ovoid to fusiform nuclei lacking significant cytologic atypia that "swirl" around small caliber vessels

reflects the chromosomal translocation t(7;17) (p15;q21) or related variant translocations frequently observed in ESS via conventional cytogenetics or FISH [89, 90] (Fig. 11.6) and is apparently more common in low-grade ESS with classic morphology than in those with variant histology. Another translocation involving *JAZF1*, t(6;7) (p21;p15), resulting in a *JAZF1–PHF1* gene fusion is present in up to 28% of ESS, as well as in an endometrial stromal sarcoma cell line [87, 91–93]. The finding of *JAZF1* rearrangement, including as the sole karyotypic abnormality in a subset of tumors, suggests that it may play a significant role in the pathogenesis of ESS. Of interest, in ESN the non-rearranged *JAZF1* allele is transcriptionally active, but in ESS it appears to be silenced [94] resulting in increased proliferation and resistance to apoptosis, suggesting that epigenetic alterations also play a role in ESS pathogenesis.

In tumors lacking *JAZF1* abnormalities, *PHF1*, a polycomb repressor gene, has been found to be recurrently involved in another chromosomal translocation and resultant gene fusion with *MEAF6* (on 1p34) [95, 96]. ESS with *PHF1* rearrangement is enriched for sex cord-like differentiation [93], but also may show myxoid morphology, smooth muscle differentiation, or typical morphology [97]. A small subset of ESS may have *PHF1* rearrangements resulting in fusion with genes other than *JAZF1* or *MEAF6*, most notably *EPC1* on 10p11 [91]. It has been reported [87] that the non-rearranged *PHF1* allele is suppressed in ESS with *PHF1* gene fusions, emphasizing that the *SUZ12* and *PHF1* polycomb genes may be functioning similarly in the pathogenesis of ESS. One ESS was shown to harbor a *BCOR-ZC3H7B* gene fusion and two cases contained a *MBTD1-CXorf67* gene fusion [98, 99]. The presence of recurrent gene fusions involving the polycomb genes *PHF1*, *EPC1*, *MBTD1*, or *SUZ12*, even in the absence of a *JAZF1* abnormality, suggests that polycomb genes likely play a significant role in the pathogenesis of ESS. While a number of other less common cytogenetic aberrations have been described in ESS, they are outside the scope of this chapter; however, there is a recent review of the literature on this subject available [100]. Furthermore, a

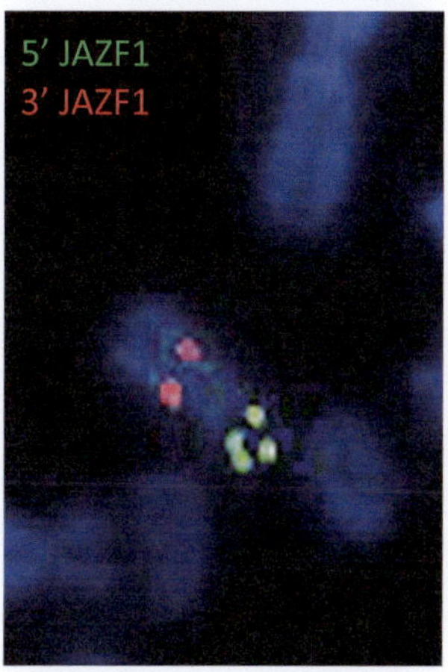

Fig. 11.6 Fluorescence in situ hybridization (*FISH*) for JAZF1. This is a break apart FISH using the 5′ end of JAZF1 (*green*) and the 3′ end of JAZF1 (*red*). When the JAZF1 locus is intact, the probes overlap producing a *yellow* signal. In the example, the signals are separated, indicating a break in the gene, consistent with a rearrangement

subset of LGESS with conventional karyotyping has no evidence of chromosomal rearrangements, as well as no evidence of *JAZF1* or *PHF1* gene fusions by RT-PCR or FISH, suggesting that some of the molecular alterations in these tumors have not yet been discovered or may be too small to detect with these methods.

It is important to remember, particularly when dealing with tumors occurring outside of the uterus, that *JAZF1* and the other described EST-associated gene rearrangements are not necessarily specific for ESS. *JAZF1* rearrangement has been documented in at least one cardiac sarcoma [101], and many of the other described gene fusions involving *PHF1*, *EPC1*, and *BCOR* have been described in a significant number of ossifying fibromyxoid tumors [102].

Other Molecular Characterizations of ESN and LGESS

Deletion of 7p has been shown in >50% of ESS by array CGH [103]. Loss of heterozygosity studies are conflicting, with some reports of loss of heterozygosity in some tumor suppressor genes (including *PTEN*, *TP53*, and *BRCA*) in at least a subset of ESS [104, 105], while others found no evidence for loss of heterozygosity in ESS.

Studies have interrogated for *APC*, *CTNNB1*, *KIT*, *EGFR*, and *PDGFR* mutations, as well as amplification of *EGFR* in ESS; none of the tumors included in the studies had any molecular aberration in these genes [106, 107]. *TP53* mutations and microsatellite instability are not features of ESS [105, 108].

High-Grade Endometrial Stromal Sarcoma (HGESS)

The discovery of recurrent *YWHAE-FAM22A/B* gene fusions in a subset of endometrial stromal sarcomas that are associated with a clinical outcome intermediate between that of LGESS and undifferentiated uterine sarcoma has led to the reintroduction of high-grade ESS (HGESS) in the most recent WHO blue book [21, 109, 110]. These tumors lack the typical morphology of EST in that they do not resemble non-neoplastic endometrium, lack CD10 expression, and have high-grade atypia (Fig. 11.7). In some cases (but not all), these tumors appear to be associated with more typical appearing areas of LGESS [111, 112]. *YWHAE* rearrangements have not been found in other gynecologic tumors and FISH, and/or RT-PCR studies may serve as a useful adjunct to the histologic diagnosis [113, 114]. CyclinD1 immunohistochemistry may be used as a marker for *YWHAE* rearrangement [88, 112], although this is not entirely sensitive or specific, particularly when considering undifferentiated endometrial carcinoma and tumors outside the gynecologic tract (clear cell sarcoma of kidney) [115–118].

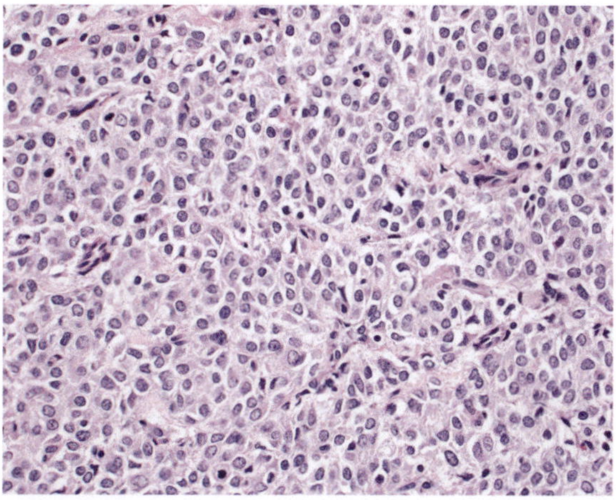

Fig. 11.7 High-grade endometrial stromal sarcoma is composed of uniform, plump, epithelioid cells

Other Molecular Features of HGESS

Based on immunohistochemical studies, there is no evidence of *TP53* mutation (via protein overexpression or complete lack of expression) in ESS. [114]

Undifferentiated Uterine Sarcoma

Undifferentiated uterine sarcoma (UUS) is a heterogeneous group of tumors, and to some degree may represent various dedifferentiated forms of specific uterine sarcomas (adenosarcoma, endometrial stromal sarcoma, carcinosarcoma, leiomyosarcoma, etc.). This is supported by the finding of small subsets of UUS harboring genetic alterations characteristic of LMS, or alternatively harboring gene fusions reported in ESS [119]. Regardless, these tumors have lost any morphologic evidence of differentiation and tend to be histologically pleomorphic and cytogenetically complex [103]. In practice, the diagnosis of UUS should only be made after extensive sampling of the tumor, to exclude a recognizable line of differentiation that aids the diagnosis. *TP53* mutations are not uncommon in UUS, in contrast to endometrial stromal neoplasms [119], suggesting that those UUS with *TP53* mutation have no relationship with ESS, or that they have acquired a secondary *TP53* mutation.

One study interrogated for *KIT*, *EGFR*, and *PDGFR* hot spot mutations, as well as amplification of *EGFR* in UUS; none of the tumors included in this study had any molecular aberration in these genes [107]. In an array CGH study on endometrial sarcomas, a large number of copy number alterations in UUS are described, including gain of 7p in a subset [103].

A small subset of what has been previously published as undifferentiated uterine sarcoma ("uniform type") may harbor *YWHAE* rearrangement, which raises the possibility that some UUS represent dedifferentiated ESS.

Uterine Tumor Resembling Ovarian Sex Cord Tumor (UTROSCT)

UTROSCT is a rare tumor of the uterus that morphologically resembles various components of sex cord stromal differentiation typically seen in the ovary [120–122] (Fig. 11.8), including Sertoli cell, granulosa cell, and Leydig cell differentiation. These tumors are typically recognizable on histologic grounds, and immunohistochemically they are positive for inhibin and CD99 among other markers [121–126]. Diagnostic difficulty with this tumor typically involves distinguishing UTROSCT from other mesenchymal tumors of the uterus with sex cord differentiation.

Little is known about the molecular features of UTROSCT. The karyotype of one case has been reported, which revealed two balanced translocations t(X;6) (p22.3, q23.2) and t(4;18) (q21.1;q21.3) [127]; however, no recurrent or specific molecular alterations have been described in this tumor. UTROSCT is known to lack *JAZF1* and *PHF1* gene fusions [128–130] and also lack *FOXL2* and *DICER1* mutations [131, 132], which are mutations found in some ovarian sex cord stromal tumors.

Mullerian Adenosarcoma

Mullerian adenosarcoma (MA) is a mixed tumor of the female genital tract, containing malignant mesenchymal and benign epithelial components (Fig. 11.9), comprising <1% of all uterine tumors [133, 134]. It most frequently occurs in the uterus, but may occur anywhere within the female genital tract and even outside of the female genital tract, presumably arising from endometriosis. Various diagnostic difficulties may be associated with MA, and broadly the differential diagnosis may include benign endometrial polyps, embryonal rhabdomyosarcoma,

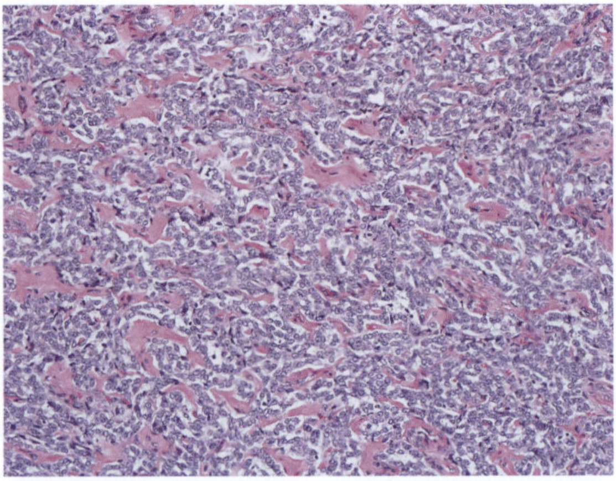

Fig. 11.8 Uterine tumor resembling ovarian sex cord tumor (*UTROSCT*) may demonstrate a variety of patterns, all mimicking various ovarian sex cord stromal tumors. In this example, the nuclei are bland, overlapping, and demonstrate nuclear grooves

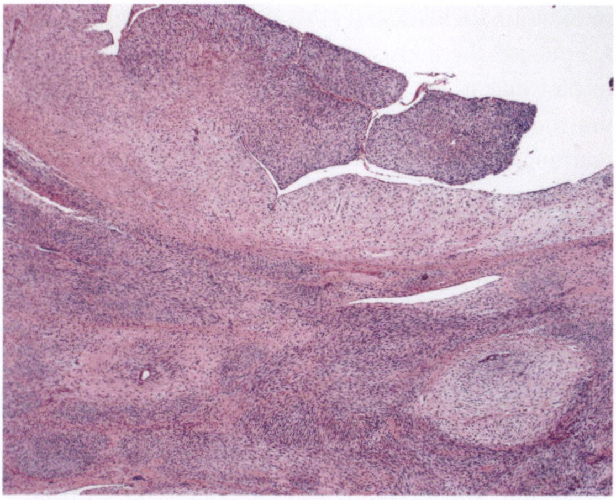

Fig. 11.9 Mullerian adenosarcoma is characterized by broad leaf-life projections into cystic spaces, stromal condensation under the epithelial component, and variable cytologic atypia and mitotic rate

carcinosarcoma, and endometrial stromal sarcoma. There have been few studies to date on the molecular features of MA, but it is known that *TP53* mutations are uncommon in MA, and when present are almost always associated with sarcomatous overgrowth, a poor prognostic indicator [135–137]. High-level copy number gains of *MYBL1* are seen in a subset of MA, most often associated with sarcomatous overgrowth. Low-level amplification of *MDM2* has also been described in MA, unrelated to sarcomatous overgrowth. *ATRX* mutations were identified in a subset of MA, which may be associated with loss of expression of ATRX by IHC. Other recurrent mutations described in MA include *FGFR2*, *KMT2C*, and *DICER1*, with *DICER1* mutations present only in MA exhibiting rhabdomyosarcoma differentiation [136]. Few gene fusions have been described in MA, but small numbers of cases with *NCOA2/3* expressed gene fusions have been described [136]. Further studies are warranted to further elucidate the molecular characteristics of MA with diagnostic and prognostic significance.

Inflammatory Myofibroblastic Tumor

Inflammatory myofibroblastic tumor (IMT) is more commonly seen in extra-uterine sites [138], but has been described in the uterus [139]. It was initially thought to represent a reactive, "pseudo-neoplastic" process, but has since been shown to be neoplastic with potential for aggressive clinical behavior. Histologically, IMT is characterized by frequent myxoid stroma and a mixture of spindled (predominant) and epithelioid tumor cells admixed with a variable number of inflammatory cells (typically plasma cells and lymphocytes). There can be significant morphologic overlap with myxoid LMS and other smooth muscle neoplasms. The molecular alteration most characteristic for IMT is rearrangement of the *ALK* gene at 2p23. This results in overexpression of ALK that may be detected by immunohistochemistry [140–143]. Although ALK-negative IMT is readily accepted outside the uterus, ALK-negative IMTs have rarely been described in the uterus, in part due to morphologic overlap and inability to reliably distinguish IMT from the much more common uterine smooth muscle tumors [140]. Similarly, *ROS1*-rearranged IMT has been described in other viscera/soft tissue sites, but has yet to be documented in the uterus [144, 145].

Embryonal Rhabdomyosarcoma

Embryonal rhabdomyosarcoma (ERMS) is an uncommon uterine tumor that most frequently occurs in the uterine cervix [146–148]. Histologically, it has similar features to embryonal rhabdomyosarcoma of soft tissue and other sites; namely, alternating hypocellular and hypercellular primitive appearing spindled cells that frequently condense underneath surface epithelium to form a "cambium" layer. Tumor cells may demonstrate striation ("strap" cells), and often islands of cartilaginous differentiation may be present. This tumor may be difficult to recognize, particularly in older women, and there can be morphologic overlap with adenosarcoma and poorly sampled carcinosarcoma, both of which may have rhabdomyosarcomatous differentiation. The only well-characterized molecular alteration in ERMS is *DICER1* mutation, which may occur as either germline or somatic inactivation [148–151]. *DICER1* is involved in miRNA processing and its inactivation is likely a key step in the pathogenesis of ERMS. No studies to date have evaluated for the presence of *DICER1* mutations in other tumors demonstrating rhabdomyosarcomatous differentiation, aside from the aforementioned adenosarcoma [136].

Other

A number of other mesenchymal tumors may occur in the uterus, such as solitary fibrous tumor [152–155], Ewings/PNET [156–167], synovial sarcoma [168], and alveolar soft part sarcoma [169–178], among others. These tumors appear to share the same molecular alterations as those occurring in soft tissue and other anatomic sites, and thus will not be discussed in greater detail.

References

1. Makinen N, Mehine M, Tolvanen J, et al. MED12, the mediator complex subunit 12 gene, is mutated at high frequency in uterine leiomyomas. Science. 2011;334:252–5.
2. Schwetye KE, Pfeifer JD, Duncavage EJ. MED12 exon 2 mutations in uterine and extrauterine smooth muscle tumors. Hum Pathol. 2014;45:65–70.

3. Bertsch E, Qiang W, Zhang Q, et al. MED12 and HMGA2 mutations: two independent genetic events in uterine leiomyoma and leiomyosarcoma. Mod Pathol. 2014;27:1144–53.
4. Zhang Q, Ubago J, Li L, et al. Molecular analyses of 6 different types of uterine smooth muscle tumors: Emphasis in atypical leiomyoma. Cancer. 2014;120:3165–77.
5. Matsubara A, Sekine S, Yoshida M, et al. Prevalence of MED12 mutations in uterine and extrauterine smooth muscle tumours. Histopathology. 2013;62:657–61.
6. Markowski DN, Huhle S, Nimzyk R, et al. MED12 mutations occurring in benign and malignant mammalian smooth muscle tumors. Genes Chromosomes Cancer. 2013;52: 297–304.
7. Mehine M, Kaasinen E, Makinen N, et al. Characterization of uterine leiomyomas by whole-genome sequencing. N Engl J Med. 2013;369:43–53.
8. Fletcher JA, Morton CC, Pavelka K, et al. Chromosome aberrations in uterine smooth muscle tumors: potential diagnostic relevance of cytogenetic instability. Cancer Res. 1990;50:4092–7.
9. Hodge JC, Morton CC. Genetic heterogeneity among uterine leiomyomata: insights into malignant progression. Hum Mol Genet. 2007;16(Spec No 1):R7-13.
10. Pandis N, Heim S, Bardi G, et al. Chromosome analysis of 96 uterine leiomyomas. Cancer Genet Cytogenet. 1991;55:11–8.
11. Nilbert M, Heim S, Mandahl N, et al. Characteristic chromosome abnormalities, including rearrangements of 6p, del(7q), +12, and t(12;14), in 44 uterine leiomyomas. Hum Genet. 1990;85:605–11.
12. Nibert M, Heim S. Uterine leiomyoma cytogenetics. Genes Chromosomes Cancer. 1990;2:3–13.
13. Levy B, Mukherjee T, Hirschhorn K. Molecular cytogenetic analysis of uterine leiomyoma and leiomyosarcoma by comparative genomic hybridization. Cancer Genet Cytogenet. 2000;121:1–8.
14. Xing YP, Powell WL, Morton CC. The del(7q) subgroup in uterine leiomyomata: genetic and biologic characteristics. Further evidence for the secondary nature of cytogenetic abnormalities in the pathobiology of uterine leiomyomata. Cancer Genet Cytogenet. 1997;98:69–74.
15. Ozisik YY, Meloni AM, Surti U, et al. Deletion 7q22 in uterine leiomyoma. A cytogenetic review. Cancer Genet Cytogenet. 1993;71:1–6.
16. Sargent MS, Weremowicz S, Rein MS, et al. Translocations in 7q22 define a critical region in uterine leiomyomata. Cancer Genet Cytogenet. 1994;77:65–8.
17. Makinen N, Vahteristo P, Kampjarvi K, et al. MED12 exon 2 mutations in histopathological uterine leiomyoma variants. Eur J Hum Genet. 2013;21:1300–3.
18. Hodge JC, Pearce KE, Clayton AC, et al. Uterine cellular leiomyomata with chromosome 1p deletions represent a distinct entity. Am J Obstet Gynecol. 2014;210(572):e571–7.
19. Moore SD, Herrick SR, Ince TA, et al. Uterine leiomyomata with t(10;17) disrupt the histone acetyltransferase MORF. Cancer Res. 2004;64:5570–7.
20. Bell SW, Kempson RL, Hendrickson MR. Problematic uterine smooth muscle neoplasms. A clinicopathologic study of 213 cases. Am J Surg Pathol. 1994;18:535–58.
21. Kurman RJ, Carcangiu ML, Herrington CS, Young RH. WHO classification of tumours of female reproductive organs. 4th ed. IARC: Lyon, France. 2014;135–150.
22. Tomlinson IP, Alam NA, Rowan AJ, et al. Germline mutations in FH predispose to dominantly inherited uterine fibroids, skin leiomyomata and papillary renal cell cancer. Nat Genet. 2002;30:406–10.
23. Joseph NM, Solomon DA, Frizzell N, et al. Morphology and immunohistochemistry for 2SC and FH aid in detection of fumarate hydratase gene aberrations in uterine leiomyomas from young patients. Am J Surg Pathol. 2015;39:1529–39.
24. Sanz-Ortega J, Vocke C, Stratton P, et al. Morphologic and molecular characteristics of uterine leiomyomas in hereditary leiomyomatosis and renal cancer (HLRCC) syndrome. Am J Surg Pathol. 2013;37:74–80.

25. Reyes C, Karamurzin Y, Frizzell N, et al. Uterine smooth muscle tumors with features suggesting fumarate hydratase aberration: detailed morphologic analysis and correlation with S-(2-succino)-cysteine immunohistochemistry. Mod Pathol. 2014;27:1020–7.
26. Alsolami S, El-Bahrawy M, Kalloger SE, et al. Current morphologic criteria perform poorly in identifying hereditary leiomyomatosis and renal cell carcinoma syndrome-associated uterine leiomyomas. Int J Gynecol Pathol. 2014;33:560–7.
27. Lehtonen R, Kiuru M, Vanharanta S, et al. Biallelic inactivation of fumarate hydratase (FH) occurs in nonsyndromic uterine leiomyomas but is rare in other tumors. Am J Pathol. 2004;164:17–22.
28. Mittal KR, Chen F, Wei JJ, et al. Molecular and immunohistochemical evidence for the origin of uterine leiomyosarcomas from associated leiomyoma and symplastic leiomyoma-like areas. Mod Pathol. 2009;22:1303–11.
29. Mittal K, Popiolek D, Demopoulos RI. Uterine myxoid leiomyosarcoma within a leiomyoma. Hum Pathol. 2000;31:398–400.
30. Quade BJ, Pinto AP, Howard DR, et al. Frequent loss of heterozygosity for chromosome 10 in uterine leiomyosarcoma in contrast to leiomyoma. Am J Pathol. 1999;154:945–50.
31. Hu J, Khanna V, Jones M, et al. Genomic alterations in uterine leiomyosarcomas: potential markers for clinical diagnosis and prognosis. Genes Chromosomes Cancer. 2001;31:117–24.
32. Packenham JP, du Manoir S, Schrock E, et al. Analysis of genetic alterations in uterine leiomyomas and leiomyosarcomas by comparative genomic hybridization. Mol Carcinog. 1997;19:273–9.
33. Agaram NP, Zhang L, LeLoarer F, et al. Targeted exome sequencing profiles genetic alterations in leiomyosarcoma. Genes Chromoso Cancer. 2016;55(2):124–30.
34. Ravegnini G, Marino-Enriquez A, Slater J, et al. MED12 mutations in leiomyosarcoma and extrauterine leiomyoma. Mod Pathol. 2013;26:743–9.
35. Liau JY, Tsai JH, Jeng YM, et al. Leiomyosarcoma with alternative lengthening of telomeres is associated with aggressive histologic features, loss of ATRX expression, and poor clinical outcome. Am J Surg Pathol. 2015;39:236–44.
36. Perot G, Croce S, Ribeiro A, et al. MED12 alterations in both human benign and malignant uterine soft tissue tumors. PLoS ONE. 2012;7:e40015.
37. Kampjarvi K, Makinen N, Kilpivaara O, et al. Somatic MED12 mutations in uterine leiomyosarcoma and colorectal cancer. Br J Cancer. 2012;107:1761–5.
38. de Graaff MA, de Jong D, Briaire-de Bruijn IH, et al. A translocation t(6;14) in two cases of leiomyosarcoma: Molecular cytogenetic and array-based comparative genomic hybridization characterization. Cancer Genet. 2015;208:537–44.
39. Liau JY, Lee JC, Tsai JH, et al. Comprehensive screening of alternative lengthening of telomeres phenotype and loss of ATRX expression in sarcomas. Mod Pathol. 2015;28: 1545–54.
40. Brewer Savannah KJ, Demicco EG, Lusby K, et al. Dual targeting of mTOR and aurora-A kinase for the treatment of uterine Leiomyosarcoma. Clin Cancer Res. 2012;18:4633–45.
41. Gibault L, Ferreira C, Perot G, et al. From PTEN loss of expression to RICTOR role in smooth muscle differentiation: complex involvement of the mTOR pathway in leiomyosarcomas and pleomorphic sarcomas. Mod Pathol. 2012;25:197–211.
42. Dhingra S, Rodriguez ME, Shen Q, et al. Constitutive activation with overexpression of the mTORC2-phospholipase D1 pathway in uterine leiomyosarcoma and STUMP: morphoproteomic analysis with therapeutic implications. Int J Clin Exp Pathol. 2011;4:134–46.
43. Dal Cin P, Quade BJ, Neskey DM, et al. Intravenous leiomyomatosis is characterized by a der(14)t(12;14) (q15;q24). Genes Chromosomes Cancer. 2003;36:205–6.
44. Quade BJ, Dal Cin P, Neskey DM, et al. Intravenous leiomyomatosis: molecular and cytogenetic analysis of a case. Mod Pathol. 2002;15:351–6.
45. Buza N, Xu F, Wu W, et al. Recurrent chromosomal aberrations in intravenous leiomyomatosis of the uterus: high-resolution array comparative genomic hybridization study. Hum Pathol. 2014;45:1885–92.

46. Ordulu Z, Nucci MR, Dal Cin P, et al. Intravenous leiomyomatosis: an unusual intermediate between benign and malignant uterine smooth muscle tumors. Mod Pathol. 2016;29:500–10.
47. Patton KT, Cheng L, Papavero V, et al. Benign metastasizing leiomyoma: clonality, telomere length and clinicopathologic analysis. Mod Pathol. 2006;19:130–40.
48. Tietze L, Gunther K, Horbe A, et al. Benign metastasizing leiomyoma: a cytogenetically balanced but clonal disease. Hum Pathol. 2000;31:126–8.
49. Nucci MR, Drapkin R, Dal Cin P, et al. Distinctive cytogenetic profile in benign metastasizing leiomyoma: pathogenetic implications. Am J Surg Pathol. 2007;31:737–43.
50. Lin J, Song X, Liu C. Pelvic intravascular leiomyomatosis associated with benign pulmonary metastasizing leiomyoma: clinicopathologic, clonality, and copy number variance analysis. Int J Gynecol Pathol. 2014;33:140–5.
51. Silva EG, Bodurka DC, Scouros MA, et al. A uterine leiomyosarcoma that became positive for HMB45 in the metastasis. Ann Diagn Pathol. 2005;9:43–5.
52. Silva EG, Tornos C, Ordonez NG, et al. Uterine leiomyosarcoma with clear cell areas. Int J Gynecol Pathol. 1995;14:174–8.
53. Silva EG, Deavers MT, Bodurka DC, et al. Uterine epithelioid leiomyosarcomas with clear cells: reactivity with HMB-45 and the concept of PEComa. Am J Surg Pathol. 2004;28: 244–9.
54. Vang R, Kempson RL. Perivascular epithelioid cell tumor ('PEComa') of the uterus: a subset of HMB-45-positive epithelioid mesenchymal neoplasms with an uncertain relationship to pure smooth muscle tumors. Am J Surg Pathol. 2002;26:1–13.
55. Simpson KW, Albores-Saavedra J. HMB-45 reactivity in conventional uterine leiomyosarcomas. Am J Surg Pathol. 2007;31:95–8.
56. Ruco LP, Pilozzi E, Wedard BM, et al. Epithelioid lymphangioleiomyomatosis-like tumour of the uterus in a patient without tuberous sclerosis: a lesion mimicking epithelioid leiomyosarcoma. Histopathology. 1998;33:91–3.
57. Michal M, Zamecnik M. Hyalinized uterine mesenchymal neoplasms with hmb-45-positive epithelioid cells: epithelioid leiomyomas or angiomyolipomas? Report of four cases. Int J Surg Pathol. 2000;8:323–8.
58. Kenerson H, Folpe AL, Takayama TK, et al. Activation of the mTOR pathway in sporadic angiomyolipomas and other perivascular epithelioid cell neoplasms. Hum Pathol. 2007;38:1361–71.
59. Ghosh I, Arun I, Sen S, et al. Metastatic perivascular epithelioid cell tumor responding to mammalian target of rapamycin inhibition. Indian J Med Paediatr Oncol. 2014;35:99–102.
60. Wagner AJ, Malinowska-Kolodziej I, Morgan JA, et al. Clinical activity of mTOR inhibition with sirolimus in malignant perivascular epithelioid cell tumors: targeting the pathogenic activation of mTORC1 in tumors. J Clin Oncol. 2010;28:835–40.
61. Benson C, Vitfell-Rasmussen J, Maruzzo M, et al. A retrospective study of patients with malignant PEComa receiving treatment with sirolimus or temsirolimus: the Royal Marsden Hospital experience. Anticancer Res. 2014;34:3663–8.
62. Dickson MA, Schwartz GK, Antonescu CR, et al. Extrarenal perivascular epithelioid cell tumors (PEComas) respond to mTOR inhibition: clinical and molecular correlates. Int J Cancer. 2013;132:1711–7.
63. Pan CC, Jong YJ, Chai CY, et al. Comparative genomic hybridization study of perivascular epithelioid cell tumor: molecular genetic evidence of perivascular epithelioid cell tumor as a distinctive neoplasm. Hum Pathol. 2006;37:606–12.
64. Bosincu L, Rocca PC, Martignoni G, et al. Perivascular epithelioid cell (PEC) tumors of the uterus: a clinicopathologic study of two cases with aggressive features. Mod Pathol. 2005;18:1336–42.
65. Conlon N, Soslow RA, Murali R. Perivascular epithelioid tumours (PEComas) of the gynaecological tract. J Clin Pathol. 2015;68:418–26.
66. Argani P, Aulmann S, Karanjawala Z, et al. Melanotic Xp11 translocation renal cancers: a distinctive neoplasm with overlapping features of PEComa, carcinoma, and melanoma. Am J Surg Pathol. 2009;33:609–19.

67. Liu F, Zhang R, Wang ZY, et al. Malignant perivascular epithelioid cell tumor (PEComa) of cervix with TFE3 gene rearrangement: a case report. Int J Clin Exp Pathol. 2014;7:6409–14.
68. Shen Q, Rao Q, Xia QY, et al. Perivascular epithelioid cell tumor (PEComa) with TFE3 gene rearrangement: clinicopathological, immunohistochemical, and molecular features. Virchows Arch. 2014;465:607–13.
69. Schoolmeester JK, Howitt BE, Hirsch MS, et al. Perivascular epithelioid cell neoplasm (PEComa) of the gynecologic tract: clinicopathologic and immunohistochemical characterization of 16 cases. Am J Surg Pathol. 2014;38:176–88.
70. Schoolmeester JK, Dao LN, Sukov WR, et al. TFE3 translocation-associated perivascular epithelioid cell neoplasm (PEComa) of the gynecologic tract: morphology, immunophenotype, differential diagnosis. Am J Surg Pathol. 2015;39:394–404.
71. Agaram NP, Sung YS, Zhang L, et al. Dichotomy of genetic abnormalities in PEComas with therapeutic implications. Am J Surg Pathol. 2015;39:813–25.
72. Malinowska I, Kwiatkowski DJ, Weiss S, et al. Perivascular epithelioid cell tumors (PEComas) harboring TFE3 gene rearrangements lack the TSC2 alterations characteristic of conventional PEComas: further evidence for a biological distinction. Am J Surg Pathol. 2012;36:783–4.
73. Rao Q, Shen Q, Xia QY, et al. PSF/SFPQ is a very common gene fusion partner in TFE3 rearrangement-associated perivascular epithelioid cell tumors (PEComas) and melanotic Xp11 translocation renal cancers: clinicopathologic, immunohistochemical, and molecular characteristics suggesting classification as a distinct entity. Am J Surg Pathol. 2015;39:1181–96.
74. Tanaka M, Kato K, Gomi K, et al. Perivascular epithelioid cell tumor with SFPQ/PSF-TFE3 gene fusion in a patient with advanced neuroblastoma. Am J Surg Pathol. 2009;33:1416–20.
75. Conklin CM, Longacre TA. Endometrial stromal tumors: the new WHO classification. Adv Anat Pathol. 2014;21:383–93.
76. Baker P, Oliva E. Endometrial stromal tumours of the uterus: a practical approach using conventional morphology and ancillary techniques. J Clin Pathol. 2007;60:235–43.
77. Dionigi A, Oliva E, Clement PB, et al. Endometrial stromal nodules and endometrial stromal tumors with limited infiltration: a clinicopathologic study of 50 cases. Am J Surg Pathol. 2002;26:567–81.
78. Tavassoli FA, Norris HJ. Mesenchymal tumours of the uterus. VII. A clinicopathological study of 60 endometrial stromal nodules. Histopathology. 1981;5:1–10.
79. McCluggage WG, Date A, Bharucha H, et al. Endometrial stromal sarcoma with sex cord-like areas and focal rhabdoid differentiation. Histopathology. 1996;29:369–74.
80. Oliva E, Clement PB, Young RH, et al. Mixed endometrial stromal and smooth muscle tumors of the uterus: a clinicopathologic study of 15 cases. Am J Surg Pathol. 1998;22:997–1005.
81. Hrzenjak A, Moinfar F, Tavassoli FA, et al. JAZF1/JJAZ1 gene fusion in endometrial stromal sarcomas: molecular analysis by reverse transcriptase-polymerase chain reaction optimized for paraffin-embedded tissue. J Mol Diagn. 2005;7:388–95.
82. Nucci MR, Harburger D, Koontz J, et al. Molecular analysis of the JAZF1-JJAZ1 gene fusion by RT-PCR and fluorescence in situ hybridization in endometrial stromal neoplasms. Am J Surg Pathol. 2007;31:65–70.
83. Koontz JI, Soreng AL, Nucci M, et al. Frequent fusion of the JAZF1 and JJAZ1 genes in endometrial stromal tumors. Proc Natl Acad Sci U S A. 2001;98:6348–53.
84. Micci F, Walter CU, Teixeira MR, et al. Cytogenetic and molecular genetic analyses of endometrial stromal sarcoma: nonrandom involvement of chromosome arms 6p and 7p and confirmation of JAZF1/JJAZ1 gene fusion in t(7;17). Cancer Genet Cytogenet. 2003;144:119–24.
85. Huang HY, Ladanyi M, Soslow RA. Molecular detection of JAZF1-JJAZ1 gene fusion in endometrial stromal neoplasms with classic and variant histology: evidence for genetic heterogeneity. Am J Surg Pathol. 2004;28:224–32.

86. Oliva E, de Leval L, Soslow RA, et al. High frequency of JAZF1-JJAZ1 gene fusion in endometrial stromal tumors with smooth muscle differentiation by interphase FISH detection. Am J Surg Pathol. 2007;31:1277–84.
87. Chiang S, Ali R, Melnyk N, et al. Frequency of known gene rearrangements in endometrial stromal tumors. Am J Surg Pathol. 2011;35:1364–72.
88. Stewart CJ, Leung YC, Murch A, et al. Evaluation of fluorescence in-situ hybridization in monomorphic endometrial stromal neoplasms and their histological mimics: a review of 49 cases. Histopathology. 2014;65:473–82.
89. Sreekantaiah C, Li FP, Weidner N, et al. An endometrial stromal sarcoma with clonal cytogenetic abnormalities. Cancer Genet Cytogenet. 1991;55:163–6.
90. Dal Cin P, Aly MS, De Wever I, et al. Endometrial stromal sarcoma t(7;17) (p15-21;q12-21) is a nonrandom chromosome change. Cancer Genet Cytogenet. 1992;63:43–6.
91. Micci F, Panagopoulos I, Bjerkehagen B, et al. Consistent rearrangement of chromosomal band 6p21 with generation of fusion genes JAZF1/PHF1 and EPC1/PHF1 in endometrial stromal sarcoma. Cancer Res. 2006;66:107–12.
92. Panagopoulos I, Mertens F, Griffin CA. An endometrial stromal sarcoma cell line with the JAZF1/PHF1 chimera. Cancer Genet Cytogenet. 2008;185:74–7.
93. D'Angelo E, Ali RH, Espinosa I, et al. Endometrial stromal sarcomas with sex cord differentiation are associated with PHF1 rearrangement. Am J Surg Pathol. 2013;37:514–21.
94. Li H, Wang J, Mor G, et al. A neoplastic gene fusion mimics trans-splicing of RNAs in normal human cells. Science. 2008;321:1357–61.
95. Panagopoulos I, Micci F, Thorsen J, et al. Novel fusion of MYST/Esa1-associated factor 6 and PHF1 in endometrial stromal sarcoma. PLoS ONE. 2012;7:e39354.
96. Micci F, Gorunova L, Gatius S, et al. MEAF6/PHF1 is a recurrent gene fusion in endometrial stromal sarcoma. Cancer Lett. 2014;347:75–8.
97. Ali RH, Al-Safi R, Al-Waheeb S, et al. Molecular characterization of a population-based series of endometrial stromal sarcomas in Kuwait. Hum Pathol. 2014;45:2453–62.
98. Panagopoulos I, Thorsen J, Gorunova L, et al. Fusion of the ZC3H7B and BCOR genes in endometrial stromal sarcomas carrying an X;22-translocation. Genes Chromosomes Cancer. 2013;52:610–8.
99. Dewaele B, Przybyl J, Quattrone A, et al. Identification of a novel, recurrent MBTD1-CXorf67 fusion in low-grade endometrial stromal sarcoma. Int J Cancer. 2014;134:1112–22.
100. Chiang S, Oliva E. Cytogenetic and molecular aberrations in endometrial stromal tumors. Hum Pathol. 2011;42:609–17.
101. Schoolmeester JK, Sukov WR, Maleszewski JJ, et al. JAZF1 rearrangement in a mesenchymal tumor of nonendometrial stromal origin: report of an unusual ossifying sarcoma of the heart demonstrating JAZF1/PHF1 fusion. Am J Surg Pathol. 2013;37:938–42.
102. Antonescu CR, Sung YS, Chen CL, et al. Novel ZC3H7B-BCOR, MEAF6-PHF1, and EPC1-PHF1 fusions in ossifying fibromyxoid tumors—molecular characterization shows genetic overlap with endometrial stromal sarcoma. Genes Chromosomes Cancer. 2014;53:183–93.
103. Halbwedl I, Ullmann R, Kremser ML, et al. Chromosomal alterations in low-grade endometrial stromal sarcoma and undifferentiated endometrial sarcoma as detected by comparative genomic hybridization. Gynecol Oncol. 2005;97:582–7.
104. Moinfar F, Kremser ML, Man YG, et al. Allelic imbalances in endometrial stromal neoplasms: frequent genetic alterations in the nontumorous normal-appearing endometrial and myometrial tissues. Gynecol Oncol. 2004;95:662–71.
105. Amant F, Dorfling CM, Dreyer L, et al. Microsatellite instability in uterine sarcomas. Int J Gynecol Cancer. 2001;11:218–23.
106. Kurihara S, Oda Y, Ohishi Y, et al. Coincident expression of beta-catenin and cyclin D1 in endometrial stromal tumors and related high-grade sarcomas. Mod Pathol. 2010;23:225–34.

107. Sardinha R, Hernandez T, Fraile S, et al. Endometrial stromal tumors: immunohistochemical and molecular analysis of potential targets of tyrosine kinase inhibitors. Clin Sarcoma Res. 2013;3:3.
108. Liu FS, Kohler MF, Marks JR, et al. Mutation and overexpression of the p53 tumor suppressor gene frequently occurs in uterine and ovarian sarcomas. Obstet Gynecol. 1994;83:118–24.
109. Lee CH, Nucci MR. Endometrial stromal sarcoma—the new genetic paradigm. Histopathology. 2015;67:1–19.
110. Lee CH, Ou WB, Marino-Enriquez A, et al. 14-3-3 fusion oncogenes in high-grade endometrial stromal sarcoma. Proc Natl Acad Sci U S A. 2012;109:929–34.
111. Sciallis AP, Bedroske PP, Schoolmeester JK, et al. High-grade endometrial stromal sarcomas: a clinicopathologic study of a group of tumors with heterogenous morphologic and genetic features. Am J Surg Pathol. 2014;38:1161–72.
112. Lee CH, Ali RH, Rouzbahman M, et al. Cyclin D1 as a diagnostic immunomarker for endometrial stromal sarcoma with YWHAE-FAM22 rearrangement. Am J Surg Pathol. 2012;36:1562–70.
113. Isphording A, Ali RH, Irving J, et al. YWHAE-FAM22 endometrial stromal sarcoma: diagnosis by reverse transcription-polymerase chain reaction in formalin-fixed, paraffin-embedded tumor. Hum Pathol. 2013;44:837–43.
114. Croce S, Hostein I, Ribeiro A, et al. YWHAE rearrangement identified by FISH and RT-PCR in endometrial stromal sarcomas: genetic and pathological correlations. Mod Pathol. 2013;26:1390–400.
115. O'Meara E, Stack D, Lee CH, et al. Characterization of the chromosomal translocation t (10;17) (q22;p13) in clear cell sarcoma of kidney. J Pathol. 2012;227:72–80.
116. Fehr A, Hansson MC, Kindblom LG, et al. YWHAE-FAM22 gene fusion in clear cell sarcoma of the kidney. J Pathol. 2012;227:e5–7.
117. Mirkovic J, Calicchio M, Fletcher CD, et al. Diffuse and strong cyclin D1 immunoreactivity in clear cell sarcoma of the kidney. Histopathology. 2015;67:306–12.
118. Shah VI, McCluggage WG. Cyclin D1 does not distinguish YWHAE-NUTM2 high-grade endometrial stromal sarcoma from undifferentiated endometrial carcinoma. Am J Surg Pathol. 2015;39:722–4.
119. Kurihara S, Oda Y, Ohishi Y, et al. Endometrial stromal sarcomas and related high-grade sarcomas: immunohistochemical and molecular genetic study of 31 cases. Am J Surg Pathol. 2008;32:1228–38.
120. Clement PB, Scully RE. Uterine tumors resembling ovarian sex-cord tumors. A clinicopathologic analysis of fourteen cases. Am J Clin Pathol. 1976;66:512–25.
121. Bakula-Zalewska E, Danska-Bidzinska A, Kowalewska M, et al. Uterine tumors resembling ovarian sex cord tumors, a clinicopathologic study of six cases. Ann Diagn Pathol. 2014;18:329–32.
122. de Leval L, Lim GS, Waltregny D, et al. Diverse phenotypic profile of uterine tumors resembling ovarian sex cord tumors: an immunohistochemical study of 12 cases. Am J Surg Pathol. 2010;34:1749–61.
123. Hurrell DP, McCluggage WG. Uterine tumour resembling ovarian sex cord tumour is an immunohistochemically polyphenotypic neoplasm which exhibits coexpression of epithelial, myoid and sex cord markers. J Clin Pathol. 2007;60:1148–54.
124. Irving JA, Carinelli S, Prat J. Uterine tumors resembling ovarian sex cord tumors are polyphenotypic neoplasms with true sex cord differentiation. Mod Pathol. 2006;19:17–24.
125. Oliva E, Young RH, Amin MB, et al. An immunohistochemical analysis of endometrial stromal and smooth muscle tumors of the uterus: a study of 54 cases emphasizing the importance of using a panel because of overlap in immunoreactivity for individual antibodies. Am J Surg Pathol. 2002;26:403–12.
126. Krishnamurthy S, Jungbluth AA, Busam KJ, et al. Uterine tumors resembling ovarian sex-cord tumors have an immunophenotype consistent with true sex-cord differentiation. Am J Surg Pathol. 1998;22:1078–82.

127. Wang J, Blakey GL, Zhang L, et al. Uterine tumor resembling ovarian sex cord tumor: report of a case with t(X;6) (p22.3;q23.1) and t(4;18) (q21.1;q21.3). Diagn Mol Pathol. 2003;12:174–80.
128. Staats PN, Garcia JJ, Dias-Santagata DC, et al. Uterine tumors resembling ovarian sex cord tumors (UTROSCT) lack the JAZF1-JJAZ1 translocation frequently seen in endometrial stromal tumors. Am J Surg Pathol. 2009;33:1206–12.
129. Umeda S, Tateno M, Miyagi E, et al. Uterine tumors resembling ovarian sex cord tumors (UTROSCT) with metastasis: clinicopathological study of two cases. Int J Clin Exp Pathol. 2014;7:1051–9.
130. Nucci MRSJ, Sukov W, Oliva E. Uterine Tumors Resembling Ovarian Sex Cord Tumor (UTROSCT) lack rearrangement of PHF1 by FISH. Mod Pathol. 2014;27:298A.
131. Croce S, de Kock L, Boshari T, et al. Uterine tumor resembling ovarian sex cord tumor (UTROSCT) commonly exhibits positivity with sex cord markers FOXL2 and SF-1 but lacks FOXL2 and DICER1 mutations. Int J Gynecol Pathol. 2016;35(4):301–308.
132. Chiang S, Staats PN, Senz J, et al. FOXL2 mutation is absent in uterine tumors resembling ovarian sex cord tumors. Am J Surg Pathol. 2015;39:618–23.
133. Clement PB, Scully RE. Mullerian adenosarcoma of the uterus: a clinicopathologic analysis of 100 cases with a review of the literature. Hum Pathol. 1990;21:363–81.
134. McCluggage WG. Mullerian adenosarcoma of the female genital tract. Adv Anat Pathol. 2010;17:122–9.
135. Howitt BE, Sholl LM, Dal Cin P, et al. Targeted genomic analysis of Mullerian adenosarcoma. J Pathol. 2015;235:37–49.
136. Piscuoglio S, Burke KA, Ng CK, et al. Uterine adenosarcomas are mesenchymal neoplasms. J Pathol. 2016;238:381–8.
137. Blom R, Guerrieri C. Adenosarcoma of the uterus: a clinicopathologic, DNA flow cytometric, p53 and mdm-2 analysis of 11 cases. Int J Gynecol Cancer. 1999;9:37–43.
138. Coffin CM, Watterson J, Priest JR, et al. Extrapulmonary inflammatory myofibroblastic tumor (inflammatory pseudotumor). A clinicopathologic and immunohistochemical study of 84 cases. Am J Surg Pathol. 1995;19:859–72.
139. Parra-Herran C, Quick CM, Howitt BE, et al. Inflammatory myofibroblastic tumor of the uterus: clinical and pathologic review of 10 cases including a subset with aggressive clinical course. Am J Surg Pathol. 2015;39:157–68.
140. Fuehrer NE, Keeney GL, Ketterling RP, et al. ALK-1 protein expression and ALK gene rearrangements aid in the diagnosis of inflammatory myofibroblastic tumors of the female genital tract. Arch Pathol Lab Med. 2012;136:623–6.
141. Takeuchi K, Soda M, Togashi Y, et al. Pulmonary inflammatory myofibroblastic tumor expressing a novel fusion, PPFIBP1-ALK: reappraisal of anti-ALK immunohistochemistry as a tool for novel ALK fusion identification. Clin Cancer Res. 2011;17:3341–8.
142. Sukov WR, Cheville JC, Carlson AW, et al. Utility of ALK-1 protein expression and ALK rearrangements in distinguishing inflammatory myofibroblastic tumor from malignant spindle cell lesions of the urinary bladder. Mod Pathol. 2007;20:592–603.
143. Cook JR, Dehner LP, Collins MH, et al. Anaplastic lymphoma kinase (ALK) expression in the inflammatory myofibroblastic tumor: a comparative immunohistochemical study. Am J Surg Pathol. 2001;25:1364–71.
144. Hornick JL, Sholl LM, Dal Cin P, et al. Expression of ROS1 predicts ROS1 gene rearrangement in inflammatory myofibroblastic tumors. Mod Pathol. 2015;28:732–9.
145. Antonescu CR, Suurmeijer AJ, Zhang L, et al. Molecular characterization of inflammatory myofibroblastic tumors with frequent ALK and ROS1 gene fusions and rare novel RET rearrangement. Am J Surg Pathol. 2015;39:957–67.
146. Li RF, Gupta M, McCluggage WG, et al. Embryonal rhabdomyosarcoma (botryoid type) of the uterine corpus and cervix in adult women: report of a case series and review of the literature. Am J Surg Pathol. 2013;37:344–55.

147. McCluggage WG, Lioe TF, McClelland HR, et al. Rhabdomyosarcoma of the uterus: report of two cases, including one of the spindle cell variant. Int J Gynecol Cancer. 2002;12: 128–32.
148. Dehner LP, Jarzembowski JA, Hill DA. Embryonal rhabdomyosarcoma of the uterine cervix: a report of 14 cases and a discussion of its unusual clinicopathological associations. Mod Pathol. 2012;25:602–14.
149. Foulkes WD, Bahubeshi A, Hamel N, et al. Extending the phenotypes associated with DICER1 mutations. Hum Mutat. 2011;32:1381–4.
150. Heravi-Moussavi A, Anglesio MS, Cheng SW, et al. Recurrent somatic DICER1 mutations in nonepithelial ovarian cancers. N Engl J Med. 2012;366:234–42.
151. Doros L, Yang J, Dehner L, et al. DICER1 mutations in embryonal rhabdomyosarcomas from children with and without familial PPB-tumor predisposition syndrome. Pediatr Blood Cancer. 2012;59:558–60.
152. Strickland KC, Nucci MR, Esselen KM, et al. Solitary fibrous tumor of the uterus presenting with lung metastases: a case report. Int J Gynecol Pathol. 2016;35(1):25–9.
153. Yang EHB, Nucci MR. Solitary fibrous tumor of the female genital tract: a clinicopathologic analysis of 6 cases. Mod Pathol. 2015;28:316A.
154. Casanova J, Vizcaino JR, Pinto F, et al. Abdominal mass mimicking a leiomyoma: malignant uterine solitary fibrous tumor. Gynecol Oncol Case Rep. 2012;2:143–5.
155. Chu PW, Liu JY, Peng YJ, et al. Solitary fibrous tumor of the uterus. Taiwan J Obstet Gynecol. 2006;45:350–2.
156. Daya D, Lukka H, Clement PB. Primitive neuroectodermal tumors of the uterus: a report of four cases. Hum Pathol. 1992;23:1120–9.
157. Sorensen JB, Schultze HR, Madsen EL, et al. Primitive neuroectodermal tumor (PNET) of the uterine cavity. Eur J Obstet Gynecol Reprod Biol. 1998;76:181–4.
158. Ng SB, Sirrampalam K, Chuah KL. Primitive neuroectodermal tumours of the uterus: a case report with cytological correlation and review of the literature. Pathology. 2002;34:455–61.
159. Odunsi K, Olatinwo M, Collins Y, et al. Primary primitive neuroectodermal tumor of the uterus: a report of two cases and review of the literature. Gynecol Oncol. 2004;92:689–96.
160. Varghese L, Arnesen M, Boente M. Primitive neuroectodermal tumor of the uterus: a case report and review of literature. Int J Gynecol Pathol. 2006;25:373–7.
161. Mittal S, Sumana G, Gupta M, et al. Primitive neuroectodermal tumor of the uterus: a case report. Int J Gynecol Cancer. 2007;17:524–7.
162. Blattner JM, Gable P, Quigley MM, et al. Primitive neuroectodermal tumor of the uterus. Gynecol Oncol. 2007;106:419–22.
163. Park JY, Lee S, Kang HJ, et al. Primary Ewing's sarcoma-primitive neuroectodermal tumor of the uterus: a case report and literature review. Gynecol Oncol. 2007;106:427–32.
164. Yi T, Wang P, Lin L, et al. Ewing's sarcoma/peripheral primitive neuroectodermal tumors of the uterus confirmed with fluorescence in situ hybridization in a 29-year-old Chinese female: a case report and published work review. J Obstet Gynaecol Res. 2015;41:478–82.
165. Kathuria K, Gupta S, Maheshwari A, et al. Primary primitive neuroectodermal tumor of the uterus: a case report with an unusual molecular pathology finding. J Cancer Res Ther. 2011;7:488–90.
166. Ren YL, Tang XY, Li T. Ewing sarcoma-primitive neuroectodermal tumor of the uterus: a clinicopathologic, immunohistochemical and ultrastructural study of one case. Arch Gynecol Obstet. 2011;283:1139–43.
167. Majeed U, Ilyas MA, Uddin N, et al. Primary Ewing's sarcoma–primitive neuroectodermal tumour of uterus. J Obstet Gynaecol. 2009;29:73–4.
168. Dundr P, Fischerova D, Povysil C, et al. Primary synovial sarcoma of the uterus. Pathol Oncol Res. 2012;18:529–33.
169. Burch DJ, Hitchcock A, Masson GM. Alveolar soft part sarcoma of the uterus: case report and review of the literature. Gynecol Oncol. 1994;54:91–4.
170. Nolan NP, Gaffney EF. Alveolar soft part sarcoma of the uterus. Histopathology. 1990;16:97–9.

171. Gray GF Jr, Glick AD, Kurtin PJ, et al. Alveolar soft part sarcoma of the uterus. Hum Pathol. 1986;17:297–300.
172. Roma AA, Yang B, Senior ME, et al. TFE3 immunoreactivity in alveolar soft part sarcoma of the uterine cervix: case report. Int J Gynecol Pathol. 2005;24:131–5.
173. Radig K, Buhtz P, Roessner A. Alveolar soft part sarcoma of the uterine corpus. Report of two cases and review of the literature. Pathol Res Pract. 1998;194:59–63.
174. Guillou L, Lamoureux E, Masse S, et al. Alveolar soft-part sarcoma of the uterine corpus: histological, immunocytochemical and ultrastructural study of a case. Virchows Arch A Pathol Anat Histopathol. 1991;418:467–71.
175. Sahin AA, Silva EG, Ordonez NG. Alveolar soft part sarcoma of the uterine cervix. Mod Pathol. 1989;2:676–80.
176. Abeler V, Nesland JM. Alveolar soft-part sarcoma in the uterine cervix. Arch Pathol Lab Med. 1989;113:1179–83.
177. Flint A, Gikas PW, Roberts JA. Alveolar soft part sarcoma of the uterine cervix. Gynecol Oncol. 1985;22:263–7.
178. Schoolmeester JKOE, Keeney G, Carlson J, Fritchie K, Young R, Nucci MR. Alveolar soft part sarcoma of the female genital tract: an immunohistochemical and molecular cytogenetic study. Mod Pathol. 2015;28:305A.

Part IV
Cervical Carcinomas

Chapter 12
Molecular Pathology of Cervical Dysplasia and Carcinoma

Yimin Ge and Ming Guo

The incidence of cervical cancer and its associated mortality rate have declined significantly over the past 40 years in developed countries, primarily due to successful screening using the Papanicolaou test. Once the most common cancer affecting women in the USA, in 2011, the number of new cases dropped to 12,109 with 4092 deaths [1]. However, globally, cervical cancer still remains a significant threat to women's health, especially in regions with lower average income and fewer resources such as sub-Saharan Africa. Cervical cancer is the fourth most common cancer (after breast, colorectal, and lung cancers) and the fourth most common cause of cancer death for women (266,000 deaths in 2012), with 528,000 new cases diagnosed worldwide each year [2]. Most strikingly, there is an 18-fold variation in mortality rates between different regions of the world, with nearly nine of ten deaths (87%) due to cervical cancer occurring in less developed regions [3].

The majority of cervical cancers in the USA are carcinomas (98.1%), including squamous cell carcinoma (SCC, about 65%), adenocarcinoma (about 28%), and a small fraction of uncommon histologic types [4]. In the past two decades, significant advances have been made in the prevention and treatment of cervical cancers owing to landmark findings about the causative role of human papilloma virus (HPV) in cervical cancers and precancerous lesions [5]. Virtually, all cervical cancers result from persistent infection by one or more HPV genotypes, primarily those classified by the International Agency for Research on Cancer (IARC) as groups 1 and 2a (conventionally referred as high-risk HPV, hrHPV) [6–8]. Complex genetic and

Y. Ge (✉)
Department of Pathology and Genomic Medicine, Houston Methodist Hospital, Houston, TX, USA
e-mail: yge@houstonmethodist.org

M. Guo
Pathology, University of Texas MD Anderson Cancer Center, Houston, TX, USA
e-mail: MGuo@mdanderson.org

M.T. Deavers and D.M. Coffey (eds.), *Precision Molecular Pathology of Uterine Cancer*, Molecular Pathology Library,
DOI 10.1007/978-3-319-57985-6_12

epigenetic changes occur as a result of HPV infection leading to the transformation of cervical epithelial cells to precancerous lesions and eventually to cancer.

HPV vaccines promise to have a dramatic impact on the development of precancerous cervical lesions and the prevention of cervical cancer. Both bivalent (Cervarix) and quadrivalent (Gardasil) vaccines contain L1 capsid proteins from the two most prevalent genotypes of hrHPV (16 and 18), which are responsible for more than 70% of cervical cancers worldwide. High efficacies of the vaccines against cervical precancerous lesions and cancer associated with HPV16/18 have been determined in multiple trials since the FDA initially approved the vaccines in 2006 [9–12]. In 2014, the FDA approved a nonavalent HPV vaccine (Gardasil 9), which has demonstrated equivalent protection against the four genotypes in the quadrivalent vaccine (Gardasil) and has high protective efficacy against five additional hrHPV genotypes, namely 31, 33, 45, 52, and 58. Promising results also have been obtained from trials conducted with a new generation of vaccines, including L2 vaccines with the potential advantage of broad-spectrum protection, and therapeutic vaccines targeting peptides E6 and E7 that are critical in tumorigenesis [13, 14]. The data acquired from the studies demonstrated a dramatic reduction in the rates of HPV-related cervical precancerous lesions and cancer in regions with high vaccination coverage such as Australia, where a publicly funded national HPV vaccination program has been implemented [15, 16]. Worldwide, however, low vaccination coverage rates are still recorded in many regions [17] and remain a significant challenge due to health system deficiencies and the patients' attributes [18]. The implementation of the effective two-dose scheme (rather than three doses) and the extension of vaccination to men should enhance the coverage of the population and further contain HPV-associated malignancies.

The present chapter will discuss the molecular basis of the pathogenesis, diagnosis, prognosis, prevention, and treatment of cervical cancers and their precursor lesions with an emphasis on HPV-driven neoplasms of the cervix.

Molecular Biology of Cervical Cancer and Precursor Lesions

Classification of HPV

More than 40 HPV genotypes can infect the epithelial cells of the female genital tract. In 2012, the expert working group at IARC recommended the categorization of HPV genotypes into four groups based on their carcinogenicities: carcinogenic (group 1), probably carcinogenic (group 2A), possibly carcinogenic (group 2B), and not classifiable (group 3) [19]. Among HPV-positive cervical cancers, 96% are attributed to the 13 HPV genotypes (commonly referred as hrHPV) from groups 1 and 2A, and 2.6–7% of the genotypes are from group 2B [20]. Only extremely rare cases are associated with other HPV genotypes.

Natural History of HPV Infection

HPVs are small, nonenveloped double-stranded DNA viruses that commonly infect the basal cells through micro-abrasions of the cervical mucosa. The life cycle of the virus is completed by subsequent expression of viral genes leading to viral DNA replication and release of infectious virions [21, 22]. Most infections are self-limited and cleared by the host immune system within 9–12 months [23]. However, immunity is typically short-lived and ineffective in preventing future infections by the same or different HPV genotypes [24, 25]. A small fraction of women is unable to eliminate the virus and thus becomes persistently infected by HPV; this condition can lead to genetic instability and cell transformation (discussed below).

Persistent HPV Infection and Cell Transformation

HPV infection of basal cells can maintain a stable episomal form as the viral genome is replicated in conjunction with cellular DNA during the S-phase of the cell cycle (productive infection). In this form of infection, integration of viral DNA into the host genome does not occur and infection regresses primarily through cell-mediated immune responses to the viral oncoproteins E2, E6, and E7. Immune evasion, however, leads to persistent HPV infection and cervical lesions, which are crucial steps for HPV-mediated cell transformation that is characterized by an aborted normal viral life cycle and overexpression of E6 and E7 in proliferative cells. In turn, the altered expression pattern of E6 and E7 is considered to be a consequence of viral DNA integration or methylation of viral promoters [26, 27]. Integration of viral DNA into the cellular DNA leads to the destruction of the gene encoding E2, the product of which plays a crucial role in the HPV vegetative cycle by suppressing the expression of the E6 and E7 oncoproteins [28, 29].

The primary effect of deregulated E6 and E7 expression is the degradation of the tumor suppressor genes p53 and pRb leading to uncontrolled cell proliferation [27, 30]. In addition, the oncoproteins E6 and E7 were recently found to have even broader biological effects on host cells by forming complexes with other proteins resulting in chromosomal remodeling [31–34]. Furthermore, E6 and E7 can change cell functions by altering the expression of micro-RNAs (miRNAs) [35–37]. The overall effect of E6 and E7 overexpression in proliferative cells is chromosomal instability, which is a pivotal factor for the accumulation of aberrant genes that eventually lead to malignancy.

Squamo-Columnar Junction Cells

Squamo-columnar junction (SCJ) cells are considered to be highly susceptible to HPV-mediated transformation, whereas productive infections may exclusively arise in ectocervical epithelium [38, 39]. SCJ cells have a gene expression profile including keratin 7, anterior gradient 2 (AGR2), matrix metalloproteinase 7 (MMP7), and guanine deaminase (GDA) [38]. It was demonstrated that cells with an SCJ phenotype can be found on the surface of high-grade squamous intraepithelial lesions (HSIL) that share both HPV DNA and p16 immunoreactivity [40]. Studies showed this unique profile is present in cervical cancers, most cervical intraepithelial neoplasia (CIN) 2 and 3 lesions, and one-third of CIN 1 lesions [38, 41]. Therefore, the identification of transformation zone epithelium in cervical specimens is critical to ensure accurate interpretation, and effort should be made to demonstrate a well-visualized transformation zone in the specimen through additional sections, deeper levels, or re-sampling if necessary.

Genetic and Epigenetic Changes in Cervical Cancers

Chromosomal instability caused by deregulation of E6 and E7 may lead to numerous host cell aberrations. The E6 and E7 oncoproteins can bind to the tumor suppressor genes p53 and pRB with high affinity. The result of E6 binding to p53 is subsequent ubiquitination and degradation, resulting in the loss of function of p53 as a tumor suppressor [42]. The binding of E7 to pRb results in proteasomal degradation of pRb and disruption of the pRb-E2F complex, leading to a subsequent release of free E2F transcription factor and unrestricted proliferation [43]. The genomic instability may contribute to accumulation of genetic aberrations in the host cell including DNA mutations, altered copy numbers, deletions, and DNA methylation.

Chromosomal aberrations: The most frequent copy number changes in cervical SCC are 3q gain, 3p loss, and 11q loss, whereas 17q gain is most common in adenocarcinomas [44]. The common alterations in high-grade CIN are gain at 1p and 3q, and loss at 4q, 2q, 4p, 11p, and 3p (in decreasing order) [44]. In these chromosomal aberration regions, novel oncogene eye absent homologue 2 (EYA2) and tumor suppressor gene mir-375 have been identified in cervical cancers [45–47].

DNA mutations: DNA changes in the PIK3CA signaling pathway are the most common mutations identified in SCC and adenocarcinoma of the cervix [48, 49]. A lower frequency of epidermal growth factor receptor (EGFR) mutations in SCC and KRAS mutations in adenocarcinoma has been observed [48]. Other reported DNA mutations in cervical cancers include the E1a-binding protein 300 (EP300), F-box and WP repeat domain-containing 7 (FBXW7), HLAB, MAPK1, PTEN, STK11, nuclear factor erythroid 2-like 2 (NFE2L2), E74-like factor 3 (ELF-3), and the core-binding factor beta-subunit (CBFB) [49].

Aberrant DNA methylations: Increased DNA methylation of CpG-rich promoters usually represses gene transcription in humans. Aberrant methylation patterns have been observed in many tumor suppressor genes in cervical cancer and precursor lesions and are often related to cell type [50, 51]. Cell adhesion molecule 1 (CADM1) is the most frequently methylated gene in HSIL, followed by cadherin

1 (CDH1), death-associated protein kinase (DPAK1), and telomerase reverse transcriptase (TERT) [50]. In both cervical SCC and adenocarcinoma, the frequently methylated genes are CADM1, CDH1, DPAK1, EPB41L3, FAM19A4, myelin and lymphocyte (MAL), paired box 1 (PAX1), PR domain-containing 14 (PRDM14), and TERT [50]. In cervical cancer, alterations of DNA methylation in specific genes such as DAPK1, RARB, WIF1, and SLIT2 may also occur early in cervical carcinogenesis [52]. In addition, aberrant DNA methylation of DLX4 and SIM1 has been proposed as predictive markers for disease progression of cervical low-grade squamous intraepithelial lesion [53].

Recently, HPV DNA methylation has attracted attention due to its role in the development of cervical cancer. Many studies demonstrated altered methylation patterns during disease progression, commonly involving the late genes L1 and L2 [54, 55]. Methylation of the E2-binding sites (E2BSs) reduces E2 binding, thus resulting in deregulated expression of the oncoproteins E6 and E7, [7, 56] which is considered the key step for cell transformation. Gradual increase of E2BS methylation has been reportedly associated with disease progression, presumably due to further increase of E6 and E7 expression [54, 55, 57].

Altered micro-RNAs: Micro-RNAs are noncoding regulatory RNAs that are considered to play an important role in the development and progression of cervical cancer [58, 59]. Among the large number of altered miRNAs reported in cervical cancer, only a few have been consistently identified in several studies; these include up-regulation of miR-15b, miR-16, miR-146a, and miR-155, and down-regulation of miR-126, miR-143, and miR-145 [37, 60–62]. Although down-regulation of several miRNAs in cervical cancer can be associated with an increase in promoter methylation in the respective genes, [58, 63, 64] most miRNA alterations involve secondary changes of chromosomal aberrations following HPV infection. The challenges in using miRNAs as cancer biomarkers include independent validation for a large number of possibly altered miRNAs and determination of their functional relevance in the development and progression of cervical cancer. A recent study demonstrated that a significant increase in the expression of miR-27a and a lower level of miR-34a were detected in CIN2 and 3 as compared to CIN1, and in SCC as compared to CIN2 and 3 [65].

Cervical Cancer Prevention and Risk Profiling

HPV Testing in Cervical Cancer Prevention

High-risk HPV genotypes (HPV 16, 18, 31, 33, 35, 39, 45, 51, 52, 56, 58, 59, 66, 68) are responsible for the development of more than 99% of cervical cancers and 90% of cervical precancerous lesions (i.e., cervical intraepithelial neoplasia grade 2 or 3) [6, 66, 67]. In the past decade, testing for high-risk HPV genotypes in conjunction with the Papanicolaou (Pap) cytology test has been recommended and applied in the USA to increase cervical cancer screening efficacy [68–72]. Prior to HPV testing, the Pap cytology test was used for cervical cancer screening in the USA for decades. Although the sensitivity of the Pap test for detecting CIN3+ is relatively low, it has been a successful cancer screening tool and has significantly reduced the incidence of cervical cancer in the screened population. Women with a high risk of CIN2+ are referred for a diagnostic colposcopy/biopsy evaluation. Once CIN2+ is confirmed on the biopsy, the Loop Electrosurgical Excision Procedure (LEEP) or a cone excision is recommended to eliminate the CIN2+ lesion [73].

Although both HPV and Pap testing are used for cervical cancer risk prediction, the implications of the HPV test result and the Pap test result are different. A single positive HPV test result may not be clinically relevant. HPV is the most prevalent sexually transmitted pathogen, and HPV infection is very common in young women [74], but most HPV infections are transient with few clinical implications. Only a small percentage of women with a persistent high-risk HPV infection are at risk of developing CIN3+. Epidemiologically, HPV infection in women reaches a maximum in the mid-twenties and declines with age in the USA, and the incidence of cervical cancer gradually increases with age [75]. Due to the high prevalence of HPV and the low incidence of precancerous cervical lesions in young women, HPV testing is not cost-effective and has a limited predictive value for CIN3+ in women 30 years of age and younger. Consequently, cervical cancer screening via HPV/Pap co-testing as a means to predict CIN2+ is only recommended for women 30 years of age and older in the USA [69]. Additionally, HPV testing has been recommended as an adjunct to Pap cytology testing in women exhibiting mildly abnormal Pap test results in order to achieve optimal efficacy in predicting CIN2+. However, the combination of HPV and Pap cytology test results, the woman's age, and re-screening intervals results in a highly complex screening system for triage and follow-up [70]. For these reasons, HPV primary screening has been recommended as an alternative test for cervical cancer screening in the USA [72].

HPV and Pap Cytology Co-testing

HPV and Pap co-testing as a primary screening method in women aged 30 years and older was recommended by the American Cancer Society (ACS) and the American Society of Colposcopy and Cervical Pathology (ASCCP) in 2004 [76]. In 2006, the consensus guidelines issued by ASCCP for cervical cancer prevention reiterated the necessity for HPV and Pap cytology co-testing for women aged 30 years and older with a 3-year screening interval [69]. In the 2012 consensus guidelines, the screening interval was extended to 5 years [70]. Randomized clinical trials demonstrated that HPV and Pap co-testing increased detection of CIN3 + and decreased the incidence of CIN3+ during the follow-up periods, findings that permitted prolonged screening intervals [77, 78]. Women with negative HPV/Pap cytology co-testing results have a significantly lower risk of developing CIN3+ as compared to women with a sole negative Pap cytology result [79, 80]. In addition, compared to Pap cytology, HPV testing can provide a long-term prediction for the risk of cervical cancer [81, 82]. The current US guidelines with an extended 5-year screening interval recommendation are intended to reduce unnecessary follow-up testing and the associated morbidity and costs, while maintaining testing efficacy similar to that of using sole Pap cytology testing at a 3-year screening interval.

HPV16/18 Genotyping

During cervical cancer screening using HPV and Pap cytology co-testing, a small percentage of women have HPV+/Pap-test results. [83] In primary HPV screening, Pap cytology is used for women with positive HPV test results. Consequently, some women also have HPV +/Pap-test results. Women with HPV+/Pap-co-testing results have an increased risk for CIN2+ [84]. However, the risk is not great enough to require an immediate colposcopic evaluation, and current cervical cancer screening guidelines recommend the following: repeat co-testing in 12 months or HPV genotyping for HPV16 alone or both HPV16/18. If repeated HPV/Pap cytology co-testing or HPV 16/18 genotyping yields a positive result, the woman is referred for further evaluation by colposcopy [70]. This indicates that HPV16 is more clinically relevant than non-16 high-risk HPV genotypes for cervical cancer carcinogenesis.

Data from randomized clinical trials demonstrated that women with HPV16 have a significantly higher risk of developing CIN3+ than women with non-16 high-risk HPV genotypes; this indicates that HPV16 is more clinically relevant than non-16 high-risk HPV genotypes for cervical cancer carcinogenesis [66, 85–90]. In long-term follow-up studies, the risk of CIN3+ was also significantly higher in women with positive HPV16/18 genotyping than in those with non-16/18 high-risk HPV genotypes [66, 89, 91]. The clinical relevance of HPV16 justifies reflex HPV16/18 genotyping for women with HPV+/Pap-co-testing results.

HPV Testing Assays

The FDA has approved HPV testing for cervical cancer screening in the following clinical settings: reflex HPV testing in Pap cytology specimens with ASC-US, HPV/Pap co-testing in women aged 30 years and older, and HPV primary screening. Since 2003, the FDA has approved six commercially available HPV testing assays for cervical cancer screening (Table 12.1). The Hybrid Capture 2 (HC2, Qiagen, Valencia, CA) was the first FDA-approved HPV assay widely used in the USA with extensive published technical and clinical studies including several clinical trials. HC2 can detect 13 high-risk HPV types with a unique design of

Table 12.1 Major clinical applications of HPV testing assays approved by FDA

Clinical applications	2003	2009	2011	2014
Reflex for ASC-US	HC2	Cervista HR	Cobas, aptima HPV	
HPV/Pap co-testing	HC2	Cervista HR	Cobas, aptima HPV	
Reflex HPV16/18		Cervista HPV16/18	Cobas, aptima HPB16 18/45	
Primary screening				Cobas

Since Cobas HPV was approved by FDA for all of the applications of HPV testing inSurePath Pap specimens in 2016. This is the only FDA approved HPV testing assay in SurePath

Table 12.2 The US FDA-approved HPV testing assays

	HC2[a]	Cervista HPV	Aptima HPV	Cobas HPV
PCR-based	No	No	Yes	Yes
Amplification	Signal	Signal	E6, E7 RNA	E6, E7, DNA
HPV detection[b]	13 types	14 types	14 types	14 types
HPV genotyping	No	HPV16, 18	HPV16, 18, 45	HPV16, 18
Internal controls	No	Yes	Yes	Yes
Equivocal zone	Yes	No	No	No
Company	Qiagen	Hologic	Hologic	Roche

[a]Hybrid capture 2

[b]HPV types: 13 high-risk HPV types: HPV16, 18, 31, 33, 35, 39, 45, 51, 52, 56, 58, 59, 68. 14 high-risk HPV types: HPV16, 18, 31, 33, 35, 39, 45, 51, 52, 56, 58, 59, 66, 68

RNA-DNA hybridization for 13 high-risk HPV types. Therefore, it is a non-PCR-based HPV assay. Despite the fact that the HC2 HPV assay is the most widely used HPV test to date, it lacks both an internal control for specimen adequacy determination and the capability of HPV16/18 genotyping. The Cervista HPV HR and Cervista HPV16/18 assays (Hologic, Marlborough, MA) are also non-PCR-based HPV assays approved by the FDA, but have the advantage of an internal control and the capability of HPV16/18 genotyping (Table 12.2).

The Cobas HPV assay is a PCR-based test approved by the FDA for HPV/Pap cytology co-testing (2012) and HPV primary screening (2014). The Cobas HPV is the only FDA-approved HPV assay for HPV primary screening. One of the advantages of the Cobas HPV assay is its high degree of automation, which allows large quantities of Pap specimens to be processed. Another advantage of the Cobas HPV assay is that HPV16/18 genotyping results are available in the same testing platform as for high-risk HPV, which allows specific triage for women with positive HPV16 or 18 during HPV primary screening.

The only HPV testing assays designed to target HPV mRNA are Aptima HPV and Aptima HPV16 18/45 assays (Hologic, Marlborough, MA). The Aptima HPV testing assays detect HPV E6 and E7 mRNA and are considered more clinically relevant than HPV DNA in predicting CIN3+; this is the case because E6 and E7 mRNAs are indicators of active transcription of the HPV E6 and E7 oncogenes.

Aptima HPV assays are highly automated with the ability to detect HPV16, HPV18, and HPV45 genotypes.

In situ hybridization (ISH) has also been used in cervical tissue examination to determine HPV status [92, 93]. As the ISH assay is a signal-amplification based assay, it can be performed on small tissue specimens; it provides the advantage of successful testing in cases with insufficient DNA, which is not possible with PCR-based HPV testing [93]. To date, studies using ISH in Pap cytology specimens showed relatively low sensitivity [94].

Tumor Markers in Pap Cytology for Cervical Cancer Screening

High-risk HPV infection in the basal layer of cervical squamous cells can induce disruption of the cell cycle, resulting in cell proliferation and immortalization. Increased expression of the oncoproteins E6 and E7 related to high-risk HPV can be detected when HPV integration into the host genome occurs. The E7 oncoprotein can bind and inactivate pRB leading to E2F activation. These reactions induce expression of S-phase genes such as encoding minichromosome maintenance proteins (MCMs), TOP2A, Ki-67, p14, and p16, which are associated with cell proliferation; p16 is a regulatory protein controlling S-phase progression. These S-phase gene products can be detected in CIN3+ by immunostaining. In the last decade, multiple regulatory gene products have been evaluated as markers in Pap cytology specimens for predicting CIN3+ [95]. The markers that have been most frequently evaluated include p16, MIB-1 (Ki-67), and MCM2/TOP2A (ProExC, BD).

Immunostaining for P16, MIB-1, and MCM2/TOP2A (ProExC) in Pap Cytology Specimens

Immunostaining for a single marker (p16) or combined markers (p16/Ki-67, MCM2/TOP2A) has been evaluated in Pap specimens, predominantly liquid-based cytology specimens, to assist in CIN3+ prediction. Most studies were designed to compare immunostaining with HPV test results for predicting CIN2+. Because a positive result from the S-phase biomarkers is more specific than a positive HPV result in predicting the risk for CIN3 progression, these biomarkers have the potential to improve the predictive value of HPV testing or possibly replace Pap cytology for risk profiling. However, practically, it is difficult to standardize the immunostaining methods used for Pap cytology specimens and the interpretation of the results, in particular the 'cutoff' for a positive result. Interpretation of immunostains in Pap cytology specimens may be the major obstacle to using immunostaining for predicting CIN2+. Interpreting the significance of a few positively stained cells can be challenging because of the frequent occurrence of staining of nondysplastic cells, such as endocervical or metaplastic cells [96].

In cervical biopsies, p16 immunostaining is used as a surrogate marker of high-risk HPV to help confirm CIN2 or CIN3. In Pap cytology specimens, p16 is the most studied immunostain for prediction of CIN3+. Meta-analysis studies have demonstrated higher specificity, but lower or comparable sensitivity of p16 in predicting CIN2 + compared to HPV testing [95, 97]. In a recent study with a large cohort, p16 immunostaining had significantly lower sensitivity but higher specificity for CIN3+ compared to HPV assays such as HC2 and Cobas HPV [98]. To improve the efficacy of p16 immunostaining for CIN3+ prediction, MIB-1 (Ki-67) has been added as a dual test. In cervical biopsies, dual p16/Ki-67 immunostaining has been used to verify or resolve controversial morphologic interpretations of CIN2+. ProExC is a commercially available cocktail that contains two monoclonal antibodies for MCM2 and TOP2A, regulatory proteins of DNA replication. In cervical specimens, the distribution of ProExC staining is reported to be closely associated with CIN3+ [99]. Similar to p16, ProExC in Pap cytology specimens has comparable or lower sensitivity, but higher specificity than HPV testing for CIN3+ [95]. However, immunostaining with ProExC also can have nonspecific staining, potentially leading to false-positive results [96]. To date, none of these biomarkers have been used clinically for screening.

Methylation Markers

Aberrant DNA methylation during cervical carcinogenesis and in high-risk HPV has been evaluated as potential markers for prediction of CIN3. In Pap cytology specimens, multiple DNA methylation markers have been evaluated, including methylation markers in promoter regions of tumor suppressor genes (CADM1, MAL, PAX1, SOX1, and FAM19A4) [100–102]. Methylation in high-risk HPV such as HPV16, 18, 31, and 33 also has been evaluated for cervical cancer risk prediction [103, 104].

Compared to Pap cytology, combined CADM1 and MAL methylation markers have shown higher sensitivity for CIN+ [105]. Combined CADM1/MAL methylation markers have also shown efficacy comparable to Pap/HPV16/18 co-testing in predicting CIN3+ [106].

Additionally, several methylation markers have higher specificity for CIN3+ when used individually. PAX1 and SOX1 are reported to be highly specific for CIN3, and when combined they have similar sensitivity and higher specificity for CIN3+ compared to Pap/HPV co-testing [107]. High specificity for CIN3+ was also observed for FAM19A4 methylation [108]. Recently, in an HPV primary screening study, molecular triage using methylation markers was evaluated. When combined methylation markers MAL/miR124-2 were compared to Pap cytology triage results for women with positive HPV, a similar detection rate for CIN2+ was observed in women with positive HPV16 results, and methylation of the L1 and L2 genes of HPV16 was reported to be highly associated with CIN3+ [109]. In summary, these approaches hold the potential to replace Pap cytology testing as the triage tool in cervical cancer screening in the future.

Molecular Basis of Emerging Biological Treatment for Cervical Cancers

Despite efforts at prevention and early diagnosis of cervical cancer through the implementation of HPV vaccination and screening with the Papanicolaou and HPV tests, approximately 5% of women in North America have stage IV disease at the time of cervical cancer diagnosis [110]. Although the prognosis is favorable for early stage cervical cancer, the 5-year survival rate for women with cancer that has spread beyond the pelvis is only 17% [111]. During the past two decades, platinum-based chemotherapy with or without external beam radiation therapy has been the cornerstone treatment for recurrent, metastatic, or persistent cervical cancer [112]. Other cytotoxic drugs have also been studied as therapeutic agents, but the results were largely unsatisfactory. During the last decade, recognition of the carcinogenic effect of HPV and increased understanding of the biomolecular events following HPV infection have provided a strong foundation for the development of new drugs and innovative therapies. Recently, promising results have been reported from studies of molecular agents targeting critical pathways in cervical cancer [113]. Table 12.3 summarizes potential molecular therapeutic agents for cervical cancer currently under evaluation.

Anti-Angiogenic Agents

Overexpression of vascular endothelial growth factor (VEGF) is associated with advanced stage and poor prognosis in cervical cancers [114–116]. E6-mediated p53 degradation results in up-regulation of a series of pro-angiogenic activities including the increase in VEGF [117]. The VEGF pathway may be blocked through either extracellular interference with VEGF itself via antibodies (bevacizumab or aflibercept) or by intracytoplasmic inhibition of the VEGF receptor tyrosine kinase (RTK) with drugs such as pazopanib, nintedanib, cediranib, sunitinib, and sorafenib. An alternative approach is the use of a fusion protein that prevents the interaction of angiopoietin with the Tie2 receptor on endothelial cells.

Bevacizumab (Avastin) was the first clinically available humanized monoclonal antibody against VEGF-A. A phase II trial evaluating bevacizumab as a single agent in recurrent cervical SCC showed a response rate of 11%, a no-progression rate of 24% at 6 months, a median progression-free survival (PFS) of 3.4 months, and a median overall survival (OS) of 7.2 months [118]. Further phase III trials showed that addition of bevacizumab to combination chemotherapy for patients with recurrent, persistent, or metastatic cervical cancer was associated with an improvement of 3.7 months in the median OS, with beneficial effects in patients who had been previously treated with platinum or irradiation [119]. Regimens consisting of bevacizumab with irradiation and/or various cytotoxic agents are being currently evaluated and have exhibited promising preliminary results [120–123]

Table 12.3 Emerging biological treatments under evaluation for cervical cancers

Category	Agent	Target	Mechanism	References
Anti-angiogenic agents	Bevacizumab	VEGFR-A	Inhibition of VEGF-A	[118–124]
	Sunitinib, sorafenib, imatinib, pazopanib, cediranib	EGFR RTK	Inhibition of tumor angiogenesis	[124–126]
	AMG386 PF-486884	Angiopoietins	Inhibition of angiopoietins	[127–129]
EGFR inhibitors	Gefitinib, elotinib cetuximab, lapatinib, trastuzumab, panitumumab	HER1 (EGFR), HER2, HER3, and HER4	Inhibition of overexpressed EGFR function	[100–104, 130–135]
mTOR inhibitors mTOR-specific siRNA	*Temsirolimus* *mTOR siRNA*	mTOR	Inhibition of mTOR	[139, 171–173]
Demethylating agents	Decitabine (5-aza-2′ deoxycytidine)	Hypermethylated genes	Demethylation of hypermethylated genes	[140–142]
SRC kinase inhibitors	Dasatinib	SRC kinases	Down-regulation of Src kinases	[136, 137, 174]
WEE1 inhibitors	MK-1775 (AZD-1775)	WEE1	Inhibition of pro-proliferation kinase WEE1	[113, 138, 175]
Short interfering RNAs (siRNAs)	siRNA	HPV E6 and E7 oncogenes	Inhibition of E6/E7 oncogene translation	[150–154]
Histone deacetylase inhibitors	Tricostatin A, vorinostat, valproic acid, hydralazine-valproate	Histone deacetylase	Competition with HPV oncoproteins for p53 binding	[176–179]
Restoration of wild-type p53	MG132, bortezomib, lopinvir	Proteasome	Prevention of E6-induced proteasomal degradation of p53	[143, 144]
	Recombinant adenovirus-p53 (rAD-p53)	NA	Increase WT p53 production	[145–148]

(continued)

Table 12.3 (continued)

Category	Agent	Target	Mechanism	References
Poly ADP ribose polymerase inhibitors	Veliparib, olaparib		Synergism with cisplatin or radiation	[180–182]
Cyclooxygenase-2 (COX-2) inhibitors	Celecoxib	COX-2 isoform	Inhibition of arachidonic acid transformation to prostaglandin precursors	[159–165]
Antioxidant	Polyphones		Proliferation inhibition, apoptosis induction, and chemosensitivity enhancement	[155–157]
Anti-viral agent	Lopinavir Cydofovir	HPV	Inhibition of HPV oncoproteins	[154, 166–168, 170]

EGFR RTK inhibitors such as sunitinib, sorafenib, imatinib, pazopanib, and cediranib are new anti-angiogenic agents under investigation for cervical cancer. Monotherapies using sunitinib and imatinib for advanced cervical cancer showed no response with adverse side effects [124, 125]. A phase II trial conducted for pazopanib as a single agent for advanced or recurrent cervical cancer showed improved PFS and OS (median OS 50.7 weeks) with a favorable toxicity profile [126]. Various combinations of EGFR RTK inhibitors with other treatment modalities (chemotherapy and radiation therapy) are currently being evaluated [113].

Angiopoietins (ANGPTs) are ligands of the endothelial cell receptor Tie2 and play an important role in angiogenesis [127]. ANGPTs are elevated in cervical cancer patients [128] and are capable of promoting tumor angiogenesis in cervical cancer [129]. Two ANGPT traps, AMG386 and PF-486884, are under development for cervical cancer treatment [127].

Inhibitors of Epidermal Growth Factor Receptor

The epidermal growth factor receptor (EGFR) family includes HER1 (EGFR), HER2 (ErbB-2), HER3 (ErbB3), and HER4 (ErbB4). Expression of EGFR can be stimulated by hrHPV E6/E7, and EGFR is overexpressed in 85% of cervical SCCs [100, 130]. The expression of HER2 and HER4 is also elevated in cervical cancer [101]. EGFR expression and co-expression of EGFR and HER2 are associated with poor prognosis in cervical cancer patients due to modulation of tumor chemosensitivity and radiosensitivity [102, 103].

EGFR-family inhibitors that are being evaluated for the treatment of cervical cancer include gefitinib, erlotinib, cetuximab, lapatinib, trastuzumab, and panitumumab [113]. An in vitro study showed that erlotinib prevented hrHPV-induced immortalization of cultured human cervical epithelial cells and stimulated apoptosis in cells that expressed the HPV-16 E6/E7 oncoproteins [104]. However, no increase in survival was observed in trials using gefitinib, erlotinib, or cetuximab as single agents in the treatment of advanced or recurrent cervical cancer [131–133]. A study using cetuximab together with cisplatin and topotecan demonstrated an objective response rate of 32%, but concerning toxicity was also observed [134]. Various regimens involving EGFR inhibitors with cytotoxic agents and/or radiation therapy are currently under investigation [113]. Anti-HER2 treatment most likely has limited value in cervical cancer because it is rarely overexpressed and has controversial prognostic significance [135].

Inhibitors of the Mammalian Target of Rapamycin

The mammalian target of rapamycin (mTOR) is a kinase regulating cell growth and cell cycle progression. Aberrant activation of the mTOR pathway has been observed in cervical cancer as a result of multiple genetic and epigenetic abnormalities, as well as interactions between HPV oncoproteins and the mTOR pathway [136–138]. In a phase II trial using the mTOR inhibitor temsirolimus as a single agent for recurrent, locally advanced or metastatic cervical cancer, modest activity was observed with about two-thirds of the patients exhibiting disease stability [139]. Further clinical trials with or without chemoradiation are currently underway.

Demethylating Agents

Aberrant methylation of multiple genes has been linked to carcinogenesis in cervical cancer. These genes include the CpG island of p16, fragile histidine triad (FHIT) tumor suppressor gene, retinoic acid receptor beta, E-cadherin anaphase-promoting complex (APC), and Ras family of genes [140]. Aberrant hypermethylation of the mitotic checkpoint gene CHFR correlates with lack of sensitivity to taxanes in cervical cancer cells [141]. On the other hand, it has been reported that aberrant DNA hypermethylation of the WRN gene increased the sensitivity of cervical cancer cells to the topoisomerase I inhibitor CPT-11 [140]. Demethylating agents, such as decitabine (5-aza-2′ deoxycytidine) inhibiting DNA methyltransferase, have been introduced as new therapeutic agents in cervical cancer treatment aiming to restore the expression of several tumor suppressor genes and thus slow cell proliferation [142].

Proteasome Inhibitors

HPV E6-induced degradation of p53 is critical in cervical cancer oncogenesis, which is brought about by ubiquitin-mediated proteasomal degradation [143]. Functional restoration of wild-type TP53 can be achieved by conventional therapy with cisplatin or radiation treatment. A novel approach to restore wild-type TP53 is to prevent ubiquitin–proteasome degradation by proteasome inhibitors [144]. Several promising proteasome inhibitors such as MG132, bortezomib, and lopinvir have been tested on cervical cancer cell lines; the therapeutic mechanisms involve increased p53 levels and transcription, induction of apoptosis, and synergism with cisplatin. The recombinant adenovirus-p53 (rAD-p53), which was designed to increase the level of functional intracellular p53, is being evaluated with chemotherapy for locally advanced cervical cancer in a phase II trial [145–148]. The results from a recent study suggest that the effect of rAd-p53 in inhibiting HeLa cell proliferation and induction of apoptosis are mediated by down-regulation of VEGF [149].

Micro-RNAs and Short Interfering RNAs

Micro-RNAs (miRNAs) arrest translation of targeted mRNA and regulate multiple oncogenic pathways [150]. Short interfering RNAs (siRNAs), which mimic miRNAs, may also inhibit the translation of targeted mRNA. In vitro and in vivo studies showed that therapeutic siRNA specific for HPV E6 and E7 oncoproteins exerts their inhibitory effects in cervical cancer cells by silencing transcription of these genes, thus restoring p53 and Rb functions [151–154]. In light of the previous encouraging preclinical data, several technical issues related to clinical administration of siRNAs are under evaluation.

Antioxidants

Oxidative DNA damage is most likely elevated during HPV-driven carcinogenesis of the cervix, and progressive elevation of the oxidative stress marker 8-OHdG was observed during progression from normal tissue to dysplasia and cancer in the cervix [155]. Polyphenols, which are antioxidant agents, have been shown to inhibit proliferation of HPV-positive cancer cells, to induce apoptosis, and to enhance chemosensitivity in cervical cancer cells [156]. Antioxidants appear to act at several steps in the cascade of cell transformation promoted by HPV infection, and thus may hold great potential for prevention and therapy of cervical cancer [157].

Cyclooxygenase-2 Inhibitors

Cyclooxygenase (COX-2) is involved in inflammatory processes and is frequently expressed in cervical intraepithelial lymphocytes (IELs) and cancers [158]. The HPV oncoproteins E5, E6, and E7 increase transcription of COX-2, which is associated with inhibition of apoptosis, active angiogenesis, and reduced radiosensitivity [159–162]. Cervical cancer biopsies from COX-2-treated patients showed decreased COX-2, Ki-67, CD31, and microvessel density and increased prostaglandin E2 (PGE2) levels [163]. However, a phase II trial on locally advanced cervical cancer treated with chemoradiation in combination with a COX-2 inhibitor (celecoxib) recorded cardiotoxicity and fistula formation without any beneficial activity [164]. Although no significant benefits have been reported from the use of COX-2 inhibitors as radio-sensitizers in cervical cancer, their potential application in targeting cervical IELs has been proposed as this route may play a role in cancer prevention [165].

Anti-viral Agents

Anti-viral agents have been considered for therapy in cervical cancer. Their mode of action involves interruption of HPV-induced carcinogenesis via inhibition of the oncoproteins E6/E7 or interference with oncoprotein functions [154, 166, 167]. Alternatively, agents designed to interfere with oncoprotein E1/E2 functions also have shown an inhibitory effect on HPV replication. The anti-HIV drug lopinavir has been shown to inhibit cervical cancer cells by interacting with p53 [168], a result indicative of its potential clinical application. A phase II trial conducted for paclitaxel, 13-cis retinoic acid [169], and interferon alfa-2b in the treatment of advanced stage or recurrent cervical cancer showed a median PFS of 3.4 months and an OS of 11.2 months [169]. In addition, topical application of the broad-spectrum anti-viral agent cydofovir has been under evaluation for high-grade cervical dysplasia [170].

References

1. United-States-Cancer-Statistics-Working-Group. United States cancer statistics: 1999–2012 incidence and mortality web-based report. Atlanta U S Dept Health Hum Serv Centers Dis Control Prev Natl Cancer Inst. 2015.
2. WHO. Latest world cancer statistics. 2013.
3. WHO. Cervical cancer: estimated incidence, mortality and prevalence worldwide in 2012. 2015.
4. Howlader N, Noone AM, Krapcho M, Garshell J, Miller D, Altekruse SF, Kosary CL, Yu M, Ruhl J, Tatalovich Z, Mariotto A, Lewis DR, Chen HS, Feuer EJ, Cronin KA, editors. SEER cancer statistics review, 1975–2012. National Cancer Institute; 2015.
5. Crosbie EJ, Einstein MH, Franceschi S, Kitchener HC. Human papillomavirus and cervical cancer. Lancet. 2013;382:889–99.
6. Walboomers JM, Jacobs MV, Manos MM, et al. Human papillomavirus is a necessary cause of invasive cervical cancer worldwide. J Pathol. 1999;189:12–9.
7. Auger M, Khalbuss W, Nayar R, et al. Accuracy and false-positive rate of the cytologic diagnosis of follicular cervicitis: observations from the College of American Pathologists Pap Educational Program. Arch Pathol Lab Med. 2013;137:907–11.
8. Bosch FX, Lorincz A, Munoz N, Meijer CJ, Shah KV. The causal relation between human papillomavirus and cervical cancer. J Clin Pathol. 2002;55:244–65.
9. Kash N, Lee MA, Kollipara R, Downing C, Guidry J, Tyring SK. Safety and efficacy data on vaccines and immunization to human papillomavirus. J Clin Med. 2015;4:614–33.
10. Future-II-Study-Group. Prophylactic efficacy of a quadrivalent human papillomavirus (HPV) vaccine in women with virological evidence of HPV infection. J Infect Dis. 2007;196:1438–46.
11. Romanowski B, de Borba PC, Naud PS, et al. Sustained efficacy and immunogenicity of the human papillomavirus (HPV)-16/18 AS04-adjuvanted vaccine: analysis of a randomised placebo-controlled trial up to 6.4 years. Lancet. 2009;374:1975–85.
12. Julius JM, Ramondeta L, Tipton KA, Lal LS, Schneider K, Smith JA. Clinical perspectives on the role of the human papillomavirus vaccine in the prevention of cancer. Pharmacotherapy. 2011;31:280–97.

13. Gambhira R, Karanam B, Jagu S, et al. A protective and broadly cross-neutralizing epitope of human papillomavirus L2. J Virol. 2007;81:13927–31.
14. Bae SH, Park YJ, Park JB, Choi YS, Kim MS, Sin JI. Therapeutic synergy of human papillomavirus E7 subunit vaccines plus cisplatin in an animal tumor model: causal involvement of increased sensitivity of cisplatin-treated tumors to CTL-mediated killing in therapeutic synergy. Clin Cancer Res. 2007;13:341–9.
15. Gertig DM, Brotherton JM, Budd AC, Drennan K, Chappell G, Saville AM. Impact of a population-based HPV vaccination program on cervical abnormalities: a data linkage study. BMC Med. 2013;11:227.
16. Saville AM. Cervical cancer prevention in Australia: planning for the future. Cancer Cytopathol. 2015:Epub ahead of print.
17. Owsianka B, Ganczak M. Evaluation of human papilloma virus (HPV) vaccination strategies and vaccination coverage in adolescent girls worldwide. Przegl Epidemiol. 2015;69(53–8):151–5.
18. Sussman AL, Helitzer D, Bennett A, Solares A, Lanoue M, Getrich CM. Catching up with the HPV vaccine: challenges and opportunities in primary care. Ann Fam Med. 2015;13:354–60.
19. IARC. Working group on the evaluation of carcinogenic risks to humans. Biological agents. Volume 100 B. A review of human carcinogens. IARC Monogr Eval Carcinog Risks Hum. 2012;100:1–441.
20. de Sanjose S, Quint WG, Alemany L, et al. Human papillomavirus genotype attribution in invasive cervical cancer: a retrospective cross-sectional worldwide study. Lancet Oncol. 2010;11:1048–56.
21. Doorbar J, Quint W, Banks L, et al. The biology and life-cycle of human papillomaviruses. Vaccine. 2012;30(Suppl 5):F55–70.
22. Kajitani N, Satsuka A, Kawate A, Sakai H. Productive lifecycle of human papillomaviruses that depends upon squamous epithelial differentiation. Front Microbiol. 2012;3:152.
23. Ho GY, Bierman R, Beardsley L, Chang CJ, Burk RD. Natural history of cervicovaginal papillomavirus infection in young women. N Engl J Med. 1998;338:423–8.
24. Garcia-Chacon R, Velasco-Ramirez SF, Flores-Romo L, Daneri-Navarro A. Immunobiology of HPV Infection. Arch Med Res. 2009;40:443–8.
25. Bosch FX, Burchell AN, Schiffman M, et al. Epidemiology and natural history of human papillomavirus infections and type-specific implications in cervical neoplasia. Vaccine. 2008;26(Suppl 10):K1–16.
26. Duensing S, Munger K. The human papillomavirus type 16 E6 and E7 oncoproteins independently induce numerical and structural chromosome instability. Cancer Res. 2002;62:7075–82.
27. Moody CA, Laimins LA. Human papillomavirus oncoproteins: pathways to transformation. Nat Rev Cancer. 2010;10:550–60.
28. Thierry F, Yaniv M. The BPV1-E2 trans-acting protein can be either an activator or a repressor of the HPV18 regulatory region. EMBO J. 1987;6:3391–7.
29. Vinokurova S, Wentzensen N, Kraus I, et al. Type-dependent integration frequency of human papillomavirus genomes in cervical lesions. Cancer Res. 2008;68:307–13.
30. Klingelhutz AJ, Roman A. Cellular transformation by human papillomaviruses: lessons learned by comparing high- and low-risk viruses. Virology. 2012;424:77–98.
31. McLaughlin-Drubin ME, Munger K. Biochemical and functional interactions of human papillomavirus proteins with polycomb group proteins. Viruses. 2013;5:1231–49.
32. McLaughlin-Drubin ME, Crum CP, Munger K. Human papillomavirus E7 oncoprotein induces KDM6A and KDM6B histone demethylase expression and causes epigenetic reprogramming. Proc Natl Acad Sci U S A. 2011;108:2130–5.
33. Hyland PL, McDade SS, McCloskey R, et al. Evidence for alteration of EZH2, BMI1, and KDM6A and epigenetic reprogramming in human papillomavirus type 16 E6/E7-expressing keratinocytes. J Virol. 2011;85:10999–1006.

34. Au Yeung CL, Tsang WP, Tsang TY, Co NN, Yau PL, Kwok TT. HPV-16 E6 upregulation of DNMT1 through repression of tumor suppressor p53. Oncol Rep. 2010;24:1599–604.
35. Martinez I, Gardiner AS, Board KF, Monzon FA, Edwards RP, Khan SA. Human papillomavirus type 16 reduces the expression of microRNA-218 in cervical carcinoma cells. Oncogene. 2008;27:2575–82.
36. Au Yeung CL, Tsang TY, Yau PL, Kwok TT. Human papillomavirus type 16 E6 induces cervical cancer cell migration through the p53/microRNA-23b/urokinase-type plasminogen activator pathway. Oncogene. 2011;30:2401–10.
37. Zheng ZM, Wang X. Regulation of cellular miRNA expression by human papillomaviruses. Biochim Biophys Acta. 2011;1809:668–77.
38. Herfs M, Yamamoto Y, Laury A, et al. A discrete population of squamocolumnar junction cells implicated in the pathogenesis of cervical cancer. Proc Natl Acad Sci U S A. 2012;109:10516–21.
39. McNairn AJ, Guasch G. Epithelial transition zones: merging microenvironments, niches, and cellular transformation. Eur J Dermatol. 2011;21(Suppl 2):21–8.
40. Herfs M, Vargas SO, Yamamoto Y, et al. A novel blueprint for 'top down' differentiation defines the cervical squamocolumnar junction during development, reproductive life, and neoplasia. J Pathol. 2013;229:460–8.
41. Herfs M, Parra-Herran C, Howitt BE, et al. Cervical squamocolumnar junction-specific markers define distinct, clinically relevant subsets of low-grade squamous intraepithelial lesions. Am J Surg Pathol. 2013;37:1311–8.
42. Scheffner M, Huibregtse JM, Vierstra RD, Howley PM. The HPV-16 E6 and E6-AP complex functions as a ubiquitin-protein ligase in the ubiquitination of p53. Cell. 1993;75:495–505.
43. Dyson N, Howley PM, Munger K, Harlow E. The human papilloma virus-16 E7 oncoprotein is able to bind to the retinoblastoma gene product. Science. 1989;243:934–7.
44. Thomas LK, Bermejo JL, Vinokurova S, et al. Chromosomal gains and losses in human papillomavirus-associated neoplasia of the lower genital tract - a systematic review and meta-analysis. Eur J Cancer. 2014;50:85–98.
45. Bierkens M, Krijgsman O, Wilting SM, et al. Focal aberrations indicate EYA2 and hsa-miR-375 as oncogene and tumor suppressor in cervical carcinogenesis. Genes Chromosomes Cancer. 2013;52:56–68.
46. Wang F, Li Y, Zhou J, et al. miR-375 is down-regulated in squamous cervical cancer and inhibits cell migration and invasion via targeting transcription factor SP1. Am J Pathol. 2011;179:2580–8.
47. Akagi K, Li J, Broutian TR, et al. Genome-wide analysis of HPV integration in human cancers reveals recurrent, focal genomic instability. Genome Res. 2014;24:185–99.
48. Wright AA, Howitt BE, Myers AP, et al. Oncogenic mutations in cervical cancer: genomic differences between adenocarcinomas and squamous cell carcinomas of the cervix. Cancer. 2013;119:3776–83.
49. Ojesina AI, Lichtenstein L, Freeman SS, et al. Landscape of genomic alterations in cervical carcinomas. Nature. 2013;506:371–5.
50. Wentzensen N, Sherman ME, Schiffman M, Wang SS. Utility of methylation markers in cervical cancer early detection: appraisal of the state-of-the-science. Gynecol Oncol. 2009;112:293–9.
51. Szalmas A, Konya J. Epigenetic alterations in cervical carcinogenesis. Semin Cancer Biol. 2009;19:144–52.
52. Siegel EM, Riggs BM, Delmas AL, Koch A, Hakam A, Brown KD. Quantitative DNA methylation analysis of candidate genes in cervical cancer. PLoS ONE. 2015;10:e0122495.
53. Sakane J, Taniyama K, Miyamoto K, et al. Aberrant DNA methylation of DLX4 and SIM1 is a predictive marker for disease progression of uterine cervical low-grade squamous intraepithelial lesion. Diagn Cytopathol. 2015;43:462–70.
54. Johannsen E, Lambert PF. Epigenetics of human papillomaviruses. Virology. 2013;445:205–12.

55. Clarke MA, Wentzensen N, Mirabello L, et al. Human papillomavirus DNA methylation as a potential biomarker for cervical cancer. Cancer Epidemiol Biomarkers Prev. 2012;21:2125–37.
56. Thain A, Jenkins O, Clarke AR, Gaston K. CpG methylation directly inhibits binding of the human papillomavirus type 16 E2 protein to specific DNA sequences. J Virol. 1996;70:7233–5.
57. Steenbergen RD, Snijders PJ, Heideman DA, Meijer CJ. Clinical implications of (epi)genetic changes in HPV-induced cervical precancerous lesions. Nat Rev Cancer. 2014;14:395–405.
58. Gomez-Gomez Y, Organista-Nava J, Gariglio P. Deregulation of the miRNAs expression in cervical cancer: human papillomavirus implications. Biomed Res Int. 2013;2013:407052.
59. Rao Q, Shen Q, Zhou H, Peng Y, Li J, Lin Z. Aberrant microRNA expression in human cervical carcinomas. Med Oncol. 2012;29:1242–8.
60. Kaczkowski B, Morevati M, Rossing M, Cilius F, Norrild B. A decade of global mRNA and miRNA profiling of HPV-positive cell lines and clinical specimens. Open Virol J. 2012;6:216–31.
61. Saavedra KP, Brebi PM, Roa JC. Epigenetic alterations in preneoplastic and neoplastic lesions of the cervix. Clin Epigenetics. 2012;4:13.
62. Gocze K, Gombos K, Juhasz K, et al. Unique microRNA expression profiles in cervical cancer. Anticancer Res. 2013;33:2561–7.
63. Wilting SM, Verlaat W, Jaspers A, et al. Methylation-mediated transcriptional repression of microRNAs during cervical carcinogenesis. Epigenetics. 2013;8:220–8.
64. Yao T, Rao Q, Liu L, et al. Exploration of tumor-suppressive microRNAs silenced by DNA hypermethylation in cervical cancer. Virol J. 2013;10:175.
65. Gocze K, Gombos K, Kovacs K, Juhasz K, Gocze P, Kiss I. MicroRNA expressions in HPV-induced cervical dysplasia and cancer. Anticancer Res. 2015;35:523–30.
66. Monsonego J, Cox JT, Behrens C, et al. Prevalence of high-risk human papilloma virus genotypes and associated risk of cervical precancerous lesions in a large U.S. screening population: data from the ATHENA trial. Gynecol Oncol. 2015;137:47–54.
67. Smith JS, Lindsay L, Hoots B, et al. Human papillomavirus type distribution in invasive cervical cancer and high-grade cervical lesions: a meta-analysis update. Int J Cancer. 2007;121:621–32.
68. Wright TC Jr, Schiffman M, Solomon D, et al. Interim guidance for the use of human papillomavirus DNA testing as an adjunct to cervical cytology for screening. Obstet Gynecol. 2004;103:304–9.
69. Wright TC Jr, Massad LS, Dunton CJ, et al. 2006 consensus guidelines for the management of women with abnormal cervical screening tests. J Low Genit Tract Dis. 2007;11:201–22.
70. Saslow D, Solomon D, Lawson HW, et al. American cancer society, American society for colposcopy and cervical pathology, and American society for clinical pathology screening guidelines for the prevention and early detection of cervical cancer. J Low Genit Tract Dis. 2012;16:175–204.
71. Massad LS, Einstein MH, Huh WK, et al. 2012 updated consensus guidelines for the management of abnormal cervical cancer screening tests and cancer precursors. J Low Genit Tract Dis. 2013;17:S1–27.
72. Huh WK, Ault KA, Chelmow D, et al. Use of primary high-risk human papillomavirus testing for cervical cancer screening: interim clinical guidance. J Low Genit Tract Dis. 2015;19:91–6.
73. Wright TC Jr, Massad LS, Dunton CJ, et al. 2006 consensus guidelines for the management of women with cervical intraepithelial neoplasia or adenocarcinoma in situ. J Low Genit Tract Dis. 2007;11:223–39.
74. Dunne EF, Unger ER, Sternberg M, et al. Prevalence of HPV infection among females in the United States. JAMA. 2007;297:813–9.
75. Rositch AF, Nowak RG, Gravitt PE. Increased age and race-specific incidence of cervical cancer after correction for hysterectomy prevalence in the United States from 2000 to 2009. Cancer. 2014;120:2032–8.

76. Bulletins ACoP. ACOG practice bulletin: clinical management guidelines for obstetrician-gynecologists. Number 45, August 2003. Cervical cytology screening (replaces committee opinion 152, March 1995). Obstet Gynecol. 2003;102:417–27.
77. Bulkmans NW, Berkhof J, Rozendaal L, et al. Human papillomavirus DNA testing for the detection of cervical intraepithelial neoplasia grade 3 and cancer: 5-year follow-up of a randomised controlled implementation trial. Lancet. 2007;370:1764–72.
78. Naucler P, Ryd W, Tornberg S, et al. Human papillomavirus and Papanicolaou tests to screen for cervical cancer. N Engl J Med. 2007;357:1589–97.
79. Dillner J, Rebolj M, Birembaut P, et al. Long term predictive values of cytology and human papillomavirus testing in cervical cancer screening: joint European cohort study. BMJ. 2008;337:a1754.
80. Katki HA, Kinney WK, Fetterman B, et al. Cervical cancer risk for women undergoing concurrent testing for human papillomavirus and cervical cytology: a population-based study in routine clinical practice. Lancet Oncol. 2011;12:663–72.
81. Castle PE, Glass AG, Rush BB, et al. Clinical human papillomavirus detection forecasts cervical cancer risk in women over 18 years of follow-up. J Clin Oncol. 2012;30:3044–50.
82. Ronco G, Dillner J, Elfstrom KM, et al. Efficacy of HPV-based screening for prevention of invasive cervical cancer: follow-up of four European randomised controlled trials. Lancet. 2014;383:524–32.
83. Katki HA, Schiffman M, Castle PE, et al. Five-year risks of CIN3+ and cervical cancer among women who test Pap-negative but are HPV-positive. J Low Genit Tract Dis. 2013;17: S56–63.
84. Schiffman M, Burk RD, Boyle S, et al. A study of genotyping for management of human papillomavirus-positive, cytology-negative cervical screening results. J Clin Microbiol. 2015;53:52–9.
85. Schiffman M, Wentzensen N. Human papillomavirus infection and the multistage carcinogenesis of cervical cancer. Cancer Epidemiol Biomarkers Prev. 2013;22:553–60.
86. Wright TC Jr, Stoler MH, Sharma A, et al. Evaluation of HPV-16 and HPV-18 genotyping for the triage of women with high-risk HPV + cytology-negative results. Am J Clin Pathol. 2011;136:578–86.
87. Castle PE, Stoler MH, Wright TC Jr, Sharma A, Wright TL, Behrens CM. Performance of carcinogenic human papillomavirus (HPV) testing and HPV16 or HPV18 genotyping for cervical cancer screening of women aged 25 years and older: a subanalysis of the ATHENA study. Lancet Oncol. 2011;12:880–90.
88. Katki HA, Wacholder S, Solomon D, Castle PE, Schiffman M. Risk estimation for the next generation of prevention programmes for cervical cancer. Lancet Oncol. 2009;10:1022–3.
89. Kjaer SK, Frederiksen K, Munk C, Iftner T. Long-term absolute risk of cervical intraepithelial neoplasia grade 3 or worse following human papillomavirus infection: role of persistence. J Natl Cancer Inst. 2010;102:1478–88.
90. Kitchener HC, Gilham C, Sargent A, et al. A comparison of HPV DNA testing and liquid based cytology over three rounds of primary cervical screening: extended follow up in the ARTISTIC trial. Eur J Cancer. 2011;47:864–71.
91. Khan MJ, Castle PE, Lorincz AT, et al. The elevated 10-year risk of cervical precancer and cancer in women with human papillomavirus (HPV) type 16 or 18 and the possible utility of type-specific HPV testing in clinical practice. J Natl Cancer Inst. 2005;97:1072–9.
92. Guo M, Gong Y, Deavers M, et al. Evaluation of a commercialized in situ hybridization assay for detecting human papillomavirus DNA in tissue specimens from patients with cervical intraepithelial neoplasia and cervical carcinoma. J Clin Microbiol. 2008;46:274–80.
93. Kelesidis T, Aish L, Steller MA, et al. Human papillomavirus (HPV) detection using in situ hybridization in histologic samples: correlations with cytologic changes and polymerase chain reaction HPV detection. Am J Clin Pathol. 2011;136:119–27.
94. Alameda F, Marinoso ML, Bellosillo B, et al. Detection of HPV by in situ hybridization in thin-layer (ThinPrep) cervicovaginal samples. Tumour Biol. 2011;32:603–9.

95. Pinto AP, Degen M, Villa LL, Cibas ES. Immunomarkers in gynecologic cytology: the search for the ideal 'biomolecular Papanicolaou test'. Acta Cytol. 2012;56:109–21.
96. Oberg TN, Kipp BR, Vrana JA, et al. Comparison of p16INK4a and ProEx C immunostaining on cervical ThinPrep cytology and biopsy specimens. Diagn Cytopathol. 2010;38:564–72.
97. Roelens J, Reuschenbach M, von Knebel Doeberitz M, Wentzensen N, Bergeron C, Arbyn M. p16INK4a immunocytochemistry versus human papillomavirus testing for triage of women with minor cytologic abnormalities: a systematic review and meta-analysis. Cancer Cytopathol. 2012;120:294–307.
98. Szarewski A, Mesher D, Cadman L, et al. Comparison of seven tests for high-grade cervical intraepithelial neoplasia in women with abnormal smears: the Predictors 2 study. J Clin Microbiol. 2012;50:1867–73.
99. Guo M, Baruch AC, Silva EG, et al. Efficacy of p16 and ProExC immunostaining in the detection of high-grade cervical intraepithelial neoplasia and cervical carcinoma. Am J Clin Pathol. 2011;135:212–20.
100. Kim JW, Kim YT, Kim DK, Song CH, Lee JW. Expression of epidermal growth factor receptor in carcinoma of the cervix. Gynecol Oncol. 1996;60:283–7.
101. Mariani L, Vici P, Venuti A, et al. HER family expression in preneoplastic low and high-grade cervical lesions. Int J Gynaecol Obstet. 2012;119.
102. Noordhuis MG, Eijsink JJ, Ten Hoor KA, et al. Expression of epidermal growth factor receptor (EGFR) and activated EGFR predict poor response to (chemo) radiation and survival in cervical cancer. Clin Cancer Res. 2009;15:7389–97.
103. Perez-Regadera J, Sanchez-Munoz A, De-la-Cruz J, et al. Impact of epidermal growth factor receptor expression on disease-free survival and rate of pelvic relapse in patients with advanced cancer of the cervix treated with chemoradiotherapy. Am J Clin Oncol. 2011;34:395–400.
104. Woodworth CD, Diefendorf LP, Jette DF, et al. Inhibition of the epidermal growth factor receptor by erlotinib prevents immortalization of human cervical cells by Human Papillomavirus type 16. Virology. 2011;421:19–27.
105. De Strooper LM, Hesselink AT, Berkhof J, et al. Combined CADM1/MAL methylation and cytology testing for colposcopy triage of high-risk HPV-positive women. Cancer Epidemiol Biomarkers Prev. 2014;23:1933–7.
106. Hesselink AT, Heideman DA, Steenbergen RD, et al. Combined promoter methylation analysis of CADM1 and MAL: an objective triage tool for high-risk human papillomavirus DNA-positive women. Clin Cancer Res. 2011;17:2459–65.
107. Lai HC, Ou YC, Chen TC, et al. PAX1/SOX1 DNA methylation and cervical neoplasia detection: a taiwanese gynecologic oncology group (TGOG) study. Cancer Med. 2014;3:1062–74.
108. Luttmer R, De Strooper LM, Berkhof J et al. Comparing the performance of FAM19A4 methylation analysis, cytology and HPV16/18 genotyping for the detection of cervical (pre)cancer in high-risk HPV-positive women of a gynecologic outpatient population (COMETH study). Int J Cancer. 2015.
109. Lorincz AT, Brentnall AR, Vasiljevic N, et al. HPV16 L1 and L2 DNA methylation predicts high-grade cervical intraepithelial neoplasia in women with mildly abnormal cervical cytology. Int J Cancer. 2013;133:637–44.
110. Waggoner SE. Cervical cancer. Lancet. 2003;361:2217–25.
111. Jemal A, Siegel R, Ward E, et al. Cancer statistics, 2008. CA Cancer J Clin. 2008;58:71–96.
112. Hirte H, Kennedy EB, Elit L, Fung MFK. Systemic therapy for recurrent, persistent, or metastatic cervical cancer: a clinical practice guideline. Curr Oncol. 2015;22:211–9.
113. Vici P, Mariani L, Pizzuti L, et al. Emerging biological treatments for uterine cervical carcinoma. J Cancer. 2014;5:86–97.
114. Cheng WF, Chen CA, Lee CN, Wei LH, Hsieh FJ, Hsieh CY. Vascular endothelial growth factor and prognosis of cervical carcinoma. Obstet Gynecol. 2000;96:721–6.

115. Hashimoto I, Kodama J, Seki N, et al. Vascular endothelial growth factor-C expression and its relationship to pelvic lymph node status in invasive cervical cancer. Br J Cancer. 2001;85:93–7.
116. Lee JS, Kim HS, Jung JJ, Lee MC, Park CS. Expression of vascular endothelial growth factor in adenocarcinomas of the uterine cervix and its relation to angiogenesis and p53 and c-erbB-2 protein expression. Gynecol Oncol. 2002;85:469–75.
117. Willmott LJ, Monk BJ. Cervical cancer therapy: current, future and anti-angiogenesis targeted treatment. Expert Rev Anticancer Ther. 2009;9:895–903.
118. Monk BJ, Sill MW, Burger RA, Gray HJ, Buekers TE, Roman LD. Phase II trial of bevacizumab in the treatment of persistent or recurrent squamous cell carcinoma of the cervix: a gynecologic oncology group study. J Clin Oncol. 2009;27:1069–74.
119. Tewari KS, Sill MW, Long HJ 3rd, et al. Improved survival with bevacizumab in advanced cervical cancer. N Engl J Med. 2014;370:734–43.
120. Schefter TE, Winter K, Kwon JS, et al. A phase II study of bevacizumab in combination with definitive radiotherapy and cisplatin chemotherapy in untreated patients with locally advanced cervical carcinoma: preliminary results of RTOG 0417. Int J Radiat Oncol Biol Phys. 2012;83:1179–84.
121. Schefter T, Winter K, Kwon JS, et al. RTOG 0417: efficacy of bevacizumab in combination with definitive radiation therapy and cisplatin chemotherapy in untreated patients with locally advanced cervical carcinoma. Int J Radiat Oncol Biol Phys. 2014;88:101–5.
122. Zighelboim I, Wright JD, Gao F, et al. Multicenter phase II trial of topotecan, cisplatin and bevacizumab for recurrent or persistent cervical cancer. Gynecol Oncol. 2013;130:64–8.
123. Hagemann AR, Novetsky AP, Zighelboim I, et al. Phase II study of bevacizumab and pemetrexed for recurrent or persistent epithelial ovarian, fallopian tube or primary peritoneal cancer. Gynecol Oncol. 2013;131:535–40.
124. Mackay HJ, Tinker A, Winquist E, et al. A phase II study of sunitinib in patients with locally advanced or metastatic cervical carcinoma: NCIC CTG Trial IND.184. Gynecol Oncol. 2010;116:163–7.
125. Candelaria M, Arias-Bonfill D, Chavez-Blanco A, et al. Lack in efficacy for imatinib mesylate as second-line treatment of recurrent or metastatic cervical cancer expressing platelet-derived growth factor receptor alpha. Int J Gynecol Cancer. 2009;19:1632–7.
126. Monk BJ, Mas Lopez L, Zarba JJ, et al. Phase II, open-label study of pazopanib or lapatinib monotherapy compared with pazopanib plus lapatinib combination therapy in patients with advanced and recurrent cervical cancer. J Clin Oncol. 2010;28:3562–9.
127. Nasarre P, Thomas M, Kruse K, et al. Host-derived angiopoietin-2 affects early stages of tumor development and vessel maturation but is dispensable for later stages of tumor growth. Cancer Res. 2009;69:1324–33.
128. Kopczynska E, Makarewicz R, Biedka M, Kaczmarczyk A, Kardymowicz H, Tyrakowski T. Plasma concentration of angiopoietin-1, angiopoietin-2 and Tie-2 in cervical cancer. Eur J Gynaecol Oncol. 2009;30:646–9.
129. Shim WS, Teh M, Bapna A, et al. Angiopoietin 1 promotes tumor angiogenesis and tumor vessel plasticity of human cervical cancer in mice. Exp Cell Res. 2002;279:299–309.
130. Kersemaekers AM, Fleuren GJ, Kenter GG, et al. Oncogene alterations in carcinomas of the uterine cervix: overexpression of the epidermal growth factor receptor is associated with poor prognosis. Clin Cancer Res. 1999;5:577–86.
131. Goncalves A, Fabbro M, Lhomme C, et al. A phase II trial to evaluate gefitinib as second- or third-line treatment in patients with recurring locoregionally advanced or metastatic cervical cancer. Gynecol Oncol. 2008;108:42–6.
132. Schilder RJ, Sill MW, Lee YC, Mannel R. A phase II trial of erlotinib in recurrent squamous cell carcinoma of the cervix: a gynecologic oncology group Study. Int J Gynecol Cancer. 2009;19:929–33.
133. Hertlein L, Lenhard M, Kirschenhofer A, et al. Cetuximab monotherapy in advanced cervical cancer: a retrospective study with five patients. Arch Gynecol Obstet. 2011;283:109–13.

134. Kurtz JE, Hardy-Bessard AC, Deslandres M, et al. Cetuximab, topotecan and cisplatin for the treatment of advanced cervical cancer: a phase II GINECO trial. Gynecol Oncol. 2009;113:16–20.
135. Fadare O, Zheng W. HER2 protein (p 185(HER2)) is only rarely overexpressed in cervical cancer. Int J Gynecol Pathol. 2004;23:410–1; author reply 411-2.
136. Hirano S, Ito N, Takahashi S, Tamaya T. Clinical implications of insulin-like growth factors through the presence of their binding proteins and receptors expressed in gynecological cancers. Eur J Gynaecol Oncol. 2004;25:187–91.
137. Kong L, Deng Z, Shen H, Zhang Y. Src family kinase inhibitor PP2 efficiently inhibits cervical cancer cell proliferation through down-regulating phospho-Src-Y416 and phospho-EGFR-Y1173. Mol Cell Biochem. 2011;348:11–9.
138. Franko-Tobin LG, Mackey LV, Huang W, et al. Notch1-mediated tumor suppression in cervical cancer with the involvement of SST signaling and its application in enhanced SSTR-targeted therapeutics. Oncologist. 2012;17:220–32.
139. Tinker AV, Ellard S, Welch S, et al. Phase II study of temsirolimus (CCI-779) in women with recurrent, unresectable, locally advanced or metastatic carcinoma of the cervix. A trial of the NCIC clinical trials group (NCIC CTG IND 199). Gynecol Oncol. 2013;130:269–74.
140. Masuda K, Banno K, Yanokura M, et al. Association of epigenetic inactivation of the WRN gene with anticancer drug sensitivity in cervical cancer cells. Oncol Rep. 2012;28:1146–52.
141. Banno K, Yanokura M, Kawaguchi M, et al. Epigenetic inactivation of the CHFR gene in cervical cancer contributes to sensitivity to taxanes. Int J Oncol. 2007;31:713–20.
142. Tanaka T, Bai T, Toujima S, et al. Demethylation restores SN38 sensitivity in cells with acquired resistance to SN38 derived from human cervical squamous cancer cells. Oncol Rep. 2012;27:1292–8.
143. Hengstermann A, Linares LK, Ciechanover A, Whitaker NJ, Scheffner M. Complete switch from Mdm2 to human papillomavirus E6-mediated degradation of p53 in cervical cancer cells. Proc Natl Acad Sci U S A. 2001;98:1218–23.
144. Anchoori RK, Khan SR, Sueblinvong T, et al. Stressing the ubiquitin-proteasome system without 20S proteolytic inhibition selectively kills cervical cancer cells. PLoS ONE. 2011;6: e23888.
145. Stern PL, van der Burg SH, Hampson IN, et al. Therapy of human papillomavirus-related disease. Vaccine. 2012;30(Suppl 5):F71–82.
146. Miyamoto Y, Nakagawa S, Wada-Hiraike O, et al. Sequential effects of the proteasome inhibitor bortezomib and chemotherapeutic agents in uterine cervical cancer cell lines. Oncol Rep. 2013;29:51–7.
147. Hampson L, Kitchener HC, Hampson IN. Specific HIV protease inhibitors inhibit the ability of HPV16 E6 to degrade p53 and selectively kill E6-dependent cervical carcinoma cells in vitro. Antivir Ther. 2006;11:813–25.
148. Zhou J LF, Xiao J.. Recombinant adenovirus-p 53 combined with chemotherapy in treatment of locally advanced cervical cancer (a phase II study). J Clin Oncol. 2013;31(suppl): abstr5525.
149. Liu YG, Zheng XL, Liu FM. The mechanism and inhibitory effect of recombinant human P53 adenovirus injection combined with paclitaxel on human cervical cancer cell HeLa. Eur Rev Med Pharmacol Sci. 2015;19:1037–42.
150. Bermudez-Morales VH, Peralta-Zaragoza O. Madrid-Marina V [Gene therapy with cytokines against cervical cancer]. Salud Publica Mex. 2005;47:458–68.
151. Bharti AC, Shukla S, Mahata S, Hedau S, Das BC. Anti-human papillomavirus therapeutics: facts & future. Indian J Med Res. 2009;130:296–310.
152. Butz K, Denk C, Ullmann A, Scheffner M, Hoppe-Seyler F. Induction of apoptosis in human papillomaviruspositive cancer cells by peptide aptamers targeting the viral E6 oncoprotein. Proc Natl Acad Sci U S A. 2000;97:6693–7.
153. Zhou J, Li B, Peng C, et al. Inhibition of cervical cancer cell growth in vitro and in vivo by lentiviral-vector mediated shRNA targeting the common promoter of HPV16 E6 and E7 oncogenes. Antiviral Res. 2013;98:305–13.

154. Tan S, de Vries EG, van der Zee AG, de Jong S. Anticancer drugs aimed at E6 and E7 activity in HPV-positive cervical cancer. Curr Cancer Drug Targets. 2012;12:170–84.
155. Sgambato A, Zannoni GF, Faraglia B, et al. Decreased expression of the CDK inhibitor p27Kip1 and increased oxidative DNA damage in the multistep process of cervical carcinogenesis. Gynecol Oncol. 2004;92:776–83.
156. Singh M, Bhui K, Singh R, Shukla Y. Tea polyphenols enhance cisplatin chemosensitivity in cervical cancer cells via induction of apoptosis. Life Sci. 2013;93:7–16.
157. Di Domenico F, Foppoli C, Coccia R, Perluigi M. Antioxidants in cervical cancer: chemopreventive and chemotherapeutic effects of polyphenols. Biochim Biophys Acta. 2012;1822:737–47.
158. Mandic A, Usaj-Knezevic S, Kapicl TI, Nincic D, Malenkovic G. Cyclooxygenase-2 expression in cervical cancer. Vojnosanit Pregl. 2014;71:997–1005.
159. Kulkarni S, Rader JS, Zhang F, et al. Cyclooxygenase-2 is overexpressed in human cervical cancer. Clin Cancer Res. 2001;7:429–34.
160. Kim SH, Oh JM, No JH, Bang YJ, Juhnn YS, Song YS. Involvement of NF-kappaB and AP-1 in COX-2 upregulation by human papillomavirus 16 E5 oncoprotein. Carcinogenesis. 2009;30:753–7.
161. Subbaramaiah K, Dannenberg AJ. Cyclooxygenase-2 transcription is regulated by human papillomavirus 16 E6 and E7 oncoproteins: evidence of a corepressor/coactivator exchange. Cancer Res. 2007;67:3976–85.
162. Chen HH, Su WC, Chou CY, et al. Increased expression of nitric oxide synthase and cyclooxygenase-2 is associated with poor survival in cervical cancer treated with radiotherapy. Int J Radiat Oncol Biol Phys. 2005;63:1093–100.
163. Ferrandina G, Ranelletti FO, Legge F, et al. Celecoxib modulates the expression of cyclooxygenase-2, ki67, apoptosis-related marker, and microvessel density in human cervical cancer: a pilot study. Clin Cancer Res. 2003;9:4324–31.
164. Herrera FG, Chan P, Doll C, et al. A prospective phase I-II trial of the cyclooxygenase-2 inhibitor celecoxib in patients with carcinoma of the cervix with biomarker assessment of the tumor microenvironment. Int J Radiat Oncol Biol Phys. 2007;67:97–103.
165. Young JL, Jazaeri AA, Darus CJ, Modesitt SC. Cyclooxygenase-2 in cervical neoplasia: a review. Gynecol Oncol. 2008;109:140–5.
166. Liu Y, Liu Z, Androphy E, Chen J, Baleja JD. Design and characterization of helical peptides that inhibit the E6 protein of papillomavirus. Biochemistry. 2004;43:7421–31.
167. Baleja JD, Cherry JJ, Liu Z, et al. Identification of inhibitors to papillomavirus type 16 E6 protein based on three-dimensional structures of interacting proteins. Antiviral Res. 2006;72:49–59.
168. Zehbe I, Richard C, Lee KF, Campbell M, Hampson L, Hampson IN. Lopinavir shows greater specificity than zinc finger ejecting compounds as a potential treatment for human papillomavirus-related lesions. Antiviral Res. 2011;91:161–6.
169. Song M, DiPaola RS, Cracchiolo BM, et al. Phase 2 trial of paclitaxel, 13-cis retinoic acid, and interferon alfa-2b in the treatment of advanced stage or recurrent cervical cancer. Int J Gynecol Cancer. 2014;24:1636–41.
170. Van Pachterbeke C, Bucella D, Rozenberg S, et al. Topical treatment of CIN2+ by cidofovir: results of a phase II, double-blind, prospective, placebo-controlled study. Gynecol Oncol. 2009;115:69–74.
171. Contreras-Paredes A, De la Cruz-Hernandez E, Martinez-Ramirez I, Duenas-Gonzalez A, Lizano M. E6 variants of human papillomavirus 18 differentially modulate the protein kinase B/phosphatidylinositol 3-kinase (akt/PI3K) signaling pathway. Virology. 2009;383:78–85.
172. Feng W, Duan X, Liu J, Xiao J, Brown RE. Morphoproteomic evidence of constitutively activated and overexpressed mTOR pathway in cervical squamous carcinoma and high grade squamous intraepithelial lesions. Int J Clin Exp Pathol. 2009;2:249–60.
173. Ji J, Zheng PS. Activation of mTOR signaling pathway contributes to survival of cervical cancer cells. Gynecol Oncol. 2010;117:103–8.

174. Manavi M, Hudelist G, Fink-Retter A, Gschwandtler-Kaulich D, Pischinger K, Czerwenka K. Gene profiling in Pap-cell smears of high-risk human papillomavirus-positive squamous cervical carcinoma. Gynecol Oncol. 2007;105:418–26.
175. Hirai H, Iwasawa Y, Okada M, et al. Small-molecule inhibition of Wee1 kinase by MK-1775 selectively sensitizes p53-deficient tumor cells to DNA-damaging agents. Mol Cancer Ther. 2009;8:2992–3000.
176. Brehm A, Nielsen SJ, Miska EA, et al. The E7 oncoprotein associates with Mi2 and histone deacetylase activity to promote cell growth. EMBO J. 1999;18:2449–58.
177. de la Cruz-Hernandez E, Perez-Cardenas E, Contreras-Paredes A, et al. The effects of DNA methylation and histone deacetylase inhibitors on human papillomavirus early gene expression in cervical cancer, an in vitro and clinical study. Virol J. 2007;4:18.
178. Lin Z, Bazzaro M, Wang MC, Chan KC, Peng S, Roden RB. Combination of proteasome and HDAC inhibitors for uterine cervical cancer treatment. Clin Cancer Res. 2009;15:570–7.
179. Coronel J, Cetina L, Pacheco I, et al. A double-blind, placebo-controlled, randomized phase III trial of chemotherapy plus epigenetic therapy with hydralazine valproate for advanced cervical cancer. Preliminary results. Med Oncol. 2011;28(Suppl 1):S540–6.
180. Guggenheim ER, Ondrus AE, Movassaghi M, Lippard SJ. Poly(ADP-ribose) polymerase-1 activity facilitates the dissociation of nuclear proteins from platinum-modified DNA. Bioorg Med Chem. 2008;16:10121–8.
181. Shunkwiler L, Ferris G, Kunos C. Inhibition of Poly(ADP-Ribose) Polymerase Enhances Radiochemosensitivity in Cancers Proficient in DNA Double-Strand Break Repair. Int J Mol Sci. 2013;14:3773–85.
182. Kunos C, Deng W, Dawson D, et al. A phase I-II evaluation of veliparib (NSC #737664), topotecan, and filgrastim or pegfilgrastim in the treatment of persistent or recurrent carcinoma of the uterine cervix: an NRG oncology/gynecologic oncology group study. Int J Gynecol Cancer. 2015;25:484–92.

Index

Note: Page numbers followed by *f* and *t* refer to figures and tables respectively

A

Aberrant DNA methylations, 256–257, 262
Aberrant E-cadherin protein, 11
Aberrant mismatch repair protein expression patterns, 175
Aberrant p53 staining, 53, 126
ACS*See* American Cancer Society
AKT inhibitors, 101, 151, 191, 195
AKT-mTOR signal transduction pathway, 98
Alcohol intake, 204
ALK-negative IMTs, 240
Altered micro-RNAs, 257
American Cancer Society (ACS), 204, 258
American Society of Colposcopy and Cervical Pathology (ASCCP), 258
Angiogenesis, 195–197
Angiopoietins (ANGPTs), 200, 266
Anti-angiogenic agents, 263, 266
Anti-HER2 therapies, 161, 266
Anti-HIV drug lopinavir, 269
Antioxidants, 268
Antiviral agents, 269
APAM*See* Atypical polypoid adenomyoma
Aptima HPV assays, 260
ARID1A, 23–24, 53, 69, 128, 134
Array comparative genomic hybridization studies, 233
ASCCP*See* American Society of Colposcopy and Cervical Pathology
Atypical leiomyoma, 229
Atypical polypoid adenomyoma (APAM), 27
Avastin, 196, 263

B

Bariatric surgery, 206
Bax, 23, 133
Bcl-2, 133
Benign metastasizing leiomyoma (BML), 231
β-catenin immunohistochemistry, 71*f*
Bevacizumab (Avastin), 196, 263
Biphasic intermixed histologic pattern, 33
BML*See* Benign metastasizing leiomyoma
Bokhman type I tumors, 50
Bokhman type II tumors, 50
BORIS*See* Brother of the regulator of imprinted sites
BRAF mutation, 178, 194, 195
BRCA mutation, 181
Breast carcinoma, 43, 45*f*
Brother of the regulator of imprinted sites (BORIS), 162

C

Cancer Genome Atlas Research Network, 12
Carcinogenesis, dualistic model of, 7
Carcinosarcoma, 32, 33, 156*f*
CCC*See* Clear cell carcinoma
Cediranib (AZD2171), 196
Cell adhesion molecule, 11
Cellular leiomyoma, 228–229
Cervical cancers, genetic and epigenetic changes in, 256–257
Cervical dysplasia and carcinoma, molecular pathology of, 253–254
- genetic and epigenetic changes, 256–257
- HPV
  - classification, 254
  - infection, natural history of, 255
- molecular basis of emerging biological treatment, 263, 264t–265t
  - anti-angiogenic agents, 263, 266
  - antioxidants and COX-2 inhibitors, 268
  - antiviral agents, 269
  - demethylating agents and proteasome inhibitors, 267
  - EGFR, inhibitors of, 266
  - miRNAs and siRNAs, 268
  - mTOR, inhibitors of, 266–267

M.T. Deavers and D.M. Coffey (eds.), *Precision Molecular Pathology of Uterine Cancer*, Molecular Pathology Library,
DOI 10.1007/978-3-319-57985-6

Cervical dysplasia and carcinoma, molecular pathology of (*cont.*)
 persistent HPV infection and cell transformation, 255
 prevention and risk profiling
  HPV and Pap cytology co-testing, 258–259
  HPV16/18 genotyping, 259
  HPV testing, 257–261, 260t
  Pap cytology for cervical cancer screening, tumor markers, 261–262
 SCJ cells, 255–256
Cetuximab, 266
Chromodomain-helicase-DNA-binding protein 4 (CHD4), 107–108
Chromosomal aberrations, 256
Ciliated variant, 26
Clear cell carcinoma (CCC), 31, 31*f*, 123–124, 125*f*, 127*t*, 130
Clonality, 156
Cobas HPV assay, 260
Colorectal carcinomas, 44
Confirmatory testing, 180
Contraceptives, 205
Conventional leiomyoma, 227–228
Conventional leiomyosarcoma, 229–231, 230*f*
Copanlisib, 193
Copy number variations, 161–162
Cowden syndrome, 35, 36, 169, 179–181, 179*f*, 180*f*, 207
CTNNB1, 23, 71–72, 71*f*, 79, 80, 102, 131, 160
Cyclo-oxygenase-2 (COX-2), 157, 268
Cytoplasm, 124
Cytoplasmic staining, 56

D
Dasatinib, 200
Dedifferentiated type, 32
Demethylating agents, 267
Diabetes, 205
Diet, 204
DNA
 damage repair pathways, 197
 mismatch repair gene mutation analysis, 178
 MMR, 75, 206
 mutations, 256
 polymerase epsilon, 76
 sequencing, 88
Double-strand breaks (DSBs), 197
Dual inhibitor agents, 193–194
Dual tyrosine kinase inhibitor, 199
Dyslipidemia, 205

E
E2 binding sites (E2BSs), 257
E-cadherin, 11
Education, 206
EGFR/Her-1*See* Epidermal Growth Factor Receptor
EGFR RTK inhibitors, 266
Embryonal rhabdomyosarcoma (ERMS), 240
Emerging biological treatment, molecular basis of, 263, 264*t*–265*t*
 anti-angiogenic agents, 263, 266
 antioxidants and COX-2 inhibitors, 268
 antiviral agents, 269
 demethylating agents and proteasome inhibitors, 267
 EGFR, inhibitors of, 266
 miRNAs and siRNAs, 268
 mTOR, inhibitors of, 266–267
EmGD*See* Endometrial glandular dysplasia
EMT*See* Epithelial-to-mesenchymal transition
Endocervical adenocarcinoma, 146
Endocervix, microglandular hyperplasia of, 145
Endometrial biopsy, 148
Endometrial (uterine) cancer, 51, 158, 187
 molecular landscape of, 188–189, 189t, 190f
 pathways of interest in
  angiogenesis, 195–197
  EGFR pathway, 198–199
  PARP pathway, 197–198
  PI3K/AKT pathway, 190–194, 192t
  Ras/Raf pathway, 194–195
 prevention of, 201, 202t–203t
 targeted therapy for, 187–188
Endometrial carcinoma, 174*f*, 177*f*
 vs. extramüllerian primaries, 43–47
 histopathologic classification of
  clear cell carcinoma, 31, 31f
  endometrioid adenocarcinoma, 24–28, 25f, 27t, 28t
  hereditary endometrial carcinoma, 35–36
  mixed carcinoma, 32
  mucinous carcinoma, 28
  neuroendocrine tumors, 33–34
  prognostic factors, 34
  serous carcinoma, 29–31, 29f, 30t
  staging of endometrial carcinoma, 34, 35t
  undifferentiated carcinoma, 32–33, 33f
 and Lynch syndrome, 55–57
 molecular features of, 136

vs. Other Müllerian primaries, 47–50
precursor lesions and molecular profiles
Type I endometrial cancer, 3–4
uterine serous carcinoma (Type 2), 4–12
putative pathogenetic model for, 21–24
subtyping of, 50–55
Endometrial clear cell carcinomas, molecular genetic features of, 132*t*
Endometrial glands, 43
Endometrial glandular dysplasia (EmGD), 9
Endometrial hyperplasia, 47
Endometrial *POLE* mutant tumors, 78
Endometrial serous carcinoma glandular pattern, low power section from, 5*f*
Endometrial serous carcinoma, high power illustration of, 5*f*
Endometrial stromal neoplasms, 233–235
ESN and LGESS, 234–236, 234f
HGESS, 236–237, 237f
Endometrial stromal nodule (ESN), 234, 236
Endometrioid adenocarcinoma, 4, 24–28, 25*f*, 27*t*, 28*t*, 53, 65–66, 188
microsatellite instability, 75–76, 77t
PI3K/AKT pathway
ARID1A, 69
CTNNB1, 71–72
KRAS, 69–70
PIK3CA, 68
PIK3R1 and PIK3R2, 68–69
PTEN, 66–68, 67f
TP53, 72–75
POLE, 76, 78
TCGA, 79–80, 79f
Endometrioid carcinoma, molecular alterations in, 7–8
Endometrioid endometrial carcinoma, 51
Endometrium
microglandular adenocarcinoma of, 147
mucinous adenocarcinoma of, 144f
clinical features, 143
histopathologic features, 144–145
immunohistochemical profile, 146–147
papillary mucinous metaplasia, 147–148, 147f, 148–151
E7 oncoprotein, 261
Epidermal growth factor receptor (EGFR), 11, 198–199, 266
Epithelial-to-mesenchymal transition (EMT), 157
ERBB2 aberrations in SEC, 103–104
ER immunoreactivity, 31
ERMS*See* Embryonal rhabdomyosarcoma
ER/vimentin/mCEA/p16
immunohistochemical panel, 49
ESN*See* Endometrial stromal nodule
Ethanol, 204
Everolimus, 102–103
Extensive immature squamous differentiation, 24–25
Extensive keratinization, 26
Extramüllerian primaries, endometrial carcinoma *vs.*, 43–47

F

Familial breast ovarian cancer syndromes (*BRCA* mutations), 181
Familial cancer syndromes, 169
FBXW7 aberrations in SEC, 105–106, 105*f*
FGF inhibition*See* Fibroblast growth factor inhibition
FGF receptors (FGFRs), 196
Fibroblast growth factor (FGF) inhibition, 196–197
FIGO grade 2 endometrioid adenocarcinoma, with glandular and solid patterns, 25*f*
FIGO grading of endometrioid carcinoma, 27*t*
FISH*See* Fluorescence in situ hybridization
Flat negative immunostaining, 30
Fluorescence in situ hybridization (FISH), 10, 235–236, 235*f*

G

Gastric adenocarcinomas, 44
Gene fusions, 234–236
Genetics, 150
Genomic characterization of USC, 12
Germline mutations, 181
Gilotrif®, 105

H

Hallmark cancers of Lynch syndrome, 55
Hepatocyte nuclear factor-1β (HNF-1β), 126, 131, 133
HER2 (ERBB2) aberrations in SEC, 103–104
Herceptin®, 104
Hereditary cancer syndromes, 206
Hereditary endometrial carcinoma, 35–36, 169
Cowden syndrome, 179–181, 179f, 180f
familial breast ovarian cancer syndromes (BRCA mutations), 181
LFS, 181–182
Lynch syndrome
clinical features, 171
molecular basis, 170
pathologic features, 171, 172f, 173
screening and confirmatory testing, 173, 174, 174f, 175, 175f, 176, 176f, 177, 177f, 178

polymerase proofreading-(POLD1) associated syndrome, 181
Hereditary leiomyomatosis and renal cell carcinoma syndrome, 229
Hereditary non-polyposis colorectal cancer (HNPCC), 35
Her-2/neu, 10, 198
High-grade endometrial stromal sarcoma (HGESS), 236–237, 237*f*
High-risk HPV infection, 261
Histopathologic classification of endometrial carcinoma
clear cell carcinoma, 31, 31f
endometrioid adenocarcinoma, 24–28, 25f, 27t, 28t
hereditary endometrial carcinoma, 35–36
mixed carcinoma, 32
mucinous carcinoma, 28
neuroendocrine tumors, 33–34
prognostic factors, 34
serous carcinoma, 29–31, 29f, 30t
staging of endometrial carcinoma, 34, 35t
undifferentiated carcinoma, 32–33, 33f
HLRCC-associated leiomyoma, 230*f*
HMGA1, 228, 231
HMGA2, 228, 229, 231
HNPCC*See* Hereditary non-polyposis colorectal cancer
Hormone replacement therapy (HRT), 201, 203
HPV*See* Human papillomavirus
HPV16/18 genotyping, 259
HRT*See* Hormone replacement therapy
Human papillomavirus (HPV)
classification of, 254
infection, natural history of, 255
and Pap cytology co-testing, 258–259
primary screening study, 262
testing, 257–261, 260t
vaccines, 254
Hyperplasia, 4
Hypertension, 205

I
Immune evasion, 255
Immune therapy, 201
Immunohistochemical typing of endometrial carcinoma, 28*t*
Inflammatory myofibroblastic tumor (IMT), 239–240
In situ hybridization (ISH), 261
Intensive surveillance programs, 182
Intravenous leiomyomatosis (IVL), 231
ISH*See* in situ hybridization
IVL*See* Intravenous leiomyomatosis

J
JAZF1 abnormalities, 235
JAZF1–PHF1 gene fusion, 235
JAZF1–SUZ12, 234

K
Karyotypes of leiomyoma, 228
Ki-67, 26, 148
KRAS, 8, 69–70, 149*f*, 150–151, 188, 195, 199

L
Lapatinib, 104–105
Large cell neuroendocrine carcinoma (LCNEC), 34
LEEP*See* Loop Electrosurgical Excision Procedure
Leiomyoma, 227, 228*f*
Lesions, 4
Levonorgestrel-releasing intrauterine system, 205–206
LFS*See* Li-Fraumeni syndrome
LGESS*See* Low-grade endometrial stromal sarcoma
Li-Fraumeni syndrome (LFS), 181–182
Loop Electrosurgical Excision Procedure (LEEP), 258
Low-grade endometrial stromal sarcoma (LGESS), 234, 234*f*, 236
Low-grade mucinous endometrial adenocarcinoma, 145
Lynch syndrome, 35, 36, 57*f*, 169, 207
clinical features, 171
endometrial carcinoma and, 55–57
molecular basis, 170
pathologic features, 171, 172f, 173
screening and confirmatory testing, 173, 174, 174f, 175, 175f, 176, 176f, 177, 177f, 178
Lynch syndrome-related endometrial carcinomas, 171

M
MA*See* Mullerian adenosarcoma
Malignant mixed Müllerian tumor (MMMT) *See* Uterine carcinosarcoma (UCS)
Mammaglobin, 44
Mammalian target of rapamycin (mTOR), 190, 192
inhibitors of, 102, 266–267
MATH domain*See* Meprin and TRAF homology domain

MED12, 227–228
MEK inhibition, 101, 151, 195
Meprin and TRAF homology (MATH) domain, 108
Metastatic tumors, 43
Metformin, 199, 206
Methylation markers, 262
Microglandular adenocarcinoma, 145
  of endometrium, 147
Microglandular hyperplasia of endocervix, 145
Micro-RNAs (miRNAs), 162–163, 268
  expression profiles in UCS, 162
Microsatellite instability (MSI), 8, 176–177, 201
Mismatch repair (MMR)
  deficiency, 161
  immunohistochemistry, 56
  protein immunohistochemistry, 173–176, 174f–177f
Mixed carcinoma, 32
MLH1 promoter methylation analysis, 178
MMMT*See* Malignant mixed Müllerian tumor
MMR*See* Mismatch repair
Molecular alterations
  in endometrioid carcinoma, 7–8
  in serous carcinoma, 9–12
Molecular landscape of endometrial cancer, 188–189, 189*t*, 190*f*
Molecular profiles
  Type I endometrial cancer, 3–4
  uterine serous carcinoma (Type II), 4–12
Molecular signature, 7
Monomorphic type, 32
Monotherapies, 266
Morphologic clues, 43
mRNA expression profiles in UCS, 162
mTOR*See* Mammalian target of rapamycin
Mucinous adenocarcinoma of endometrium, 144*f*
  clinical features, 143
  histopathologic features, 144–145
  immunohistochemical profile, 146
    differential diagnosis, 146–147
  papillary mucinous metaplasia, 147–148, 147f
    genetics, 150
    KRAS, 150–151
    PTEN, 151
    pyloric/gastric metaplasia of endometrium, 148–150
Mucinous carcinoma, 28
Mucinous metaplasia, 148
Mullerian adenosarcoma (MA), 238–239, 239*f*
Mullerian epithelium, 7
Multifocal mucinous lesions, 148
Murine models of EC, 98
Mutated genes in UCS, 160–161

N
Napsin A, 133
NCI's National Clinical Trials Network (NCTN)—Exceptional Responders Initiative (NCT02243592), 110
Neuroendocrine growth pattern, 34
Neuroendocrine tumors, 33–34
Neutrophils, 145
Next-generation sequencing (NGS) techniques, 158
Non-endometrioid endometrial cancer, risk factors for, 201
Non-hormonal intrauterine devices, 205
Novel clinical trial designs, 109–110
NRG Oncology—Gynecologic Oncology Group (GOG), 199
Nuclear atypia, 144
Nuclear BAF250a protein, 53
Nuclear stratification, 124–125
Nuclei, 32

O
Obesity, 203
OCP*See* Oral contraceptives
Oncogenesis, precursor lesion and, 135–136
Oral contraceptives (OCP), 205
Ovarian clear cell carcinoma, molecular features of, 136
Oxidative DNA damage, 268

P
P16 (INK4a), 11–12
P53, 9, 156*f*, 158, 159*f*, 200
Pan-cancer analysis, 109
Pan-PI3K inhibitor pilaralisib, 101
Pap cytology, 258, 262
Papillary mucinous metaplasia, 147–148, 147*f*
  genetics, 150
  KRAS, 150–151
  PTEN, 151
  pyloric/gastric metaplasia of endometrium, 148–150
PARADIGM-SHIFT algorithm, 97
PCOS*See* Polycystic ovary syndrome
PCR-based hypermethylation testing, 178
PCR-based MSI testing, 176–177
PDGFR*See* Platelet-derived growth factor receptor
PEComa*See* Perivascular epithelioid cell tumor
Pembrolizumab, 201

Perivascular epithelioid cell tumor (PEComa), 232–233, 232*f*
Peutz–Jeghers syndrome (PJS), 148–150
Phase II ENDORAD trial, 102
Phosphatase and tensin homolog *(PTEN)*, 7–8, 53, 66–68, 67*f*, 135, 151
  Cleveland Clinic risk assessment tool, 180
Phosphatidylinositol 3-kinase (PI3K/AKT) pathway, 159–163, 160*f*, 161*t*, 190–194, 192*t*
  aberrations in SEC, 98–101
  ARID1A, 69
  CTNNB1, 71–72
  KRAS, 69–70
  PIK3CA, 68
  PIK3R1 and PIK3R2, 68–69
  PTEN, 66–68, 67f
  TP53, 72–75
PIK3CA, 68, 135
PIK3R1, 68–69, 99
PIK3R2, 68–69
PJS*See* Peutz–Jeghers syndrome
Platelet-derived growth factor receptor (PDGFR), 196
POLE, 76, 78, 160–161
Poly ADP-ribose polymerase (PARP) pathway, 197–198
Polycystic ovary syndrome (PCOS), 205
Polymerase proofreading-(POLD1) associated syndrome, 181
Polyphenols, 268
Populations for prevention strategies, 206–207
Postmenopausal women, 203
PPP2R1A, 134–135
  in SEC, 106–107
Precursor lesions
  and oncogenesis, 135–136
  Type I endometrial cancer, 3–4
  uterine serous carcinoma (Type II), 4–12
Prognostic factors, 34
Proteasome inhibitors, 267
Protein kinase mTOR, 192
Protein S6 kinase (pS6K), 191
Pure EIC, 6
Pyloric/gastric metaplasia of endometrium, 148–150

Q
Quasi-malignant, 231–232

R
RAD51B translocations, 233
Ras/Raf pathway, 194–195
Recombinant adenovirus-p53 (rAD-p53), 267
Reed syndrome, 229
REGgamma, 98
Ridaforolimus, phase II trials of, 103

S
SCJ cells*See* Squamo-columnar junction cells
SCNEC*See* Small cell neuroendocrine carcinoma
Screening and confirmatory testing
  microsatellite instability analysis, 176–177
  mismatch repair protein immunohistochemistry, 173–176, 174f–177f
  MLH1 promoter methylation analysis, 178
Secretory differentiation, variant with, 26
Secretory variant, 26
SEIC*See* Serous endometrial intraepithelial carcinoma
Serous adenocarcinoma, 53
Serous carcinoma, 29–31, 29*f*, 30*t*, 49, 50*f*
  molecular alterations in, 9–12
Serous endometrial cancer (SEC), 89*t*–90*t*, 91*f*, 101*f*
  CHD4 mutations in, 107–108
  clinical trials testing targeted therapies, 92t–95t
  FBXW7 aberrations in, 105–106, 105f
  HER2 (ERBB2)
    aberrations in, 103–104
    as therapeutic target in, 104–105
  molecular pathology of, 87–88, 91
  novel clinical trial designs, 109–110
  phase II clinical trial of targeted therapies, 96t–97t
  PI3K pathway aberrations, 98–101
    as therapeutic targets, 101–103
  PPP2R1A mutations in, 106–107
  SPOP mutations in, 108–109, 108f
  TAF1 mutations in, 109
  TP53 aberrations in, 97–98
Serous endometrial intraepithelial carcinoma (SEIC), 6, 30
Serum hormone-binding globulins (SHBG), 203
Short-interfering RNAs (siRNAs), 268
Signal-amplification-based assay, 261
Single-agent temsirolimus therapy, phase II trial of, 103
Small cell neuroendocrine carcinoma (SCNEC), 34
Smooth muscle tumors
  cellular leiomyoma, 228–229

conventional leiomyoma, 227–228
conventional leiomyosarcoma, 229–231, 230f
hereditary leiomyomatosis and renal cell carcinoma syndrome, 229
unusual smooth muscle neoplasms (quasi-malignant), 231–232
Somatic gene mutational analysis, 178
Somatic mutations, 107
Speckle-type BTB/POZ protein (SPOP), 108–109, 108*f*
SPOP*See* Speckle-type BTB/POZ protein
Squamo-columnar junction (SCJ) cells, 255–256
Squamous differentiation, 24, 25*f*
Squamous morules, 47
Staging of endometrial carcinoma, 34, 35*t*
Stroma, 32
STUMP, 232
Substrate proteins, 108*f*
Sunitinib, 196
Surgery, 206

T

TAF1*See* TBD-associated factor 1
Tamoxifen, 203
Targeted therapy for endometrial cancer, 187–188
TBD-associated factor 1 (TAF1), 109
TCGA*See* The Cancer Genome Atlas
TCGA Research Network, 158
TFIID*See* Transcription factor IID
The Cancer Genome Atlas (TCGA), 51, 71, 79–80, 79*f*, 90*t*, 91, 150, 188
Therapeutic target in SEC, HER2, 104–105
Tobacco intake, 204
Transcription factor IID (TFIID), 109
Trastuzumab, 198
Trebananib (AMG-386), 200
Tumor cells, 45*f*, 124
Tumor markers in Pap cytology for cervical cancer screening, 261–262
Tumor protein 53 (*TP53,* P53), 9–10, 72–75, 134, 163, 231
aberrations in SEC, 97–98
Type I endometrial cancer, 3–4, 7
Type II tumors, 7

U

UCS*See* Uterine carcinosarcoma
Ultramutated tumors, 76
Undifferentiated carcinoma, 32–33, 33*f*
Undifferentiated component, 32
Undifferentiated endometrial adenocarcinoma, 172
Undifferentiated uterine sarcoma (UUS), 237
Unopposed estrogen exposure, 201, 203
Unusual smooth muscle neoplasms (quasi-malignant), 231–232
USCs*See* Uterine serous carcinomas
Uterine carcinosarcoma (UCS), 155–157
clinicopathologic features, 155–157
genetic alterations
PI3K/AKT pathway, 159–163, 160f, 161t
p53 pathway, 156f, 158, 159f
molecular types, 163–164
Uterine clear cell carcinoma, 123–124
biological function of immunohistochemical and genetic markers
ARID1A, 134
Bax and bcl-2, 133
hepatocyte nuclear factor-1b, 131, 133
Napsin A, 133
PIK3CA and PTEN, 135
PPP2R1A, 134–135
TP53, 134
genetic features, 130–131, 132t
histopathologic features, 124–125, 125f
immunophenotypic features, 126, 127t, 128, 129, 129f, 130
precursor lesion and oncogenesis, 135–136
Uterine mesenchymal tumors, molecular pathology of
endometrial stromal neoplasms, 233–234
ESN and LGESS, 234–236, 234f
HGESS, 236–237, 237f
perivascular epithelioid cell tumor (PEComa), 232–233, 232f
smooth muscle tumors
atypical leiomyoma, 229
cellular leiomyoma, 228–229
conventional leiomyoma, 227–228
conventional leiomyosarcoma, 229–231, 230f
hereditary leiomyomatosis and renal cell carcinoma syndrome, 229
unusual smooth muscle neoplasms (quasi-malignant), 231–232
UTROSCT, 238, 238f
ERMS, 240
IMT, 239–240
MA, 238–239, 239f
UUS, 237
Uterine serous carcinomas (Type 2), 3–12, 200

Uterine tumor resembling ovarian sex cord tumor (UTROSCT), 238, 238*f*
  ERMS, 240
  IMT, 239–240
  MA, 238–239, 239f
UUS*See* Undifferentiated uterine sarcoma

V
Variant with secretory differentiation, 26
Vascular endothelial growth factor (VEGF), 195–196, 263
VEGFR inhibition, 196
Villoglandular variant, 26

Y
YWHAE-FAM22A/B gene fusions, 236

MIX
Papier aus verantwortungsvollen Quellen
Paper from responsible sources
FSC® C105338

If you have any concerns about our products,
you can contact us on
ProductSafety@springernature.com

In case Publisher is established outside the EU,
the EU authorized representative is:
Springer Nature Customer Service Center GmbH
Europaplatz 3, 69115 Heidelberg, Germany

Printed by Libri Plureos GmbH
in Hamburg, Germany